Student Study Guide

to accompany

Kinn's # The Clinical Medical Assistant

An Applied Learning Approach

Tammy B. Morton, MS, RN, CS, CMA

Formerly Department Head, Medical Assisting Program
TriCounty Technical College
Pendleton, South Carolina

SAUNDERS
An Imprint of Elsevier Science

SAUNDERS
An Imprint of Elsevier Science
11830 Westline Industrial Drive
St. Louis, Missouri 63146

Student Study Guide to Accompany
Kinn's The Clinical Medical Assistant: An Applied Learning Approach

0-7216-0276-2

This Study Guide is dedicated to
my family, friends, and former students
who have encouraged and supported me
throughout my teaching career.

Many thanks to Karen Sorrow, Kathy Duncan, Mary Heyer, Adrianne Cochran, Christine Ambrose, and Jeanne Genz for helping make the project a success.

Executive Editor: Adrianne Cochran
Developmental Editor: Christine Ambrose
Publishing Services Manager: Gayle May
Designer: Mark Oberkrom

Printed in the United States of America

CE/MV-B

Last digit is print number: 9 8 7 6 5 4 3 2 1

To the Student

This study guide was created to assist you in achieving the objectives of each chapter in *The Clinical Medical Assistant* and in establishing a solid base of knowledge in medical assisting. Completing the exercises in each chapter in this guide will help to reinforce the material studied in the textbook and learned in class.

Study Hints for All Students

Ask Questions!

There are no stupid questions. If you do not know something or are not sure about it, you need to find out. Other people may be wondering the same thing but may be too shy to ask. The answer could mean life or death to your patient. That is certainly more important than feeling embarrassed about asking a question.

Chapter Objectives

At the beginning of each chapter in the textbook are learning objectives that you should have mastered when you finish studying that chapter. Write these objectives in your notebook, leaving a blank space after each. Fill in the answers as you find them while reading the chapter. Review to make sure your answers are correct and complete. Use these answers when you study for tests. This should also be done for separate course objectives that your instructor has listed in your class syllabus.

Vocabulary

At the beginning of each chapter in the textbook are vocabulary terms that you will encounter as you read the chapter. These vocabulary terms are in bold the first time they appear in the chapter.

Summary of Learning Objectives

Use the Summary of Learning Objectives at the end of each chapter in the textbook to help with review for exams.

Reading Hints

When reading each chapter in the textbook, look at the subject headings to learn what each section is about. Read first for the general meaning. Then reread parts you did not understand. It may help to read those parts aloud. Carefully read the information given in each table and study each figure and its legend.

Concepts

While studying, put difficult concepts into your own words to determine whether you understand them. Check this understanding with another student or the instructor. Write these concepts in your notebook.

Class Notes

When taking lecture notes in class, leave a large margin on the left side of each notebook page and write only on right-hand pages, leaving all left-hand pages blank. Look over your lecture notes soon after each class, while your memory is fresh. Fill in missing words; complete sentences and ideas; and underline key phrases, definitions, and concepts. At the top of each page, write the topic of that page. In the left margin, write the key word for that part of your notes. On the opposite left-hand page, write a summary or outline that combines material from both the textbook and the lecture. These can be your study notes for review.

Study Groups

Form a study group with some other students so you can help one another. Practice speaking and reading aloud. Ask questions about material you are not sure about. Work together to find answers.

References for Improving Study Skills

Good study skills are essential for achieving your goals in medical assisting. Time management, efficient use of study time, and a consistent approach to studying are all beneficial. There are various methods for reading a textbook and for taking class notes. Some methods that have proven helpful can be found in *Saunders Health Professional's Planner*.

Additional Study Hints for English as a Second Language (ESL) Students

Vocabulary

If you find a nontechnical word you do not know (e.g., drowsy), try to guess its meaning from the sentence (e.g., *With electrolyte imbalance, the patient may feel fatigued and drowsy*). If you are not sure of the meaning or if it seems particularly important, look it up in the dictionary.

Vocabulary Notebook

Keep a small alphabetized notebook or address book in your pocket or purse. Write down new nontechnical words you read or hear along with their meanings and pronunciations. Write each word under its initial letter so you can find it easily, as in a dictionary. For words you do not know or for words that have a different meaning in medical assisting, write down how they are used and how they sound. Look up their meanings in a dictionary or ask your instructor or first-language buddy. Then write the different meanings or usages that you have found in your book, including the medical assisting meaning. Continue to add new words as you discover them.

First-Language Buddy

ESL students should find a first-language buddy—another student who is a native speaker of English and who is willing to answer questions about word meanings, pronunciations, and culture. Maybe, in turn, your buddy would like to learn about your language and culture. This could be useful for his or her medical assisting experience as well.

Introduction

This student study guide is designed with Learning Style Icons to help you identify exercises that will appeal to your strengths and weaknesses. Over time you have developed a method for perceiving and processing information. This pattern of behavior is called your learning style. There are many different ways of examining learning styles but professionals agree that success of students has more to do with their ability to "make sense" of the information rather than whether or not they are "smart". Education that is based on attention to individual learning styles is sensitive to the different ways students learn and approach new material with a wide variety of methods so that all students have the opportunity to learn. Determining your individual learning style and understanding how it applies to your ability to learn new material is the first step to becoming a successful student.

To learn new material, two things have to happen. First is your perception of the information. This is the method you have developed over time that helps you examine the material and recognize it as real. The next step is to process the information. Processing the information is how you internalize it and make it your own. Investigating various learning styles tells you how you can combine different methods of perceiving and processing information. In his book *Becoming a Master Student*, David Ellis discusses these different methods of information perception, processing, and learning.*

Information perception involves how you go about examining new material and making it real. There are two ways learners perceive new material. Some people are concrete perceivers who learn information through direct experience by doing, acting, sensing, or feeling. Concrete learners prefer to learn things that have a personal meaning or things they feel are relevant and important to them. Other learners are abstract perceivers who take in information through analysis, observation, and reflection. Abstract learners like to think things through. They analyze the new material and build theories to help understand it. They prefer structured learning situations and use a step-by-step approach to problem solving.

Information processing is how you internalize the new information and make it your own. There are also two different methods for processing material. Active processors prefer to jump in and start doing things immediately. They make sense of the new material by immediately using it. They look for practical ways to apply the new material and typically don't mind taking risks to get the desired results. They learn best with practice and hands-on activities. Reflective processors, however, have to think about the information before they can internalize it. They prefer to observe and consider what is going on. The only way they can make sense of new material is to spend time thinking about it and learning a great deal of information about it before acting.

*Ellis D: Becoming a master student, ed 10, Boston, 2002, Houghton Mifflin.

None of us fall completely into one or the other of these categories. However, by being aware of how we generally prefer to first perceive information and then process it, we can be more sensitive to our learning style and approach new learning situations with a plan for learning the material in a way that best suits our learning preferences. Your preferred perceiving/processing learning profile will fall into one of the following stages.

Learners in Stage 1 have a concrete/reflective style. and These students want to know the purpose of the information and have a personal connection to the content. They like to consider a situation from many different points of view, observe others, and plan before taking action. Their strengths are in understanding people, brainstorming, and recognizing and creatively solving problems. If you fall into this stage you enjoy small group activities and learn well in study groups.

Stage 2 learners have an abstract/reflective style. and These students are eager to learn just for the sheer pleasure of learning rather than because the material relates to their personal lives. They like to learn lots of facts and arrange new material in a logical and clear manner. Stage 2 learners plan studying and like to create ways of thinking about the material but don't always make the connection with the practical application of the material. If you are a Stage 2 learner you prefer organized, logical presentations of material and, therefore, enjoy lectures and generally dislike group work. You also need time to process and think about the new material before applying it.

Learners in Stage 3 have an abstract/active style. and Learners with this combination of learning style want to experiment and test the knowledge they are learning. If you are a Stage 3 learner you want to know how techniques or ideas work buy you also want to practice what you are learning. Your strengths are in problem solving and making decisions but you may tend to lack focus and be hasty in your decision-making. You learn best with hands-on practice by doing experiments, projects, and lab activities. You also enjoy working alone or in small groups.

Stage 4 is made up of concrete/active learners. and Students in this stage are concerned about how they can use what they learn to make a difference in their lives. If you fall into this stage, you like to relate new material to other areas of your life. You have leadership capabilities, can create on your feet, and are usually vocal in a group but you may have difficulty getting your work done completely and on time. Stage 4 learners enjoy teaching others and working in groups and learn best when they can apply the new information to real-world problems.

To get the most out of knowing your learning profile you need to apply this knowledge to how you approach learning. There are plusses and minuses to all four of the learning stages. When faced with a learning situation that does not match your learning preference, see how you can adapt your individual learning to make the best of the information. For example, if you are bored by lectures, look for an opportunity to apply the information being presented into a real-world problem you are facing in the classroom or at home. When learning new material, if you are an abstract perceiver, take time outside of class to think about the information so you are ready to process it into your learning system. If you benefit from learning in a group, then make the effort to organize review sessions and study groups with other interested students. If you learn best by teaching others offer to assist your peers with their learning. Take time now to investigate your preferred method of learning and it will help you perceive and process information more effectively throughout your school career.

Contents

Procedure Checklists

CHAPTER 1

Becoming a Successful Student

Part I. Vocabulary

A. **Directions:** Match the following terms and definitions.

1. _____ The constant practice of considering all aspects of a situation when deciding what to believe or what to do.

2. _____ Those actions that identify the medical assistant as a member of a healthcare profession, including dependability, respectful patient care, initiative, positive attitude, and teamwork.

3. _____ How an individual looks at information and sees it as real.

4. _____ The way that an individual perceives and processes information to learn new material.

5. _____ How an individual internalizes new information and makes it his or her own.

6. _____ The process of considering new information and internalizing it to create new ways of examining information.

7. _____ Sensitivity to the individual needs and reactions of patients.

A. learning style

B. reflection

C. professional behaviors

D. processing

E. empathy

F. perceiving

G. critical thinking

B. **Directions:** Complete the following sentences by using the vocabulary words from the previous section correctly.

1. Jo uses _____ _____ when she decides which information to use when she instructs patients with newly diagnosed diabetes.

2. _____ _____ should always be displayed during the student externship experience.

3. Instructors attempt to design lessons that appeal to different _____

_____.

4. Amanda shows _____ when she expresses concern about a patient's illness.

5. Sam enjoys "hands-on" learning activities. He uses an active style of _____ information.

6. Concrete and abstract are two ways of _____ new information.

Part II. Learning Style Inventory

Directions: Using the descriptions of various learning styles from Chapter 1, insert the correct Learning Style Stage Number into the diagram below by correlating the processing and perceiving style. In his book, *Becoming a Master Student,* Ellis discusses these different methods of information perception, processing, and learning.*

	Processing	
	Watching (Reflective)	Doing (Active)
Perceiving		
Feeling (Concrete)	Stage _____	Stage _____
Thinking (Abstract)	Stage _____	Stage _____

Part III. Time Management

1. List five time management skills.

   a. _____

   b. _____

   c. _____

   d. _____

   e. _____

2. Describe five strategies for breaking the cycle of procrastination.

   a. _____

   b. _____

   c. _____

   d. _____

   e. _____

*Ellis D: Becoming a master student, ed 10, Boston, 2002, Houghton Mifflin.

Part IV. Conflict Resolution

Directions: Indicate which statements are true (T) and which statements are false (F).

1. _____ The best way to deal with conflict situations is through open, honest, assertive communication.

2. _____ The first step in conflict resolution is examination of pros and cons.

3. _____ Conflicts should be resolved immediately.

4. _____ Sometimes you will not be able to solve problems or a conflict may not be important enough for you to act to change it.

5. _____ It is best if you attempt to solve the conflict in a private place at a prescheduled time.

6. _____ You need to understand the problem and gather as much information about the situation as possible before you decide to act.

7. _____ As a future member of the healthcare team, you will frequently face problems and conflict.

Part V. Workplace Applications

Scenario: Connie is the manager of a busy family practice office. The insurance clerk has complained that the receptionist takes too many smoking breaks and accepts too many personal calls while at work.

Step One: Think about this situation and how you believe it should be handled. Record your ideas.

_____

_____

_____

_____

_____

Step Two: Pair up with a classmate and discuss your ideas. Record ideas on which you agree and compare them with those in the text.

_____

_____

_____

_____

_____

Step Three: Share your ideas with your classmates. Make notes of any ideas that you did not think of before.

_____

_____

_____

_____

_____

Part VI. Study Skills

Examine your own note-taking ability. Review the note-taking strategies in Chapter 1, and record the ideas that you plan to incorporate into your academic goals for this term.

_____

_____

_____

_____

_____

_____

_____

_____

_____

Directions: Complete the following success checklist.

	Yes	No
1. I am prepared for class.		
2. My notebook is organized.		
3. I read my assignments before coming to class.		
4. I attend all classes.		
5. I listen most of the time.		
6. I arrive early to class.		
7. I date notes in my notebook.		
8. I save all papers and course materials for review.		
9. I try to connect what I read in the text with what I learn in class.		
10. My schoolwork is a high priority.		

If you answered "No" to any of the items on the checklist, write a short plan for improvement in this area.

_____

_____

_____

_____

_____

Part VII. Test-Taking Strategies

Directions: Complete the following sentences.

1. The first step of taking charge of your academic success is to

_____

_____.

2. Before you begin a test _____.

Chapter 1 Quiz

Name: _____

1. List three examples of professional behaviors.

   a. _____

   b. _____

   c. _____

2. _____ is showing sensitivity to the individual needs and reactions of patients.

3. The process of considering new information and internalizing it to create new ways of examining information is called

   _____.

4. Initial confrontations regarding conflicts in the office should be done in

   _____.

5. True or False: Concrete learners enjoy theories and facts.

6. True or False: Active learning involves "hands-on" experiences.

7. List Two ways to use effective time management.

   a. _____

   b. _____

8. Give an example of a mind map.

   _____

CHAPTER 2

Infection Control

Part I. Vocabulary

Directions: Define the following terms in your own words.

1. anaphylaxis

_____

_____

2. antibody

_____

_____

3. antigen

_____

_____

4. antiseptic

_____

_____

5. autoimmune

_____

_____

6. contaminated

_____

_____

7. germicides

_____

_____

8. pathogenic

_____

_____

9. permeable

_____

_____

10. relapse

_____

_____

11. remission

_____

_____

12. vector

_____

_____

Part II. Chain of Infection

Directions: Label the diagram below with the following terms.

A. Reservoir host

B. Exit mode (mouth, skin, rectum, body fluid)

C. Transmission mode (air, food, hand, insects, body fluid)

D. Entry (any body opening)

E. Susceptible host

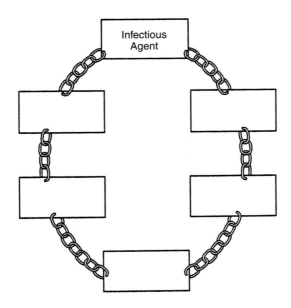

Part III. Inflammation

A. Describe the first four stages of inflammation in response to pathogenic invasion.

1. _____

_____

_____

2. _____

_____

_____

3. _____

_____

_____

4. _____

_____

_____

B. Describe the conditions that may result if the pathogen continues to invade the entire body.

1. Pus formation

_____

_____

2. Enlarged lymph nodes

_____

_____

3. Septicemia

_____

_____

C. List four types of infection and describe them.

1. _____

2. _____

3. _____

4. _____

Part IV. Pathogens and Barriers

A. List five groups of infectious organisms.

1. _____

2. _____

3. _____

4. _____

5. _____

B. Complete the table with information about various viruses.

Disease	Organism	Description	Transmission	Symptoms	Specimens	Tests
HIV-positive acquired	HIV	DNA retrovirus				
Immuno-deficiency syndrome (AIDS)						
Hepatitis A	HAV	RNA virus				
Hepatitis B	HBV	DNA virus				
Hepatitis delta	HDV	RNA virus				
Hepatitis C	HCV	RNA flavivirus				
Herpes simplex	HSV	Exhibits latency				
Chicken pox or shingles	Varicella zoster virus (VZV)	Exhibits latency, may cause shingles (herpes zoster) in patients who have had chicken pox				

C. List three types of bacteria and describe their shapes.

1. _____

2. _____

3. _____

D. List several barriers or types of personal protective equipment that are commonly used in physicians' offices.

1. _____

2. _____

3. _____

4. _____

5. _____

6. _____

E. Hypersensitivity to latex products may include the following symptoms:

1. _____

2. _____

3. _____

4. _____

5. _____

6. _____

Part V. Exposure Control

Employers with workers who are at risk for occupational exposure to blood or other infectious materials must implement an Occupational Safety and Health Administration (OSHA) Exposure Control Plan that details employee protection procedures. List seven items that should be included in the plan.

1. _____

2. _____

3. _____

4. _____

5. _____

6. _____

7. _____

Part VI. Asepsis

Directions: Define the following terms.

1. Disinfection

_____

_____

2. Medical asepsis

_____

_____

3. Surgical asepsis

_____

_____

4. Proper hand washing (two factors)

_____

_____

5. Sanitization

_____

_____

6. Sterilization

_____

_____

Part VII. Hand Washing

Directions: Review Procedure 2.1: Performing Medical Aseptic Hand Washing in your textbook. What did you learn? Practice proper hand washing for the next 24 hours. Note any new habits you have formed. Do you see any improvement? Have you noticed hand washing behaviors of others?

_____

_____

_____

Chapter 2 Quiz

Name: _____

1. The relief of systems is called

   _____.

2. Viruses form a substance called

   a. interferon

   b. spores

3. List three potentially infectious fluids.

   a. _____

   b. _____

   c. _____

4. CDC stands for _____.

5. True or False: Cocci bacteria are rod-shaped.

6. Name a symptom or sign of latex allergy.

   _____

7. True or False: Hepatitis A can be food borne.

8. Instruments in surgery are

   _____.

9. OSHA stands for

   _____.

10. Rhinitis means

    _____.

CHAPTER 3

Patient Assessment

Part I.

List five components of the medical history.

1. _____

2. _____

3. _____

4. _____

5. _____

Part II.

Describe things that influence someone's value system.

_____

_____

_____

Do you think these things have influenced your values?

_____

_____

_____

Part III.

List and describe three processes of active listening.

_____

_____

_____

The receiver of a message attaches meaning to a message based on:

_____

_____

_____

Part VI.

Directions: Complete the diagram below by including examples of nonverbal communication.

Area Observed	Observation
Breathing patterns	
Eye patterns	
Hands	
Arm placement	
Leg placement	

List four important rules to remember in preparing the appropriate environment for patient interaction.

1. _____
2. _____
3. _____
4. _____

Part V.

Directions: Label the following questions as either open-ended or closed-ended.

1. _____ How have you been getting along?
2. _____ Do you have a headache?
3. _____ Have you ever broken a bone?
4. _____ What brings you to the doctor?
5. _____ Are you feeling better?.
6. _____ Do you have high blood pressure?
7. _____ Tell me about your back pain?
8. _____ When did the nausea start?
9. _____ Did your mother have a history of cancer?
10. _____ Do you smoke?

Part VI.

Consider the following interview barriers. Give an example of each.

1. Providing unwarranted assurance

_____

_____

2. Giving advice

_____

_____

3. Using professional terms

_____

_____

4. Leading questions

_____

_____

Part VII.

List some of the important guidelines to follow in obtaining the health history of a child.

1. _____

2. _____

3. _____

4. _____

5. _____

Part VIII.

Directions: Label the following as "Subjective" (symptom) or "Objective" (sign).

1. Pain _____

2. Nausea _____

3. Dizziness _____

4. Elevated blood pressure _____

5. Labored respirations _____

6. Headache _____

7. Temperature of skin _____

8. Back pain _____

9. Color of skin _____

10. Abdominal pain _____

Part IX. _____

Directions: Review the correct method of charting in your textbook and answer the following questions.

1. What is the first step in charting? _____

_____

_____

2. What color ink do you use? _____

3. What appears on every entry? _____

4. What three things do you include about symptoms?

_____

_____

5. How do you chart intensity of pain? _____

_____

_____

6. How do you correct an error? _____

_____

_____

7. How do you add additional information at a later time? _____

_____

_____

8. Why are neatness and legibility important? _____

_____

_____

Part X. Charting Methods

A. List four components of the POMR.

1. _____

2. _____

3. _____

4. _____

B. The first letter of each part of the progress note makes up the word *SOAPE*. Describe what each of these letters stands for.

S _____

O _____

A _____

P _____

E _____

C. What is an SOMR? _____

_____

_____

D. What are some of the sections in an SOMR?

1. _____

2. _____

3. _____

4. _____

E. What is a CMR? _____

_____

Part XI. Workplace Applications _____

Directions: Document the following four scenarios by using the POMR method.

1. The patient c/o chest with pain of 4 on a 1-10 scale and sweating for 2 hours. He has been taking NTG for relief of symptoms. His VS are T-99, P-68, R-24. He also has an irregular pulse and left arm pain.

S: _____

O: _____

_____

_____

2. The patient c/o a sore throat with pain of 7 on a 1-10 scale and fever for 2 days. He has been taking OTCs and gargling with warm salt water for relief of symptoms. His VS are T-102.4, P-108, R-20. He also has an erythematous papular rash across his chest. He was exposed to strep last week.

S: _____

O: _____

_____

_____

3. The patient c/o a headache with pain of 8 on a 1-10 scale and nausea for 3 days. She has been taking Lortab 5 for relief of symptoms. Her VS are T-97.6, P-110, R-20. She also has dizziness and her eyes hurt. She is pale and her skin is damp.

S: _____

O: _____

_____

_____

4. The patient fell off a ladder 2 days ago and c/o low back pain of 5 on a 1-10 scale. He has been taking Advil for relief of symptoms. His VS are T-98.7, P-98, R-20. He also has an ecchymosis across his flank and c/o blood in his urine.

S: _____

O: _____

_____

_____

Chapter 3 Quiz

Name: _____

1. True or False: An example of pain quality is "stabbing."

2. True or False: An earache is a symptom.

3. True or False: SOAPE is part of a POMR.

4. True or False: Objective data are signs.

5. _____ complaint is the reason for seeking medical care.

6. _____ is a relationship of harmony between the patient and healthcare personnel.

7. Health insurance information is part of the

   _____ .

8. Smoking is part of the _____ history.

9. Age of a parent at death is part of the

   _____ history.

10. True or False: Open-ended questions often provide better data.

CHAPTER 4

Patient Education

Part I. Vocabulary

Directions: Fill in the blanks with the appropriate terms.

1. The holistic model suggests that patient education should take into consideration all aspects of

   patient life including patients' _____, _____, _____,

   _____, _____, and _____ needs.

Part II.

Directions: List six guidelines for patient education.

1. _____
2. _____
3. _____
4. _____
5. _____
6. _____

Part III.

Directions: List seven factors that influence learning.

1. _____
2. _____
3. _____
4. _____
5. _____
6. _____
7. _____

Part IV.

Directions: Identify eight approaches to language barriers.

1. _____

2. _____

3. _____

4. _____

5. _____

6. _____

7. _____

8. _____

Part V.

Directions: Fill in the blanks with the appropriate terms.

1. One of the most important aspects of patient teaching is to be _____ and provide
   information about _____ patients want to know _____ patients want to
   know it.

Part VI.

Directions: List 10 barriers to patient learning.

1. _____

2. _____

3. _____

4. _____

5. _____

6. _____

7. _____

8. _____

9. _____

10. _____

Part VII.

Directions: Identify five guidelines for ordering educational materials.

1. _____

2. _____

3. _____

4. _____

5. _____

Part VIII.

Directions: Complete the statement.

The role of the medical assistant educator includes:

1. _____

2. _____

3. _____

4. _____

5. _____

6. _____

7. _____

8. _____

Part IX.

Directions: Fill in the blanks with the appropriate terms.

Teaching methods that are effective include use of _____ materials, videos, and

approved _____ sites to gather information; referral to community _____

and experts; _____ demonstration of medical skills; examination of patients' records of

events; and involving _____ in the education process.

Part X. Teaching Plan Checklist

Directions: Use the following checklist to design and present a patient education program for a patient during your externship, or role play with a fellow classmate.

1. Conduct patient assessment.

   - Consider pertinent patient factors.
   - Identify barriers to learning.
   - Prioritize patient information.
   - Determine immediate and long-term needs.
   - Decide on appropriate teaching materials and methods.

     Complete _____

2. Prepare the teaching area and assemble necessary equipment and materials.

   - Use supplies and equipment the patient will use at home.
   - Provide positive feedback for correct display of skills.

     Complete _____

3. Maintain adequate, not too fast, pace.

     Complete _____

4. Repeatedly ask for patient feedback to confirm understanding.

   - Eliminate barriers to learning.
   - Address immediate learning needs.
   - Use repetition and rephrasing to promote understanding.

     Complete _____

5. Summarize the material learned or the skill mastered at the end of each teaching interaction.

     Complete _____

6. Outline a plan for the next meeting.

     Complete _____

7. Evaluate the teaching plan.

   - Was there enough time to complete the lesson?
   - Was the patient physically and psychologically ready for the information?
   - Were the goals for the session reached?

     Complete _____

8. Document the teaching intervention.

   - Material covered
   - Patient response or level of skill performance
   - Plans for next session
   - Community referrals

     Complete _____

CHAPTER 5

Nutrition and Health Promotion

Part I. _____

A. **Directions:** Describe the dietary imbalances that contribute to each of these health problems.

1. Anemia _____

2. Cancer _____

3. Constipation _____

4. Diabetes _____

5. Hypercholesterolemia _____

6. Hypertension _____

7. Osteoporosis _____

B. **Directions:** Fill in the blanks with the appropriate terms.

1. Dietary fiber is commonly called _____.

2. _____ are chemical organic compounds composed of carbon, hydrogen, and oxygen and are primarily plant products in origin. They are divided into three groups based on the complexity of their molecules: simple sugars, complex carbohydrates (starch), and dietary fiber.

3. _____ is a storage form of fuel that is used to supplement carbohydrates as an available energy source.

4. Naturally occurring _____ are found in many fruits, vegetables, and certain seasonings.

5. _____ are composed of units known as amino acids, which are the materials that our bodies use to build and repair tissues.

6. Vitamins are divided into two groups: _____-soluble (A, D, E, and K) and _____-soluble (B complex and C).

7. _____ present in the largest amounts include sodium, potassium, calcium, chlorine, phosphorus, and magnesium.

Part II.

A. **Directions:** Examine the nomogram below and answer the following questions.

   1. How much does this patient weigh in pounds? _____

      In kilograms? _____

   2. What is the height in inches? _____ In centimeters? _____

   3. What is the body surface area (BSA)? _____

   4. Use the nomogram to calculate your own BSA. _____

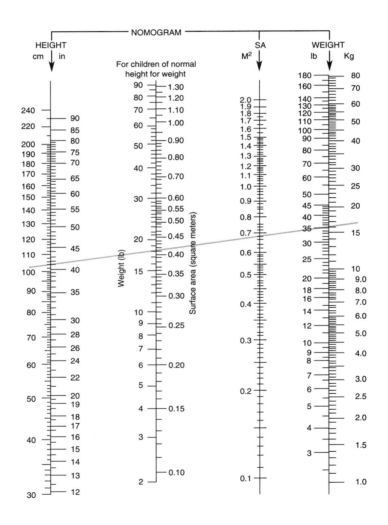

B. **Directions:** List four functions of water.

   1. _____

   2. _____

   3. _____

   4. _____

Part III.

A. **Directions:** Label each food group.

A

B ← →D

C ← →E

←F

B. **Directions:** Examine the nutrition facts label below and answer the following questions.

1. What is the normal serving size?

   _____

2. How many calories are in one serving without milk? _____

3. How many grams of fiber are present in one serving? _____

4. This food is high in _____ and _____.

NUTRITION FACTS

Services size 1¼ cups (30 g)
Servicing per container about 16

Amount per serving		Cereal	Cereal with ½ cup skim milk
Calories		110	190
Calories from fat		0	0
		% Daily value**	
Total fat 9 g*		0%	0%
Saturated fat 0 g		0%	1%
Cholesterol 0 mg		0%	1%
Sodium 270 mg		11%	14%
Total carbohydrate 26 g		9%	11%
Dietary fiber less than 1 g		0%	0%
Sugars 3 g			
Other carbohydrate 22 g			
Protein 2 g			
Vitamin A		0%	6%
Vitamin C		10%	10%
Calcium		0%	15%
Iron		50%	50%
Thiamin		25%	25%
Niacin		25%	25%
Vitamin B6		25%	25%
Folate		25%	25%
Vitamin B12		25%	30%

Amount per serving		Cereal	Cereal with ½ cup skim milk
	Calories	**2000**	**2500**
Total fat	Less than	65 g	60 g
Saturated fat	Less than	20 g	25 g
Cholesterol	Less than	300 mg	300 mg
Sodium	Less than	2400 mg	2400 mg
Total carbohydrate		300 g	375 g
Dietary fiber		25 g	30 g
Calories per gram:			
Fat 9 –			
Carbohydrate 4 –			
Protein 4			

*Amount in cereal. One half cup skim milk an additional 40 calories. Less than 5 mg cholesterol, 65 mg sodium, 6 g total carbohydrate (6 g sugars) and 4 g protein.
**Percent daily values are based on 2000 calorie diet. Your daily values may be higher may be higher or lower depending on your calorie needs.

Part IV.

Directions: Record your dietary intake for the next 24 hours. Save nutrition labels from packages so that you can examine your caloric intake. Any surprises?

	Foods	Calories	Grams of Fat
Breakfast			
Snack Water			
Lunch			
Snack Water			
Dinner			
Snack Water			
Totals			

CHAPTER 6

Vital Signs

Part I. Vocabulary

Directions: Define the following medical terms.

1. apnea

_____

_____

2. arrhythmia

_____

_____

3. bradycardia

_____

_____

4. bradypnea

_____

_____

5. dyspnea

_____

_____

6. febrile

_____

_____

7. hyperlipidemia

_____

_____

8. hypertension

_____

_____

9. hyperventilation

_____

_____

10. hypotension

_____

_____

11. orthopnea

_____

_____

12. rales

_____

_____

13. rhonchi

_____

_____

14. syncope

_____

_____

15. tachycardia

_____

_____

16. tachypnea

_____

_____

17. vertigo

_____

_____

Part II.

Directions: Complete the statement.

The cardinal four vital signs are:

1. _____

2. _____

3. _____

4. _____

Part III.

Directions: Complete the statement.

Anthropometric measurements include:

1. _____

2. _____

3. _____ _____

4. _____ and _____ _____

Part IV.

Directions: Indicate which statements are true (T) and which statements are false (F).

1. _____ A change in one or more of the patient's vital signs may indicate a change in general health.

2. _____ It sometimes is necessary to obtain some measurements a second time, after the patient is calmer or more comfortable.

3. _____ The body temperature is regulated by the hypothalamus.

4. _____ The body temperature ranges from being highest in the morning to lowest in the late afternoon.

Part V.

Directions: Complete the table of normal ranges for vital signs.

Age Group	Pulse	Respirations	Blood Pressure
Newborn			
Toddlers (1-3 yr)			
Preschool (4-6 yr)			
School Age (7-11 yr)			
Adolescent (12-16 yr)			
Adult			

Part VI. Temperatures

A. **Directions:** Use the correct terms to fill in the blanks.

1. A _____ fever rises and falls only slightly during the 24-hour period. It remains above the patient's average normal range and is called *continuous* because that is exactly what the pattern shows.

2. A _____ fever comes and goes, or it spikes and then returns into average range.

3. A _____ fever has great fluctuation but never gets back into the average range. It is a constant fever with fluctuating levels and thus is remittent.

4. _____ temperatures, when taken accurately, are approximately 1° F or 0.6° C higher than oral readings.

5. _____ temperatures are approximately 1° F or 0.6° C lower than accurate oral readings.

6. _____ readings are close to the core body temperature because the mucous membrane lining with which the thermometer comes in contact is not exposed to the air.

7. _____ thermometers are battery-operated and are available in both Fahrenheit and Celsius scales. One type is a unit equipped with two probes: a _____ one for oral use and a red one for _____ use only.

8. The _____ measurement system consists of a hand-held processor unit equipped with a probe that is covered with a disposable speculum that is placed at the opening of the ear canal. It should not be used for patients with _____ _____ or impacted _____.

9. _____ temperatures take the longest to register.

10. Water-soluble lubrication jelly is needed for obtaining _____ temperatures. The patient should be placed in the _____ position.

B. **Directions:** Document temperatures that are considered febrile.

1. Rectal or aural (ear) temperatures higher than _____° F (38° C)

2. Oral temperatures higher than _____° F (37.5° C)

3. Axillary temperatures higher than _____° F (37° C)

4. Fever of unknown origin (FUO) is a fever higher than _____° F (38.3° C) for _____ _____ in adults and _____ in children without a known diagnosis.

C. Converting Temperatures

$$C = (F - 32) \times 5/9$$

$$F = \frac{9 \times C}{5} + 32$$

Directions: Using the above formulas, convert the following temperatures from one system to the other.

1. 98.6° F = _____ C

2. 37° C = _____ F

3. 97.6° F = _____ C

4. 38° C = _____ F

5. 99.4° F = _____ C

6. 36° C = _____ F

7. 104° F = _____ C

8. 42° C = _____ F

9. 101° F = _____ C

10. 41° C = _____ F

11. 102° F = _____ C

12. 43° C = _____ F

Part VII. Pulses

A. **Directions:** List eight pulse sites and label their correct locations on the figure below.

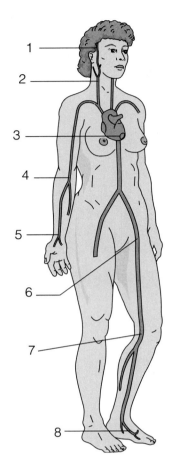

1. _____
2. _____
3. _____
4. _____
5. _____
6. _____
7. _____
8. _____

Part VIII. Respirations

Directions: Complete the sentences with the correct terms.

1. When Grace counts respirations, she understands that one respiration includes

   _____

2. Geri is documenting the three characteristics of respirations, which include _____,

   _____, and _____.

3. Dianne counts eight respirations for 30 seconds and multiplies by _____.

   She documents the rate as _____ per minute.

Part IX. Blood Pressure

Directions: Complete the sentences with the correct terms.

1. Blood pressure is a reflection of the pressure of the blood against the walls of _____.

2. The difference between the systolic and diastolic pressures is the _____

   _____.

3. Blood pressure is recorded as a fraction, with the _____ reading the numerator (top)

   and the _____ reading the denominator (bottom).

Directions: Review the process of taking a blood pressure and complete the chart below.

The sphygmomanometer must be used with a stethoscope. The objective of the procedure is to use the inflatable cuff to obliterate (cause to disappear) circulation through an artery. The stethoscope is placed over the artery just below the cuff, and then the cuff is slowly deflated to allow the blood to flow again. As blood flow resumes, cardiac cycle sounds (Korotkoff sounds) are heard through the stethoscope, and gauge readings are taken when the first (systolic) and the last (diastolic) sounds are heard.

Phase I: This is the first sound heard as the cuff deflates. The blood is resurging into the patient's artery and can be heard quite clearly as a sharp, tapping sound. Note the gauge reading when this **first** sound is heard. **Record this as the systolic pressure.**

Phase V: All sounds disappear in this phase. Note the gauge reading when the **last** sound is heard. **Record this as the diastolic pressure.**

Phase I	Phase V	Document Blood Pressure
110	80	
204	114	
116	72	
98	56	
142	88	

Part X. Workplace Applications

Directions: Vital signs are documented with temperature (T) first, pulse (P) second, and respirations (R) last; the blood pressure is recorded after the TPR. Correctly document the following vital signs in the boxes provided. Date and sign each entry as you would on a patient record.

1. Oral temperature of 98.7, apical pulse of 60, respirations 22, and orthostatic blood pressure of 152/98 supine and 114/76 standing.

2. Tympanic temperature of 96.8, radial pulse of 86, respirations 18, and bilateral blood pressure of 132/76 in the left arm and 128/80 in the right arm.

3. Rectal temperature of 101.2, pulse of 100, respirations 20, and blood pressure 126/70.

4. Axillary temperature of 97.5, carotid pulse of 78, respirations 20, and palpated blood pressure of 120.

Chapter 6 Quiz

Name: _____

1. The first tapping heard when taking a blood
   pressure is the _____.

2. Respirations that are counted as 9 for
   30 seconds are documented as

   _____ per minute.

3. A _____ blood pressure is
   done without a stethoscope.

4. Convert 146 pounds to kilograms.

5. Convert 73 kilograms to pounds.

6. True or False: Head circumference is an
   anthropometric measurement.

7. True or False: An apical pulse is taken with
   a stethoscope and counted for one full
   minute.

8. True or False: The dorsalis pedis is behind
   the knee.

9. The _____ pulse is located on
   the side of the head.

10. True or False: The radial pulse is best
    found on the thumb side of the wrist,
    1 inch above the base of the thumb.

CHAPTER 7

Assisting with the Primary Physical Examination

Part I. Vocabulary

Directions: Use the appropriate vocabulary word to complete each sentence.

1. The physician uses _____ to assess the sinuses.

2. A patient undergoing dialysis may have _____.

3. During jaundice, the _____ of the eyes turn yellow.

4. A faulty heart valve creates a _____.

5. A _____ is a small lump, lesion, or swelling felt when the skin is palpated.

6. When the carotid arteries fill with plaque, a _____ can be heard on the neck.

Part II.

A. Histology is the study of tissues. List four types of tissue in the human body.

1. _____

2. _____

3. _____

4. _____

B. What are the differences among tissue, organs, and body systems?

_____

_____

_____

C. List the 11 systems of the body and name two organs in each system.

Body System	Organs

Part III.

The medical assistant's duties can be divided into three areas:

1. _____

2. _____

3. _____

Part IV. Instruments and Equipment Needed for Physical Exam _____

Identify the instruments shown in the following figures.

1. _____

2. _____

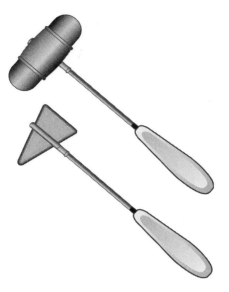

3. _____

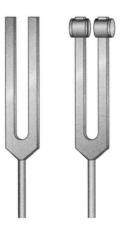

4. _____

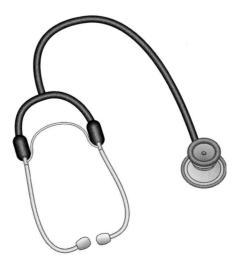

5. _____

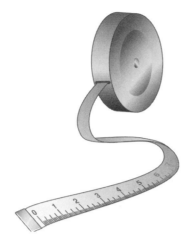

6. _____

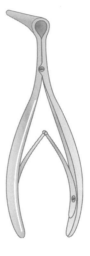

7. _____

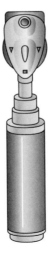

8. _____

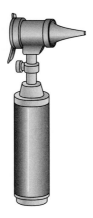

Part V.

Directions: Describe the following methods of assessment.

1. Inspection _____

2. Palpation _____

3. Percussion _____

4. Auscultation _____

5. Mensuration _____

6. Manipulation _____

Part VI. Positions for Examination

Directions: Label each position shown in the following figures.

1. _____

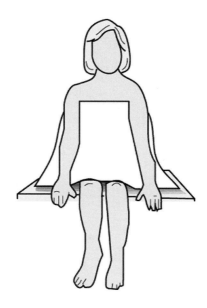

2. _____

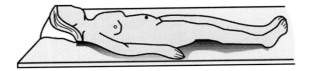

3. _____

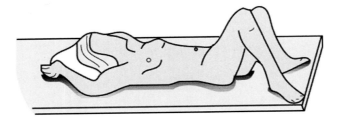

4. _____

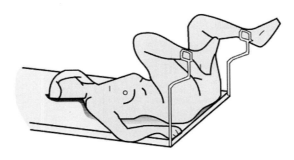

5. _____

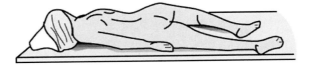

6. _____

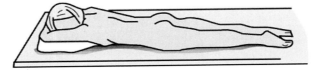

7. _____

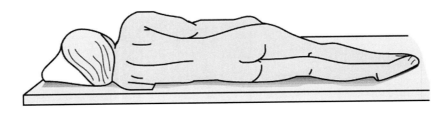

8. _____

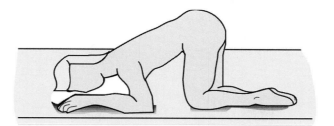

Part VII. Extra for Experts _____

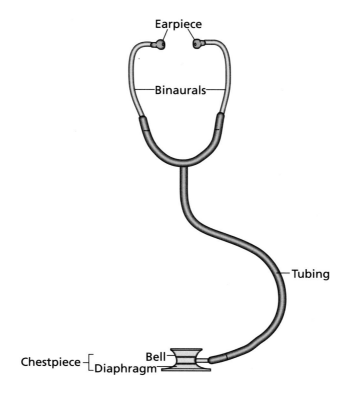

Directions: Examine the diagram of the stethoscope. Describe the function of the following.

1. Diaphragm _____

2. Bell _____

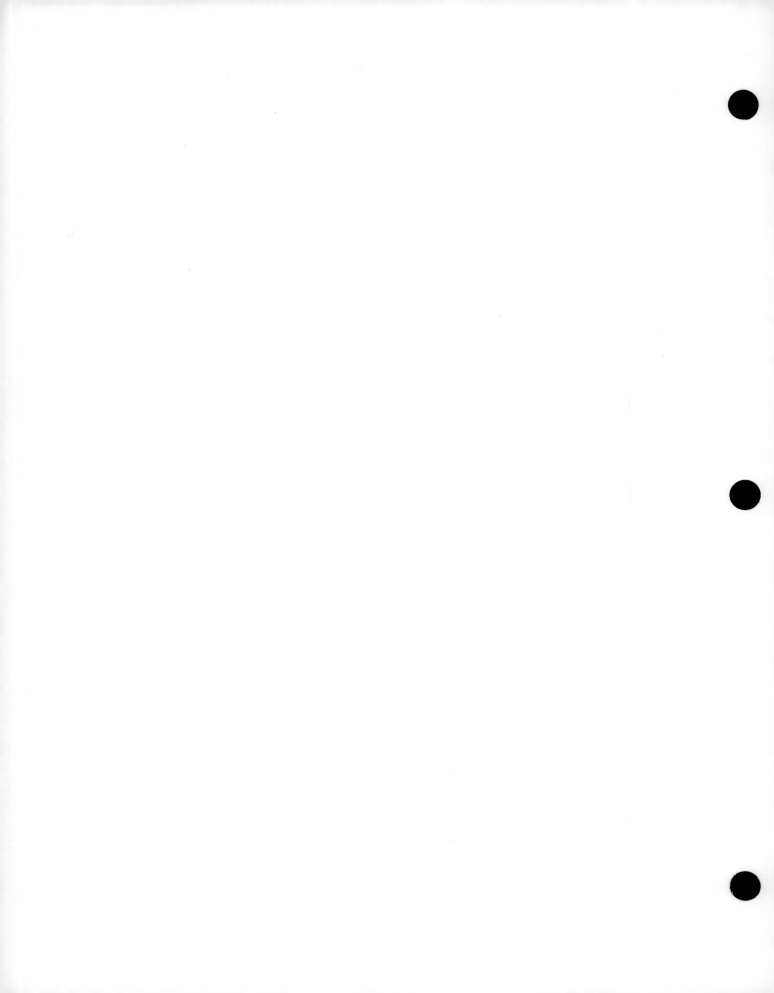

Chapter 7 Quiz

Name: _____

1. The kidneys are part of the

   _____ system.

2. The otoscope is used to examine the

   _____.

3. A tape measure is used for:

   a. palpation

   b. auscultation

   c. manipulation

   d. mensuration

4. The spinal cord is part of the

   _____ system.

5. Ligaments are included in the

   _____ system.

6. The liver is in the _____
   system.

7. Blood cells belong to the

   _____ system.

8. Rectal medications are usually
   administered with the patient in the

   _____ position.

9. True or False: The dorsal recumbent
   position includes having the patient's feet
   in stirrups.

10. True or False: Supine is flat on the back.

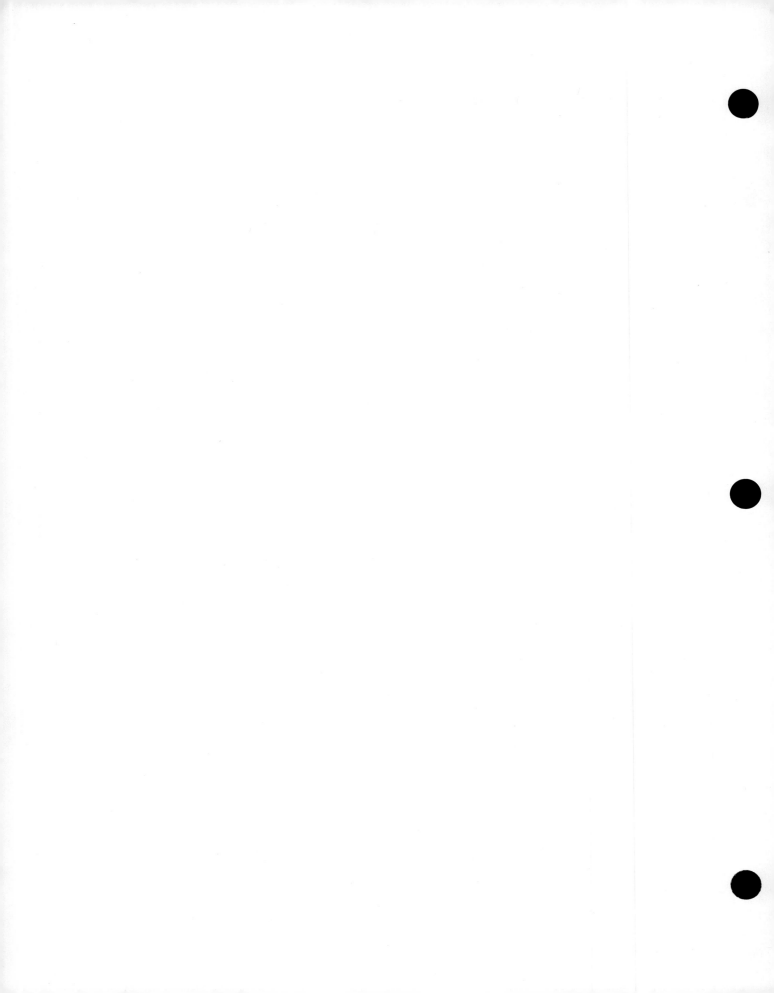

CHAPTER 8

Principles of Pharmacology

Part I. Vocabulary

Directions: Match the following terms with their definitions.

1. _____ Medications sold without a prescription.

2. _____ Drugs that are not protected by trademark

3. _____ Pertaining to a glue-like substance

4. _____ Denoting any medication route other than the gastrointestinal (oral) route

5. _____ Space within a vessel or tube

6. _____ Drug formulation in which tablets are coated with a special compound that does not dissolve until the tablet is exposed to the fluids of the small intestine

A. parenteral

B. colloidal

C. generic

D. enteric-coated

E. over-the-counter

F. lumen

Part II. Government Regulation

A. **Directions:** Complete the following statements.

1. The FDA is the _____

_____

2. The DEA is the _____

_____

3. The FTC is the _____

_____

B. **Directions:** Fill in the blank with DEA, FDA, or FTC.

1. The _____ regulates over-the-counter drug advertising.

2. The _____, a division of the Department of Health and Human Services, was created in 1936 to regulate the development and sale of all prescription and over-the-counter drugs.

3. The _____ was established in 1973 as part of the Department of Justice to enforce federal laws regarding the use of illegal drugs.

4. Every medical practice should have a copy of the controlled substances regulations. The medical assistant may secure this list from a regional office of the _____.

5. Besides approving new drugs for the marketplace, the _____ is also responsible for establishing standards for their purity and strength during the manufacturing process and for ensuring that generic brands are effective and safe.

6. Each physician who prescribes or who has controlled substances on site must register with the

_____ for a Controlled Substance Registration Certificate and will receive a specific registration number that must be included on all controlled substance prescriptions.

C. **Directions:** List six specific guidelines for prescription orders of controlled substances.

1. _____

2. _____

3. _____

4. _____

5. _____

6. _____

Part III. _____

Directions: Use your text to complete the table of classification of controlled substances.

Schedule	Guidelines	List Three Drug Examples
I	_____ medical use _____ potential for abuse Possession of these drugs is illegal.	
II	Accepted for medical use _____ restrictions _____ potential for abuse May cause severe psychological or physical dependence	

III	Accepted for medical use
	Potential for abuse less than I or II
	
	May cause _____ physical dependence or high
	  psychological dependence
	Includes combination drugs that contain limited amounts
	  of narcotics or stimulants	

IV	Accepted for medical use _____ potential for abuse May cause limited physical or psychological dependence in comparison with schedule III drugs Includes minor tranquilizers and hypnotics	
V	Accepted for medical use _____ potential for abuse May cause limited physical or psychological dependence in comparison with schedule IV drugs Includes drug mixtures containing limited amounts of narcotics	

Part IV. Conflict Resolution

Directions: Indicate which statements are true (T) and which statements are false (F).

1. _____ The chemical name represents the drug's exact formula.

2. _____ The generic drug name is assigned by the manufacturer and is protected by copyright.

3. _____ Brand names are capitalized.

4. _____ The *PDR* is the most commonly used drug reference book.

5. _____ A prescription is an order written by the physician for the compounding or dispensing and administration of drugs to a particular patient.

Directions: Fill in the blanks by choosing the correct terms from the list below.

1. _____ drugs are used to treat the disorder and cure it; antibiotics cure bacterial infections.

2. _____ drugs do not cure but provide relief from pain or symptoms related to the disorder; an example is the use of an antihistamine for allergic symptoms.

3. _____ drugs prevent the occurrence of a condition; vaccines prevent the occurrence of specific infectious diseases.

4. _____ drugs help determine the cause of a particular health problem; an example is injection of antigen serum for allergy testing.

5. _____ drugs provide patients with substances needed to maintain health; examples are estrogen replacement therapy for menopausal women and administration of insulin to patients with diabetes.

A. Prophylactic
B. Therapeutic
C. Replacement
D. Palliative
E. Diagnostic

Part V. Pharmacokinetic Terms

Directions: Complete each sentence

Excretion

Distribution

Metabolism

Absorption

1. How a drug is absorbed into the body's circulating fluids, which depends on the route by which it is administered, is called _____.

2. How a drug is transported from the site of administration to the various points in the body is called _____.

3. How a drug is inactivated, including the time it takes for the drug to be detoxified and broken down into by-products, is called _____.

4. The route by which a drug is excreted, or eliminated, from the body and the amount of time such a process requires is called _____.

Part VI. Workplace Applications

Routes of Absorption

Oral route

Topical absorption

Mucous membrane absorption

Parenteral route

Step One: Think of an example of each of the listed routes of absorption. Record your ideas.

_____

_____

_____

_____

Step Two: Pair up with a classmate and discuss your examples.

_____

_____

_____

Step Three: Share your ideas with your classmates. Make notes of any examples that you did not think of before.

_____

_____

_____

_____

List six of the factors that can affect drug action.

1. _____

2. _____

3. _____

4. _____

5. _____

6. _____

Part VII. Extra for Experts

Directions: Complete the table below by describing the action of each type of drug and giving an example of each type.

Type of Drug	Action and Example
Analgesic	
Anesthetic	
Antibiotic	
Antidepressant	
Antihistamine	
Antihypertensive	
Anti-inflammatory	
Antineoplastic	
Antitussive	

Part VIII. Self-Awareness

My biggest concern about giving medications is _____

_____

_____

_____

I look forward to _____

_____

_____

_____

I dread _____

_____

_____

_____

Chapter 8 Quiz

Name: _____

1. List three factors that affect drug action.

   a. _____

   b. _____

   c. _____

2. A _____ increases peristaltic activity of the large intestine.

3. True or False: Pharmacology is the broad science that deals with the origin, nature, chemistry, effects, and uses of drugs.

4. True or False: Pharmaceutical companies developing new medications must first gain DEA approval before the drugs can be sold to consumers.

5. True or False: A diuretic increases urinary output and decreases blood pressure.

6. True or False: Schedule II drugs are closely monitored and controlled.

7. List three types of drug names.

   a. _____

   b. _____

   c. _____

8. PDR stands for _____

   _____ _____ .

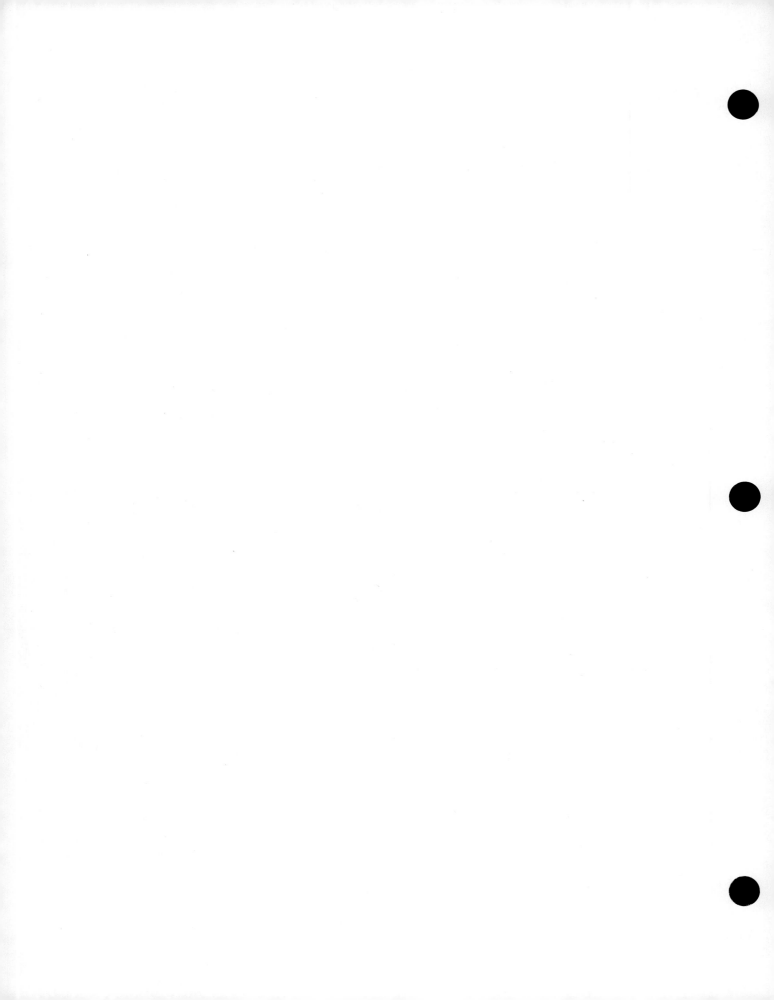

Pharmacology Math

Part I. Drug Labels

Directions: Visit a local pharmacy or grocery store that has a variety of over-the-counter (OTC) medications. Locate containers of aspirin, Tylenol, and Advil in both tablet and liquid forms for children. Complete the following table.

Drug Brand Name	Generic Name	Strength (weight in mg)	Dosage (per tablet or teaspoon)
Aspirin			
Baby aspirin tablets			
Tylenol tablets			
Tylenol liquid			
Advil or Motrin			
Advil liquid			

Part II. Metric System

Consider the following fundamental units of the metric system:

Mass or weight: gram (g) *always lowercase*

Volume: liter (L) *always capitalized*

Length: meter (m) *always lowercase*

Consider the following equivalents:

Mass and weight

1 kg = 1000 g

1 g = 1000 mg

1 mg = 1000 ig

1 dg = 0.1 g or 1/10 g

1 cg = 0.01 g or 1/100 g

1 mg = 0.001 g or 1/1000 g

Volume

1 kl = 1000 liters

1 L = 1000 ml (or cc)

1 ml (or 1 cc) = 1000 il

1 dl = 0.1 L or 1/10 L

1 cl = 0.01 L or 1/100 L

1 ml (or 1 cc) = 0.001 L or 1/1000 L

A. **Directions:** Write the prefix for the following (remember to write them in lowercase).

1. _____ one hundredth of a unit

2. _____ one tenth of a unit

3. _____ one thousandth of a unit

4. _____ one millionth of a unit

5. _____ ten units

6. _____ one hundred units

7. _____ one thousand units

B. **Directions:** Convert the following by moving the decimals or by multiplication or division.

1. 1.5 L = _____ ml   Show your work here.

2. 500 mg = _____ g

3. 3 g = _____ mg

4. 2000 mg = _____ g

5. 2.5 g = _____ mg

6. 0.5 g = _____ mg

7. 500 ml = _____ L

8. 0.75 g = _____ mg

9. 1 kg = _____ g

10. 1000 mg = _____ g

Part III. Apothecary System and Household Measurements

A. **Directions:** Insert roman numerals for use with the apothecary system.

Arabic	Roman	Arabic	Roman
1	I	15	
2		20	
3		30	
4		40	
5	V	50	L
6		60	
7		70	
8		80	
9		90	XC
10	X	100	C

Directions: Supply the abbreviations or symbols for these metric, apothecary system, and common household units.

1. ounce symbol _____

2. teaspoon _____

3. milligram _____

4. grain _____

5. pint _____

6. dram symbol _____

7. tablespoon _____

Directions: Use the conversions to complete the questions below.

1 cup = 8 oz

1 oz = 2 tablespoons

1 tablespoon = 3 teaspoons

1 teaspoon = 60 drops

1 teaspoon = 5 ml (cc)

1 tablespoon = 15 ml (cc)

1 fluid ounce = 30 ml (cc)

1 grain = 60 mg

1. A standard teaspoon equals 5 ml. If a liquid drug has 100 mg per teaspoon, how many

   milligrams are in each milliliter? _____

   How did you determine your answer?

   _____

   _____

2. You are asked to give 2 teaspoons of cough medicine to a child. How many milliliters will you give? _____

3. How many teaspoons are in one ounce? _____

4. Now that you know that 5 ml is the same as one teaspoon, how many milliliters are in one ounce? _____

Part IV. Conversions Between Systems of Measurement _____

Conversions between units of measurements can also be done by using the following formula:

$$\text{Have} \times \frac{\text{Wanted}}{\text{Have (conversion)}} = \text{Unit Wanted in New System}$$

Using the 15 gr/g conversion, convert 30 grains to milligrams:

$$30\ \text{gr} \times \frac{1.0\ \text{g}}{15\ \text{gr}} = \text{Unit Wanted}$$

Cross-multiply the problem and the gr unit cancels out to give:

$$2 \times \frac{1.0\ \text{g}}{1} = 2.0\ \text{g}$$

Directions: Convert pounds to kilograms. The conversion factor is 2.5 lb/kg.

1. 150 lb = _____ kg   Show your work here.

2. 78 lb = _____ kg

3. 22 lb = _____ kg

4. 210 lb = _____ kg

5. 64 lb = _____ kg

6. 198 lb = _____ kg

7. 112 lb = _____ kg

8. 163 lb = _____ kg

9. 13 lb = _____ kg

10. 4.4 lb = _____ kg

Directions: Convert inches to centimeters. There are 2.2 cm per inch.

1. 62 inches = _____ cm   Show your work here.

2. 34 inches = _____ cm

3. 97 inches = _____ cm

4. 5'0" = _____ inches = _____ cm

5. 6'2" = _____ inches = _____ cm

Part V. Decimals and Percents

The act of dividing a fraction results in a decimal number. Decimal numbers can then be converted to percentages by moving the decimal two spaces to the right:

0.25 = 25.0%, commonly written 25%

Directions: Convert these decimals to percentages.

1. 0.75 = _____ %

2. 0.33 = _____ %

3. 0.25 = _____ %

4. 1.0 = _____ %

5. 0.50 = _____ %

Show your work here.

Part VI. Ratio and Proportion

A proportion is written as follows:

$$\frac{4}{16} = \frac{1}{4} \text{ or } 4:16::1:4$$

The preceding proportion example has all the answers in it; there is nothing to solve. In calculating dosages, mathematical proportions are used, but with one element unknown. We must solve for that unknown, or x. For example:

$$\frac{4}{16} = \frac{1}{x}$$

Always in a proportion, we solve the problem by *cross-multiplication.* Do not confuse this with plain multiplication. If you see an equals sign (=) between two fractions, it indicates that the equation is to be *cross-multiplied.*

$$4 \times x = 16 \times 1$$

Therefore

$$4x = 16$$

We know what $4x$ equals, but next we must find what $1x$, or x, equals. To determine the value of x, we must find a way to leave x (or $1x$) alone on one side of the equation. We can change $4x$ to $1x$ by dividing the number 4 by itself:

$$4x \div 4 = 1x$$

But what we do on one side of an equation, we must do on the other side, or the equation will not be equal anymore. Therefore we divide 16 by 4:

$16 \div 4 = 4$ Therefore $x = 4$ and $\frac{4}{16} = \frac{1}{4}$

Directions: Solve for x and compare the two fractions.

1. $3:4 = x:12$

2. $1:2 = x:6$

3. $2:5 = x:100$

Show your work here.

4. $2 : 6 = x : 12$

5. $1 : 3 = x : 75$

Part VII. Calculating Dosages

Standard Formula:

$$\frac{\text{Available strength}}{\text{Ordered strength}} = \frac{\text{Available amount}}{\text{Amount to give}}$$

Procedure: Rewrite the formula, replacing unknown values with known quantities from the label and the doctor's order. The unknown, when you solve for x, will be the amount you actually give.

Let's Practice: The doctor orders 200 mg of medication. The label reads 100 mg per tablet. How many tablets do you give?

$$\frac{100 \text{ mg}}{200 \text{ mg}} = \frac{1 \text{ tablet}}{x}$$

Cross-multiply: 100 mg times x = 200 mg times 1 tablet

Divide both sides by 100 to leave x by itself on the left side.

What is the result? How many tablets do you give?

Another way to complete the same problem is to use a formula:

$$\frac{\text{Dose Desired (Doctor's Order)}}{\text{Dose on Hand}} \times \text{Quantity or Unit on Hand}$$

$$\frac{200 \text{ mg}}{100 \text{ mg}} \times 1 \text{ tablet}$$

What is the result? How many tablets do you give?

Practice calculations

Directions: Calculate the following:

Doctor's Order	Label Reads	Amount to Give	Practice Charting
Keflex 500 mg	250-mg capsule		
Lasix 40	20-mg tablet		
Zoloft 75 mg	25-mg tablet		
Claritin 30 mg	10-mg tablet		
Prilosec 40 mg	10-mg capsule		
Celebrex 150	100-mg tablet		
Vioxx 12.5	50 mg		
Lanoxin .125 mg	.25-mg tablet		

Doctor's Order	Label Reads	Amount to Give	Practice Charting
Coumadin 20 mg	5-mg tablet		
Augmentin 250	500 mg per 5 ml		
Prednisone 40 mg	5-mg tablet		
Prozac 20 mg	10-mg capsule		
Synthroid .44 mg	88 µg per tablet		
Zocor 60 mg	20-mg tablet		
Glucophage 1 g	500-mg tablet		
Zestril 2.5 mg	5-mg tablet		
Norvasc 10 mg	2.5-mg tablet		
Cipro 750 mg	250-mg tablet		
Zyrtec syrup 4 mg	5 mg/5 ml		
Zovirax 200 mg	400-mg tablet		

Part VIII. Pediatric Dosages

Directions: Complete the following:

Fried's Law

$$\text{Pediatric Dose} = \frac{\text{Child's Age in Months}}{150 \text{ months}} \times \text{Adult Dose}$$

Order	Adult Dose	Child's Age	Amount to Give
Penicillin	100,000 U	18 mo	
Benadryl	50 mg	5 yr	
Tylenol	500 mg	2 yr	
Sudafed	60 mg	10 mo	

Clark's Rule

Pediatric Dose = $\frac{\text{Child's Weight in Pounds}}{150 \text{ pounds}} \times$ Adult Dose

Order	Adult Dose	Child's Weight	Amount to Give
Penicillin	100,000 U	22 lb	
Benadryl	50 mg	13 lb	
Tylenol	500 mg	54 lb	
Sudafed	60 mg	37 lb	

West's Nomogram

Pediatric Dose = $\frac{\text{Body Surface Area (BSA) of Child in Square Meters} \times \text{Adult Dose}}{1.7 \text{ m}^2 \text{ (Average Adult BSA)}}$

Order	Adult Dose	Child's BSA	Amount to Give
Penicillin	100,000 U	.5 m^2	
Benadryl	50 mg	.3 m^2	
Tylenol	500 mg	.6 m^2	
Sudafed	60 mg	.7 m^2	

Part IX. Putting It All Together

Directions: Use Fried's Law, Clark's Rule, or West's Nomogram to answer the following questions.

1. A child weighs 42 lb. The doctor orders 1 mg of medication per kilogram. How many kilograms does the child weigh? How many milligrams of medication do you need to give? _____

2. A 5-year-old needs cough medicine. The adult dose is 20 mg. According to Fried's Law, what is the pediatric dose? _____

3. An infant weighs 14 lb. The adult dose is 100 mg. When Clark's Rule is used, how much is the pediatric dose? _____

4. The doctor orders 5 mg of medication per kilogram of body weight. The patient weighs 145 lb. How many milligrams do you give? _____

5. The child has a BSA of .9 m^2 and the adult dose is 200 mg. According to West's nomogram, what is the pediatric dose? _____

6. The nurse practitioner orders 250 mg of Rocephin to be given by injection. The vial contains Rocephin at a concentration of 500 mg/ml. How much medication will the medical assistant draw into the syringe? _____

7. The patient takes 5000 U of heparin by injection each day. The vial contains heparin, 10,000 U/ml. How much heparin does the home health nurse need to draw up into the syringe?

   _____

8. The patient weighs 163 lb. The order is for 2 mg/kg. How much medicine does the patient need? _____

9. The doctor orders Phenergan 12.5 mg by mouth. You have Phenergan syrup that has a concentration of 25 mg/5 ml. How many milliliters will you give? _____

10. You need to give a 500 injection of vitamin B$_{12}$. You have on hand vitamin B$_{12}$ at a concentration unit of 1000 unit/ml. How much will you measure in the syringe? _____

Part X. Extra for Experts

Directions: Use the Internet or a drug reference book to collect information and make index cards for the drugs that were discussed in Chapters 8 and 9.

BRAND NAME:

GENERIC NAME:

TYPE OF DRUG:

USUAL DOSE:

USES:

Chapter 9 Quiz

Name: _____

1. One cup equals _____ ounces.

2. One teaspoon equals _____ ml.

3. There are _____ ml in one ounce.

4. A grain is part of the _____ system.

   a. metric

   b. household

   c. apothecary

5. A liter is a unit of

   a. weight

   b. volume

   c. length

6. Milliliters are sometimes called

   _____.

7. The Roman numeral for four is

   _____.

8. There are _____ teaspoons in one tablespoon.

9. True or False: Clark's rule uses a child's age to calculate dosage.

10. There are _____ pounds in one kilogram.

CHAPTER 10

Administering Medications

Part I. Vocabulary

Directions: Match the following terms and definitions.

1. _____ Angled tip of a needle

2. _____ Narrowing of the bronchiole tubes

3. _____ Abnormal accumulation of fluid in the interstitial spaces of tissues

4. _____ A coating added to an oral medication that resists the effects of stomach juices; designed so medicine is absorbed in the small intestine

5. _____ Sealed so that no air is allowed to enter

6. _____ Low blood pressure

7. _____ Administering repeated injections of diluted extracts of the substance that causes an allergy; also called *desensitization*

8. _____ An abnormally hard, inflamed area

9. _____ Administering a double dose for the first dose of the medication; usually done with antibiotic therapy to reach therapeutic blood levels quickly

10. _____ Surgical removal of the breast; usually includes excision of lymph nodes in the axillary region

11. _____ The curved formation of liquids in a container

12. _____ Excretion of an unusually large amount of urine

13. _____ Drug in pill form manufactured with an indentation for division through the center

14. _____ Increase in the diameter of a blood vessel

15. _____ The quality of being thick; property of resistance to flow in a fluid

16. _____ Referring to an explosive substance's capacity to vaporize at a low temperature

17. _____ Localized area of edema or a raised lesion

A. bevel

B. scored tablet

C. hypotension

D. polyuria

E. volatile

F. wheal

G. viscosity

H. vasodilation

I. immunotherapy

J. loading dose

K. edema

L. meniscus

M. bronchoconstriction

N. induration

O. enteric-coated

P. mastectomy

Q. hermetically sealed

Part II.

Directions: List the seven rights of drug administration.

1. _____
2. _____
3. _____
4. _____
5. _____
6. _____
7. _____

Solid Oral Forms

Directions: Define the following.

1. Scored _____
2. Tablet _____
3. Buffered _____
4. Capsule _____
5. Caplet _____
6. Time-released _____

Liquid Oral Forms

Directions: Define the following.

1. Syrup _____
2. Aromatic waters _____
3. Liquors _____
4. Suspension _____
5. Emulsion _____
6. Gel/magma _____
7. Tinctures _____
8. Elixirs _____

Mucous Membrane Forms

Directions: List the site of absorption for the following.

1. Buccal _____
2. Sublingual _____
3. Inhalation _____

Topical Forms

Directions: Describe the following.

1. Lotion _____

2. Liniment _____

3. Ointment _____

4. Trandermal _____

Parenteral Forms

Directions: Define the following.

1. Vial _____

2. Ampule _____

3. Multi-use _____

4. Prefilled _____

5. Cartridge system _____

Directions: Indicate whether each item in the figure below is a vial or an ampule.

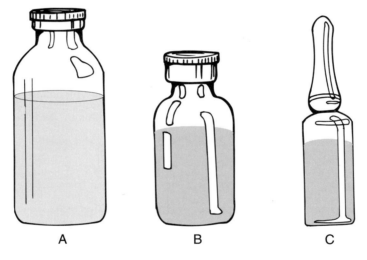

A   B   C

A. _____

B. _____

C. _____

Directions: Label the following statements as either "ampule" or "vial."

1. _____ Has a rubber stopper.

2. _____ Has sharp edges after it is opened.

3. _____ Is always single-use.

4. _____ Must have air injected into it before medicine can be removed.

5. _____ Can be multi-use.

6. _____ A filtered needle should be used to avoid getting glass in the syringe.

7. _____ Has a vacuum after it is opened.

8. _____ Extra care must be taken to avoid contamination.

9. _____ Always disposed of in a sharps container.

10. _____ Gauze or an unopened alcohol prep should be used to prevent injury as the neck breaks away.

Directions: List four routes of parenteral administration. Include approved abbreviations.

1. _____

2. _____

3. _____

4. _____

Parenteral Medication Equipment

Directions: Indicate which statements about needles are true (T) and which statements are false (F).

1. _____ Needles may be purchased separately or as part of a needle-syringe unit.

2. _____ The diameter or lumen size of a needle is called its *gauge,* and needle gauges range in size from 14 (the largest) to 28 (the smallest).

3. _____ The larger the gauge number, the smaller is the diameter of the needle.

4. _____ Gauges 25 and 26 are commonly used for subcutaneous injections.

5. _____ Larger needles (gauges 20 to 23) are usually necessary for intramuscular injections when the medication is thick (e.g., penicillin).

6. _____ Needles that are ½ or 5/8 inch long are used for intramuscular injections.

7. _____ Needles that are ½ or 5/8 inch long are used for subcutaneous injections.

8. _____ The contaminated needle should be immediately placed in a sharps container.

9. _____ The parts of the needle are the barrel, calibrated scale(s), plunger, and tip.

10. _____ Longer needles are necessary for depositing drugs intradermally.

Directions: Label the syringes in the figure below.

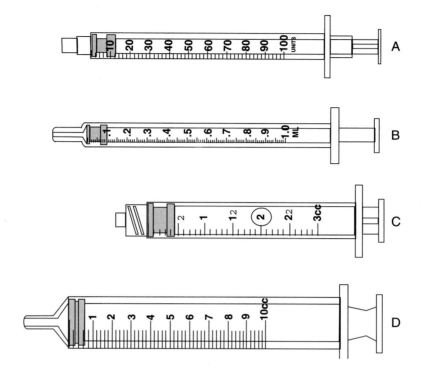

1. On the 10-cc slip-tip syringe, draw a line at 4.8 cc.

2. On the insulin syringe, draw a line at 62 units.

3. On the tuberculin syringe, draw a line at .3 cc.

4. On the 3-cc Luer-Lok syringe, draw a line at ½ cc.

Part III. Injection Sites

Directions: On the figure on p. 78, label the intramuscular, intradermal, and subcutaneous injection sites correctly.

A. Deltoid

B. Ventrogluteal

C. Vastus lateralis

D. Gluteal (dorsogluteal)

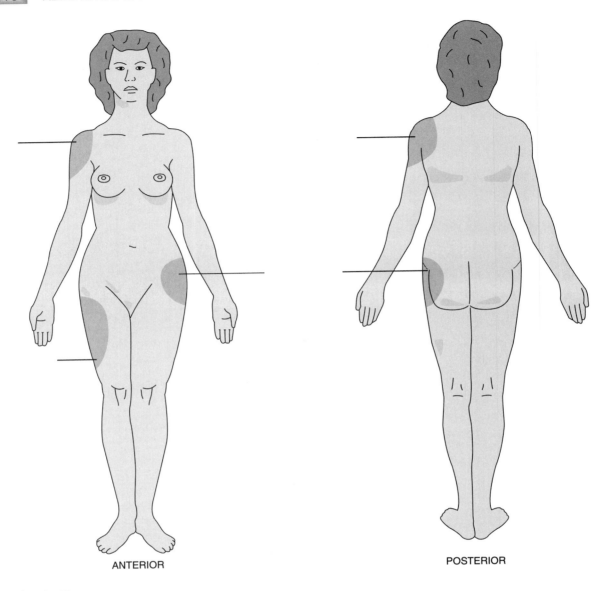

ANTERIOR   POSTERIOR

Pediatric Sites

Directions: On the figure below, label and name the appropriate injection site for a small child who is too young to walk.

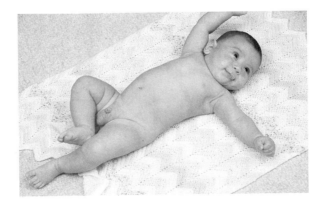

When instilling ear drops into an infant's ear, you must straighten the ear canal. On the figure below, draw an arrow to show which direction you pull the pinna.

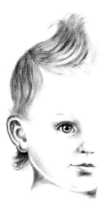

Part IV.

How do you feel about giving your first injection? How will you prepare for that experience? Discuss your thoughts with a classmate. Share your concerns with your instructor.

_____

_____

_____

_____

_____

_____

Extra for Experts

Directions: Visit a pharmacy and find out about each section of a written prescription. Label each part of the sample prescription below.

Superscription

Inscription

Subscription

Sig

Refills

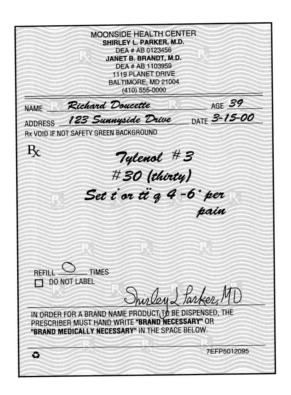

MOONSIDE HEALTH CENTER
SHIRLEY L. PARKER, M.D.
DEA # AB 0123456
JANET B. BRANDT, M.D.
DEA # AB 1103959
1119 PLANET DRIVE
BALTIMORE, MD 21004
(410) 555-0000

NAME *Richard Doucette* AGE *39*

ADDRESS *123 Sunnyside Drive* DATE *3-15-00*

Rx VOID IF NOT SAFETY GREEN BACKGROUND

℞

Tylenol # 3
 # 30 (thirty)
Set i or ii q 4-6° per
pain

REFILL _____ TIMES
☐ DO NOT LABEL

Shirley L Parker, MD

IN ORDER FOR A BRAND NAME PRODUCT TO BE DISPENSED, THE
PRESCRIBER MUST HAND WRITE **"BRAND NECESSARY"** OR
"BRAND MEDICALLY NECESSARY" IN THE SPACE BELOW.

7EFP5012095

Your patient asks you to explain what the doctor has written on the prescription. Explain the directions for taking Tylenol #3.

_____

_____

_____

_____

Spell out the following abbreviations.

1. q4h _____

2. tid _____

3. qid _____

4. bid _____

5. q3h _____

6. hs _____

7. ac _____

8. pc _____

9. prn _____

10. po _____

11. npo _____

12. pr _____

13. IV _____

14. SC (SQ) _____

15. IM _____

16. SL _____

17. qd _____

18. qod _____

19. qam _____

20. qpm _____

Chapter 10 Quiz

Name: _____

1. True or False: An 18-gauge needle is larger than a 23-gauge needle.

2. A tuberculin syringe holds _____ ml (cc).

3. True or False: An ampule is multi-use.

4. One site of a subcutaneous injections is:

   a. Vastus lateralis

   b. Deltoid

   c. Gluteal (dorsogluteal)

   d. Abdomen

5. The safest site for an intramuscular injection on a small child is the:

   a. Vastus lateralis

   b. Deltoid

   c. Gluteal (dorsogluteal)

6. Milliliters are sometimes called _____ on syringes.

7. The _____ is the slanted part of a needle.

8. _____ is the route for heparin and insulin.

9. True or False: Z-track is used for an intramuscular injection of an irritating substance.

10. True or False: Intradermal medication is usually given at a 90-degree angle.

CHAPTER 11

Assisting with Medical Emergencies

Part I. Vocabulary

A. **Directions:** Define the following.

1. cyanosis _____

2. dyspnea _____

3. ecchymosis _____

4. emetic _____

5. fibrillation _____

6. hematuria _____

7. mediastinum _____

8. myocardium _____

9. necrosis _____

10. photophobia _____

11. polydipsia _____

12. polyuria _____

13. transient ischemic attack _____

B. **Directions:** Fill in the blanks with the correct terms.

1. _____ _____ is defined as the immediate care given to a person who has been injured or has suddenly taken ill.

2. AED stands for _____.

3. CPR stands for _____.

4. CVA stands for _____.

5. TIA stands for _____.

6. MI stands for _____.

7. A heart attack, or _____, is usually caused by a blockage of the coronary arteries, which decreases the amount of blood being delivered to the myocardium. The most common signal of a heart attack is an uncomfortable pressure, squeezing, fullness, or pain in the center of the chest.

C. List five other symptoms of a heart attack.

1. _____

2. _____

3. _____

4. _____

5. _____

D. List seven types of shock.

1. _____

2. _____

3. _____

4. _____

5. _____

6. _____

7. _____

E. Sprains and strains are treated with:

1. _____

2. _____

3. _____

F. Give five examples of situations in which patients with abdominal pain should be seen immediately.

1. _____

2. _____

3. _____

4. _____

5. _____

Part II. Heat-Related Illnesses

Directions: Fill in the blanks with the correct terms.

1. _____ _____ is the most dangerous form of heat-related injury and results in a shutdown of body systems.

2. _____ are the initial signs of a heat-related emergency, and heat exhaustion is a more serious condition.

3. Patients with _____ _____ appear flushed and report headaches, nausea, vertigo, and weakness.

Part III. Emergency Situations

Directions: Complete the table with appropriate triage questions and home care advice.

Situation	Triage Questions	Home Care Advice
Syncope	1. 2.	1. 2. 3.
Animal bites	1. 2. 3.	1. 2. 3.
Insect bites and stings	1. 2.	1. 2. 3.
Asthma	1. 2.	1.
Burns	1. 2. 3.	1. 2. 3. 4.

Situation	Triage Questions	Home Care Advice
Wounds	1. 2. 3. 4.	1. 2. 3. 4.
Head injury	1.	1.

Chapter 11 Quiz

Name: _____

1. AED stands for _____

_____ _____.

2. A _____ _____
seizure involves uncontrolled muscular
contractions.

3. List three symptoms of a heart attack.

a. _____

b. _____

c. _____

4. Syncope means to _____.

5. List three causes of shock.

a. _____

b. _____

c. _____

6. True or False: Epinephrine is a
vasoconstrictor.

7. True or False: Accidental poisoning is the
leading cause of death in children.

8. List two ways to treat lacerations.

a. _____

b. _____

9. During a life-threatening emergency,

always call _____.

10. _____ means to sort patients.

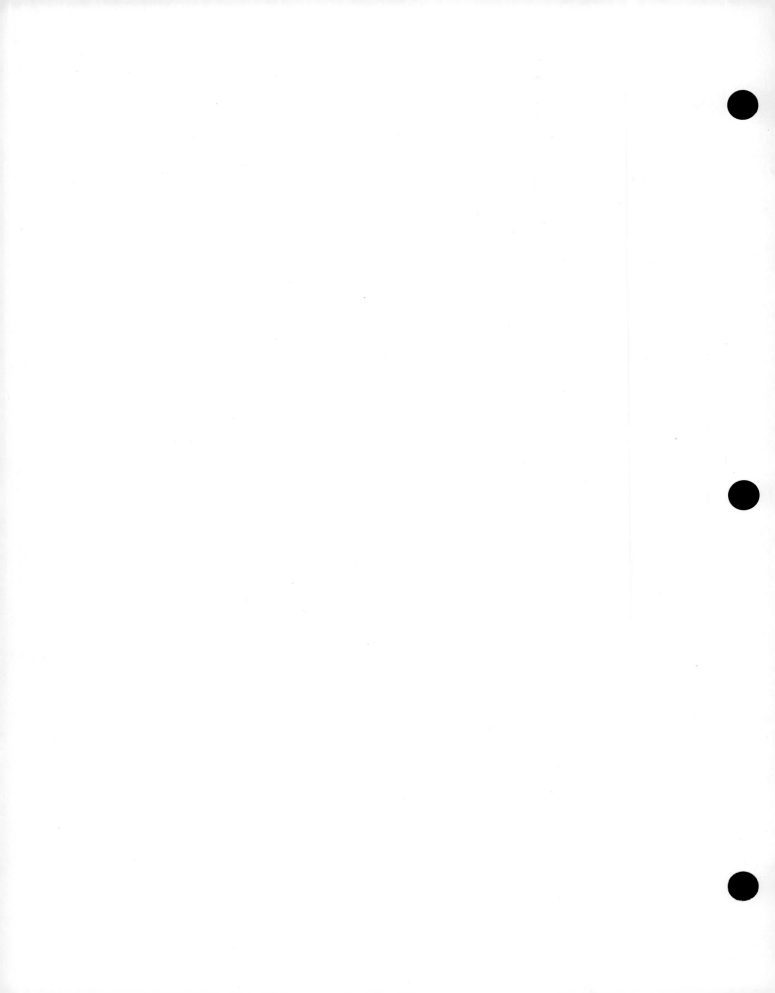

Assisting in Ophthalmology and Otolaryngology

Part I. Medical Terminology

Directions: Match the following terms and definitions.

1. _____ Adjustment of the eye for seeing various sizes of objects at different distances

2. _____ Reduction or dimness of vision with no apparent organic cause; often referred to as *lazy eye syndrome*

3. _____ An allied healthcare professional specializing in evaluation of hearing function, detection of hearing impairment, and determination of the anatomic site of impairment

4. _____ Structures found in the retina that make the perception of color possible

5. _____ A small pit in the center of the retina that is considered the center of clearest vision

6. _____ Any substance or medication that causes constriction of the pupil

7. _____ Region at the back of the eye where the optic nerve meets the retina; considered the blind spot of the eye because it contains only nerve fibers and no rods or cones and thus is insensitive to light

8. _____ Second cranial nerve that carries impulses for the sense of sight

9. _____ Formation of spongy bone in the labyrinth of the ear, often causing the auditory ossicles to become fixed and unable to vibrate when sound enters the ear

10. _____ A substance or medication that damages the eighth cranial nerve or the organs of hearing and balance

11. _____ Abnormal sensitivity to light

A. cones

B. accommodation

C. seborrhea

D. psoriasis

E. rods

F. audiologist

G. amblyopia

H. photophobia

I. optic nerve

J. otosclerosis

K. ototoxic

L. fovea centralis

M. optic disc

N. miotic

12. _____ Usually chronic, recurrent skin disease marked by bright red patches covered with silvery scales

13. _____ Structures located in the retina of the eye and forming the light-sensitive elements

14. _____ Excessive discharge of sebum from the sebaceous glands, forming greasy scales or cheesy plugs on the body

Part II. Spelling

1. Spell the name of the color blindness test. _____

2. Spell the name of the chart that is used for testing far vision. _____

3. Spell the name of the chart used for testing near vision. _____

Part III. Anatomy and Physiology

A. **Directions:** On the figure below, label the structures of the outer eye.

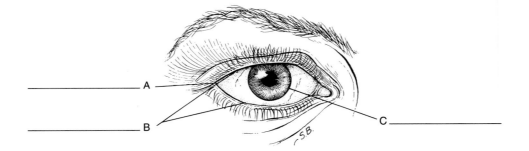

B. **Directions:** On the figure below, label the structures of the outer ear.

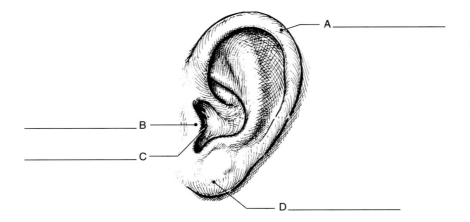

Part IV. Theory/Triage

A. **Directions:** Name the two disorders of the outer eye that are pictured below.

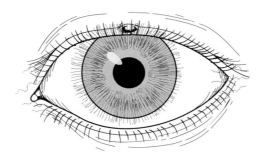

1. _____

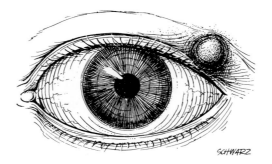

2. _____

Part V. Documentation

Directions: Refer to the charts in the figure below to answer the questions.

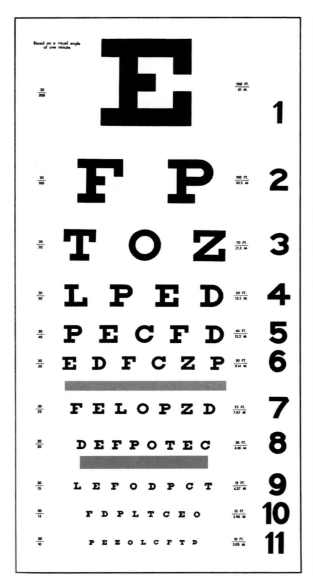

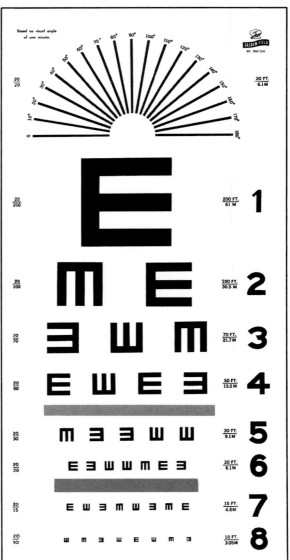

A. Your patient can read line number 8 with the right eye, number 9 with the left eye, and number 8 with both eyes on the Snellen chart. Document your findings on p. 95. Use appropriate abbreviations. Be sure to include the date and your signature. Correct mistakes by drawing one line. Use black ink.

Documentation

B. Your patient cannot read English. He indicates that he can see line number 6 with the right eye, number 5 with the left eye, and number 6 with both eyes on the **E** chart. How will you have your patient respond so that you know your findings are accurate?

Document your findings below. Use appropriate abbreviations. Be sure to include the date and your signature. Correct mistakes by drawing one line. Use black ink.

Documentation

Part VI. Drugs to Know

Directions: Use a drug reference book or the Internet to make drug cards for the following.

1. carbamide peroxide (Debrox)

2. Cortisporin otic

3. Pilocarpine ophthalmic

4. Betaoptic

5. Diamox

6. Acular

7. Livostin

8. Tobrex

9. Bleph-10

10. Timoptic

Part VII. Laboratory Tests and Diagnostic Tools to Know

A. **Directions:** Label the drawings with the names of these two hearing tests.

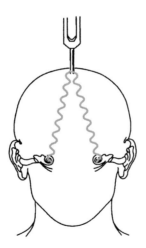

1. _____

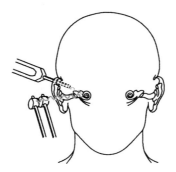

2. _____

B. **Directions:** Hold the workbook 14 inches from your eyes and look at the figure below. What is the smallest line you can read clearly? On p. 98 document your near acuity in both eyes separately and together.

ROSENBAUM POCKET VISION SCREENER

95

distance equivalent

$\frac{20}{800}$

874

Point   Jaeger

$\frac{20}{400}$

2843

26 16 $\frac{20}{200}$

638 ЕШЭ XOO   14 10 $\frac{20}{100}$

8745 ЭmШ OXO   10 7 $\frac{20}{70}$

63925 mEЭ XOX   8 5 $\frac{20}{50}$

4 2 8 3 6 5 ШEm O X O   6 3 $\frac{20}{40}$

3 7 4 2 5 8 Э Ш Э X X O   5 2 $\frac{20}{30}$

9 3 7 8 2 6 Ш m E X O O   4 1 $\frac{20}{25}$

4 2 8 7 3 9 E Ш m O O X   3 1+ $\frac{20}{20}$

Card is held in good light 14 inches from eye. Record vision for each eye separately with and without glasses. Presbyopic patients should read thru bifocal segment. Check myopes with glasses only.

DESIGN COURTESY J. G. ROSENBAUM, M.D.

PUPIL GAUGE (mm.)

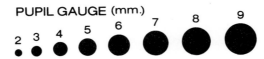

2 3 4 5 6 7 8 9

Documentation

Part IX. Transdisciplinary Skills

ICD-9 Coding

You have looked up *otitis* in the index of diseases, and you are confirming codes in the tabular index.

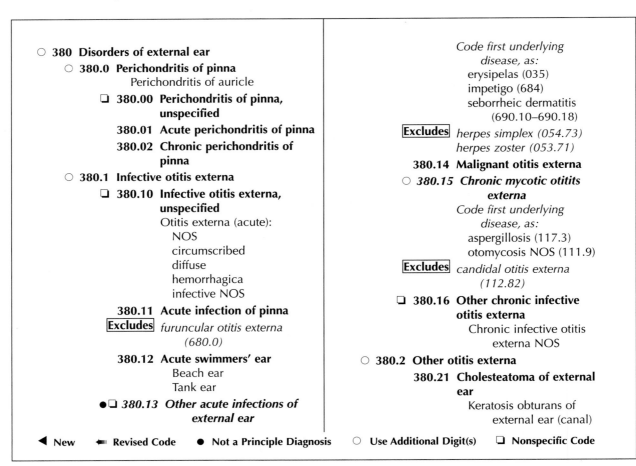

○ **380 Disorders of external ear**
  ○ **380.0 Perichondritis of pinna**
      Perichondritis of auricle
    ❑ **380.00 Perichondritis of pinna, unspecified**
      380.01 Acute perichondritis of pinna
      380.02 Chronic perichondritis of pinna
  ○ **380.1 Infective otitis externa**
    ❑ **380.10 Infective otitis externa, unspecified**
        Otitis externa (acute):
          NOS
          circumscribed
          diffuse
          hemorrhagica
          infective NOS
      380.11 Acute infection of pinna
      Excludes *furuncular otitis externa (680.0)*
      380.12 Acute swimmers' ear
        Beach ear
        Tank ear
    ●❑ *380.13 Other acute infections of external ear*

Code first underlying disease, as:
  erysipelas (035)
  impetigo (684)
  seborrheic dermatitis (690.10–690.18)
Excludes *herpes simplex (054.73) herpes zoster (053.71)*
    380.14 Malignant otitis externa
  ○ *380.15 Chronic mycotic otitis externa*
    Code first underlying disease, as:
      aspergillosis (117.3)
      otomycosis NOS (111.9)
    Excludes *candidal otitis externa (112.82)*
    ❑ **380.16 Other chronic infective otitis externa**
        Chronic infective otitis externa NOS
  ○ **380.2 Other otitis externa**
      380.21 Cholesteatoma of external ear
        Keratosis obturans of external ear (canal)

◀ **New**   ⬅ **Revised Code**   ● **Not a Principle Diagnosis**   ○ **Use Additional Digit(s)**   ❑ **Nonspecific Code**

Excludes *cholesteatoma NOS
(385.30–385.35)
postmastoidectomy (383.32)*

❏ **380.22 Other acute otitis externa**
Acute otitis externa:
actinic
chemical
contact
eczematoid
reactive

❏ **380.23 Other chronic otitis externa**
Chronic otitis externa NOS

○ **380.3 Noninfectious disorders of pinna**

❏ **380.30 Disorder of pinna,
unspecified**

**380.31 Hematoma of auricle or
pinna**

**380.32 Acquired deformities of
auricle or pinna**
Excludes *cauliflower ear (738.7)*

❏ **380.39 Other**
Excludes *gouty tophi of ear (274.81)*

380.4 Impacted cerumen
Wax in ear

○ **380.5 Acquired stenosis of external ear
canal**
Collapse of external ear canal

❏ **380.50 Acquired stenosis of external
ear canal, unspecified as to
cause**

380.51 Secondary to trauma

380.52 Secondary to surgery

380.53 Secondary to inflammation

○ **380.8 Other disorders of external ear**

**380.81 Exostosis of external ear
canal**

❏ **380.89 Other**

❏ **380.9 Unspecified disorder of external ear**

○ **381 Nonsuppurative otitis media and
Eustachian tube disorders**

○ **381.0 Acute nonsuppurative otitis media**
Acute tubotympanic catarrh
Otitis media, acute or subacute:
catarrhal
exudative
transudative
with effusion
Excludes *otitic barotrauma (993.0)*

❏ **381.00 Acute nonsuppurative otitis
media, unspecified**

381.01 Acute serous otitis media
Acute or subacute
secretory otitis media

381.02 Acute mucoid otitis media
Acute or subacute
seromucinous otitis
media
Blue drum syndrome

**381.03 Acute sanguinous otitis
media**

**381.04 Acute allergic serous otitis
media**

**381.05 Acute allergic mucoid otitis
media**

**381.06 Acute allergic sanguinous
otitis media**

○ **381.1 Chronic serous otitis media**
Chronic tubotympanic catarrh

**381.10 Chronic serous otitis media,
simple or unspecified**

❏ **381.19 Other**
Serosanguinous chronic
otitis media

○ **381.2 Chronic mucoid otitis media**
Glue ear
Excludes *adhesive middle ear disease
(385.10–385.19)*

**381.20 Chronic mucoid otitis
media, simple or unspecified**

❏ **381.29 Other**
Mucosanguinous chronic
otitis media

❏ **381.3 Other and unspecified chronic nonsuppurative otitis media**
Otitis media, chronic:
allergic   seromucinous
exudative   transudative
secretory   with effusion

❏ **381.4 Nonsuppurative otitis media, not
specified as acute or chronic**
Otitis media:
allergic   seromucinous
catarrhal   serous
exudative   transudative
mucoid   with effusion
secretory

◀ **New**   ◀━ **Revised Code**   ● **Not a Principle Diagnosis**   ○ **Use Additional Digit(s)**   ❏ **Nonspecific Code**

Code the following diagnoses.

1. Swimmer's ear _____

2. Acute serous otitis media _____

3. Chronic fungal otitis externa _____

4. Chronic serous otitis media _____

5. Impacted ear wax _____

Part IX. Certification Review

A. Refractive errors include:

1. _____

2. _____

3. _____

B. Eye disorders can range from problems with eye movement, as in strabismus and nystagmus, to infections of the eye including:

1. _____

2. _____

3. _____

4. _____

C. Disorders of the eyeball include:

1. _____

2. _____

3. _____

4. _____

D. Examination of the nose and throat begins with examination of the nasal cavity and then visual examination of the throat and the nasopharynx.

1. In the drawing below, the physician is examining the _____.

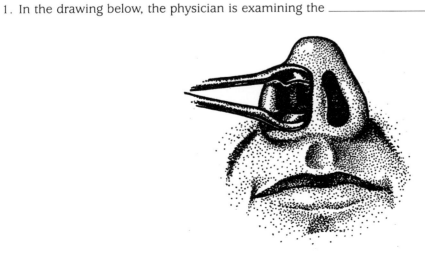

2. Name two instruments that would be needed for this exam.

   a. _____

   b. _____

E. Differentiate between otitis media and otitis externa.

_____

_____

_____

_____

F. Differentiate between hyperopia and myopia.

_____

_____

_____

_____

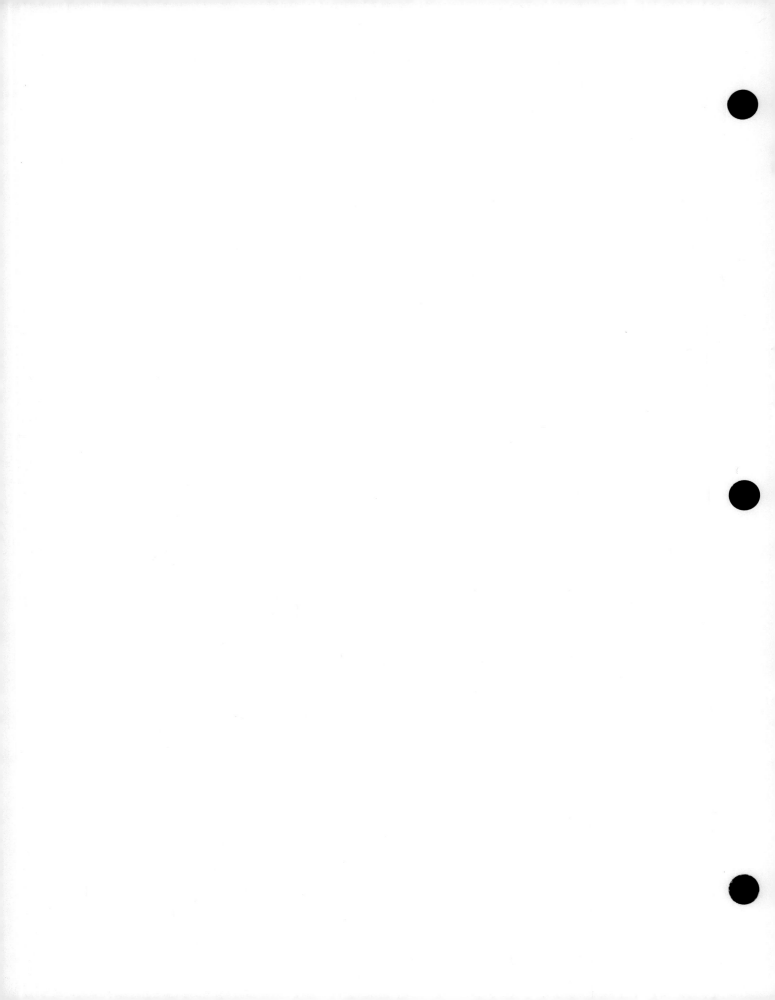

Chapter 12 Quiz

Name: _____

1. Nearsightedness is called _____.

2. OD means _____
   _____.

3. What is the name of the color blindness test?
   _____

4. OS means _____
   _____.

5. List three types of glaucoma:
   a. _____
   b. _____
   c. _____

6. Hyperopia means _____
   _____.

7. True or False: Another name for a stye is
   hordeolum.

8. List three refractive errors.
   a. _____
   b. _____
   c. _____

9. Otic means _____.

10. _____ test air versus bone
    conduction of sound.

CHAPTER 13

Assisting in Dermatology

Part I. Medical Terminology

Directions: Define the following.

1. bilirubin _____

2. cryosurgery _____

3. debridement _____

4. ecchymosis _____

5. electrodesiccation _____

6. exacerbation _____

7. hyperplasia _____

8. jaundice _____

9. keratin _____

10. leukoderma _____

11. opaque _____

12. remission _____

Part II. Spelling

Phone-etics Game

Directions: Use the telephone keypad on p. 106 to spell out the missing words.

1. Sebaceous glands release 7-3-2-8-6, an oily substance that lubricates the skin. _____

2. The epidermis is the thin uppermost layer, and the 3-3-7-6-4-7 is the thicker layer beneath.

   _____

3. A variety of microorganisms called *normal* or *resident* 3-5-6-7-2 are found on the skin and may increase the risk for integumentary system infections. _____

4. 4-6-7-8-4-4-6 impetigo is a common contagious, superficial infection caused by streptococci or *Staphylococcus aureus.* _____

5. 2-2-6-3 is a disorder of the hair follicle and sebaceous gland unit. _____

6. 3-2-z-3-6-2 is characterized by a vesicular rash located on the face, neck, elbows, posterior knees, and behind the ears. _____

	ABC	DEF
1	2	3
GHI	JKL	MNO
4	5	6
PRS	TUV	WXY
7	8	9
*	0	#

Part III. Anatomy and Physiology

Directions: Label the three layers of the skin in the drawing below.

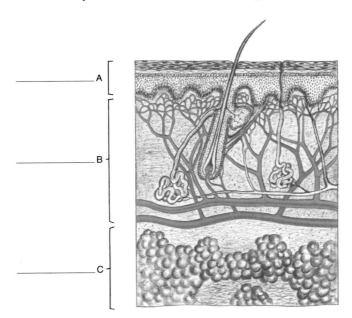

_____ A

_____ B

_____ C

Part IV. Theory/Triage

Directions: Give a common name for each of these fungal (mycotic) infections.

1. tinea pedis _____

2. tinea cruris _____

3. tinea corporis _____

4. tinea unguium _____

5. scabies _____

6. pediculosis _____

7. verrucae _____

8. erysipelas _____

Part V. Documentation

A. Your patient has a red, flat rash with itching. Use the correct medical terminology to chart your findings. Use appropriate abbreviations. Be sure to include the date and your signature. Correct mistakes by drawing one line. Use black ink.

Documentation

B. Your patient has a red, raised rash with small blisters. Use the correct medical terminology to
   chart your findings. Use appropriate abbreviations. Be sure to include the date and your signature.
   Correct mistakes by drawing one line. Use black ink.

Documentation

Part VI. Drugs to Know

Directions: Fill in the blanks with the correct terms.

1. Antiacne medications include topical tretinoin (_____) gel and antibacterial creams
   such as _____ peroxide.

2. Oral antibiotics, such as _____ and erythromycin, at a maintenance dose of 250 mg
   once or twice daily, can be prescribed to control comedones and pustules.

3. Severe cystic acne can be treated with _____, but it is a strong teratogen and should
   never be prescribed for pregnant women or those not using contraceptives.

4. Skin parasites are treated with 5% permethrin cream (_____) or 1% lindane lotion
   (_____).

5. Prednisone or methylprednisolone (Medrol) is used to treat _____.

6. Supply a brand name for each of the following antifungal topical agents: clotrimazole
   (_____), ketoconazole (_____), Spectazole, or nystatin
   (_____).

7. An antiviral drug is acyclovir (_____).

8. Zyrtec and Allegra are used to treat _____.

Part VII. Laboratory Tests and Diagnostic Tools to Know _____

A. Telephone Triage

A patient calls and states there is redness on her upper arm. What questions do you need to ask before scheduling the appointment?

_____

_____

_____

_____

_____

B. List four ways to perform allergy testing.

1. _____

2. _____

3. _____

4. _____

C. Early warning signs of malignant melanoma are:

1. A _____

2. B _____

3. C _____

4. D _____

Part VIII. ICD-9 Coding

You have looked up *herpes* in the index of diseases, and you are confirming codes in the tabular index.

Code the following diagnoses.

1. Chicken pox _____

2. Herpes zoster _____

3. Varicella _____

4. Herpes simplex virus type I _____

○ **052 Chickenpox**

052.0 Postvaricella encephalitis
Postchickenpox encephalitis

052.1 Varicella (hemorrhagic) pneumonitis

❏ **052.7 With other specified complications**

❏ **052.8 With unspecified complication**

052.9 Varicella without mention of complication
Chickenpox NOS
Varicella NOS

○ **053 Herpes zoster**

Includes: shingles
zona

053.0 With meningitis

○ **053.1 With other nervous system complications**

❏ **053.10 With unspecified nervous system**

053.11 Geniculate herpes zoster
Herpetic geniculate ganglionitis

053.12 Postherpetic trigeminal neuralgia

053.13 Postherpetic polyneuropathy

❏ **053.19 Other**

○ **053.2 With ophthalmic complications**

053.20 Herpes zoster dermatitis of eyelid
Herpes zoster ophthalmicus

053.21 Herpes zoster kerato-conjunctivitis

053.22 Herpes zoster iridocyclitis

❏ **053.29 Other**

○ **053.7 With other specified complications**

053.71 Otitis externa due to herpes zoster

❏ **053.79 Other**

❏ **053.8 With unspecified complication**

053.9 Herpes zoster without mention of complication
Herpes zoster NOS

○ **054 Herpes simplex**

Excludes *congenital herpes simplex (771.2)*

054.0 Eczema herpeticum
Kaposi's varicelliform eruption

○ **054.1 Genital herpes**

❏ **054.10 Genital herpes, unspecified**
Herpes progenitalis

054.11 Herpetic vulvovaginitis

054.12 Herpetic ulceration of vulva

054.13 Herpetic infection of penis

❏ **054.19 Other**

054.2 Herpetic gingivostomatitis

054.3 Herpetic meningoencephalitis
Herpes encephalitis
Simian B disease

○ **054.4 With ophthalmic complications**

❏ **054.40 With unspecified ophthalmic complication**

054.41 Herpes simplex dermatitis of eyelid

054.42 Dendritic keratitis

054.43 Herpes simplex disciform keratitis

054.44 Herpes simplex iridocyclitis

❏ **054.49 Other**

054.5 Herpetic septicemia

054.6 Herpetic whitlow
Herpetic felon

○ **054.7 With other specified complications**

054.71 Visceral herpes simplex

054.72 Herpes simplex meningitis

054.73 Herpes simplex otitis externa

❏ **054.79 Other**

❏ **054.8 With unspecified complication**

054.9 Herpes simplex without mention of complication

◀ **New**   ⬅ **Revised Code**   ● **Not a Principle Diagnosis**   ○ **Use Additional Digit(s)**   ❏ **Nonspecific Code**

5. Shingles _____

6. Genital herpes _____

7. Herpetic conjunctivitis and keratitis _____

8. Herpes zoster of the external ear _____

9. Simean B disease _____

10. Herpes whitlow L index finger _____

Part IX. Certification Review _____

A. **Directions:** Define and give an example of the following. Consult a medical dictionary and your text.

1. Macule

_____

_____

2. Papule

_____

_____

3. Plaque

_____

_____

4. Fissure

_____

_____

5. Pustule

_____

_____

6. Vesicle

_____

_____

7. Bulla

_____

_____

8. Cyst

_____

_____

9. Ulcer

_____

_____

10. Wheal

_____

_____

B. Name four bacterial infections of the skin.

1. _____

2. _____

3. _____

4. _____

C. List six inflammatory disorders of the skin.

1. _____

2. _____

3. _____

4. _____

5. _____

6. _____

List the seven warning signs of cancer.

1. C _____

2. A _____

3. U _____

4. T _____

5. I _____

6. O _____

7. N _____

List three procedures for appearance modification.

1. _____

2. _____

3. _____

Chapter 13 Quiz

Name: _____

1. Herpes zoster is also called

   _____.

2. HPV stands for _____

   _____ _____.

3. Tinea is another name for a

   _____ infection.

4. Pruritus means _____

   _____.

5. List three common fungal infections.

   a. _____

   b. _____

   c. _____

6. Kwell is used to treat _____

   and _____.

7. Another name for a bruise is

   _____.

8. List three depths of burns.

   a. _____

   b. _____

   c. _____

9. SLE is an abbreviation for _____

   _____ _____.

10. _____ degree burns have blisters.

Assisting in Gastroenterology

Part I. Medical Terminology

Directions: Supply the correct term for each definition.

1. _____ The surgical joining together of two normally distinct organs.

2. _____ A hard, impacted mass of feces in the colon.

3. _____ Narrow slits or clefts in the abdominal wall.

4. _____ Gas expelled through the anus.

5. _____ Abnormal enlargement of the liver.

6. _____ _____ Valve guarding the opening between the ileum and cecum; also called *the ileocolic valve.*

7. _____ Surgical formation of an opening of the ileum on the surface of the abdomen through which fecal material is emptied.

8. _____ Black, tarry stool containing digested blood; usually caused by bleeding in the upper gastrointestinal tract.

9. _____ Tumors on stems frequently found in the mucosal lining of the colon.

Part II. Spelling

Directions: Correct the misspelled words.

1. Obturater

2. Perastalsis

3. Lithitripsy

Part III. Anatomy and Physiology

A. **Directions:** Complete the following sentences.

1. The _____ _____ _____ delivers enzymes from the pancreas and bile from the liver to the duodenum where digestion is completed.

2. The _____ intestine is made up of the duodenum, jejunum, and ileum.

3. The small intestine is lined with transverse folds of tissue called _____.

B. **Directions:** List seven parts of the large intestine; start with the vermiform appendix.

1. _____

2. _____

3. _____

4. _____

5. _____

6. _____

7. _____

C. **Directions:** Define the following terms.

1. peritoneum

_____

_____

2. mesentery

_____

_____

3. omentum

_____

_____

4. adhesions

_____

_____

D. **Directions:** Label the structures of the upper abdominal cavity on the figure below.

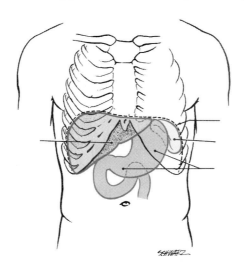

Part IV. Theory/Triage

Directions: Fill in the blanks with the correct terms.

1. _____ are concerned with the diseases and disorders involving the stomach, small intestine, large intestine (colon), appendix, and the accessory organs of the liver, gallbladder, and pancreas.

2. List three disorders of the esophagus and stomach.

    a. _____

    b. _____

    c. _____

3. List 10 disorders of the intestines.

    a. _____

    b. _____

    c. _____

    d. _____

    e. _____

    f. _____

    g. _____

    h. _____

    i. _____

    j. _____

4. List two disorders of the liver and gallbladder.

    a. _____

    b. _____

Directions: Complete the table below by listing the causes of each gastrointestinal complaint.

Gastrointestinal Complaint	
Vomiting (emesis)	Caused by:

Diarrhea	Caused by:
Constipation	Caused by:

Part V. Documentation

Directions: Complete the table below by listing the characteristics of abdominal pain that the medical assistant should report and record. Hint: Review Table 14-1 in your textbook.

Abdominal Pain	Important Characteristics That Should Be Reported and Recorded

Directions: Complete the table below by listing common sources of food poisoning.

Microorganism	Source
Staphylococcus aureus	
Escherichia coli	
Salmonella species	
Clostridium botulinum	

Part VI. Drugs to Know

Directions: Use a drug reference book or the Internet to make drug cards for the following.

1. Imodium

2. Lomotil

3. Phenergan

4. Tigan

5. Anzemet

6. Zofran

7. Kytril

8. Bentyl

9. Levsin

10. Axid

11. Preacid

12. Prilosec

13. Tagamet

14. Zantac

15. Nexium

16. Protonix

Part VII. Laboratory Tests and Diagnostic Tools to Know

A. List four tests performed for patients with ulcers.

1. _____

2. _____

3. _____

4. _____

B. Complete this chart.

Hepatitis Type	Mode of Transmission	Incubation Period
A (Infectious hepatitis)		
B (Serum hepatitis)		
C (Non-A-non-B)		

Part VIII. Transdisciplinary Skills

A. You are making follow-up phone calls after scheduling patients for the following diagnostic tests. List the instructions that you will provide for each patient.

Patient	Test	Description and Purpose	Patient Preparation
Terry Smith	Barium swallow	X-ray or fluoroscopic examination of the pharynx and esophagus after swallowing of barium sulfate; used to diagnose hiatal hernia, esophageal varices, strictures, or tumors.	
Jill Fields	Upper gastrointestinal and small-bowel series	X-ray and fluoroscopic examination of esophagus, stomach, and small intestine after swallowing of barium sulfate; used to diagnose ulcers, tumors, regional enteritis, and malabsorption syndrome.	
Pam Gibbs	Barium enema	X-ray examination of large intestine after rectal instillation of barium sulfate; used to diagnose colorectal cancer; inflammatory disease of the colon; and to detect polyps, diverticula, or obstructions.	
Vince Wells	Oral cholecystography	X-ray examination of gallbladder after ingestion of contrast medium; x-ray films are obtained before and after ingestion of high-fat meal to visualize biliary system; used to detect cholelithiasis and diagnose cholecystitis or tumors.	

Patient	Test	Description and Purpose	Patient Preparation
Suzette Yi	Sigmoidoscopy	Endoscopic examination of distal sigmoid colon, rectum, and anal canal; used to diagnose inflammatory, infectious, and ulcerative bowel disease and tumors and to detect hemorrhoids, polyps, fissures, fistulas, abscesses in the rectum and anal canal. Biopsy specimens may be collected.	
Bobby Day	Colonoscopy	Endoscopic examination of the large intestine; used to detect or monitor inflammatory or ulcerative disease, to locate site of gastrointestinal bleeding, and to identify tumors or strictures.	

B. *ICD-9* Coding

You have looked up *diverticulitis* in the index of diseases, and you are confirming codes in the tabular index.

○ **562.0 Small intestine**
    562.00 Diverticulosis of small intestine (without mention of hemorrhage)
        Diverticulosis:
           duodenum without mention of diverticulitis
           ileum without mention of diverticulitis
           jejunum without mention of diverticulitis
    562.01 Diverticulitis of small intestine (without mention of hemorrhage)
        Diverticulitis (with diverticulosis):
           duodenum
           ileum
           jejunum
           small intestine
    562.02 Diverticulosis of small intestine with hemorrhage
    562.03 Diverticulitis of small intestine with hemorrhage

○ **562.1 Colon**
    562.10 Diverticulosis of colon (without mention of hemorrhage)
        Diverticulosis without mention of diverticulitis:
           NOS
           intestine (large) without mention of diverticulitis
        Diverticular disease (colon) without mention of diverticulitis
    562.11 Diverticulitis of colon without mention of hemorrhage
        Diverticulitis (with diverticulosis):
           NOS
           colon
           intestine (large)
    562.12 Diverticulosis of colon with hemorrhage
    562.13 Diverticulitis of colon with hemorrhage

◀ **New**   ◀▦ **Revised Code**   ● **Not a Principle Diagnosis**   ○ **Use Additional Digit(s)**   ❑ **Nonspecific Code**

Code the following diagnoses.

1. Diverticulosis of small intestine with hemorrhage _____

2. Diverticulitis of small intestine _____

3. Diverticulosis of colon with hemorrhage _____

4. Diverticulitis of ileum _____

5. Diverticulosis of colon _____

Part IX. Certification Review

Directions: Fill in the blanks with the correct terms.

A. Groups at Risk for Hepatitis A, B, and C

    1. Hepatitis _____: intravenous drug users, homosexual men, patients undergoing hemodialysis, patients with hemophilia, healthcare personnel, persons with multiple sexual partners.

    2. Hepatitis _____: children and employees in day care centers, institutionalized residents, individuals traveling to infected areas.

    3. Hepatitis _____: patients who receive frequent blood transfusions, homosexual men, intravenous drug users, and hospital personnel.

B. Abdominal Regions

    1. The gallbladder is located in the _____ region of the abdomen.

    2. The appendix is located in the _____ region of the abdomen.

    3. The stomach is located in the _____ region of the abdomen.

    4. The liver is located in the _____ region of the abdomen.

    5. The pancreas is located in the _____ region of the abdomen.

C. The organism related to ulcer formation is _____.

D. True or False: Biaxin and Zithromax are antibiotics used to treat ulcers. _____

E. The patient in the figure below is placed in _____ _____ position. What are the major concerns when this position is used?

_____

_____

_____

_____

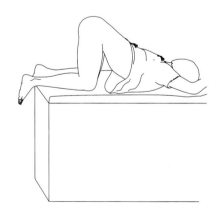

F. Name the position shown in the figure. _____

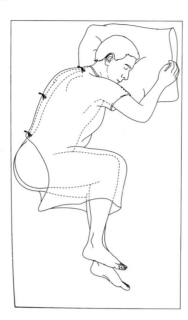

Chapter 14 Quiz

Name: _____

1. The liver is located in the

   _____ region.

2. The appendix is part of the

   _____ .

3. _____ _____,
   which is the narrowing and hardening of
   the pyloric sphincter at the distal end of the
   stomach, is typically seen as a congenital
   defect in infants.

4. Diverticulosis means:

   _____ .

5. List two foods to avoid before an occult
   blood screening.

   a. _____

   b. _____

6. Hepatitis _____ is food-borne.

7. True or False: Hepatitis B is blood-borne.

8. List two causes of ulcers.

   a. _____

   b. _____

9. Cholelithiasis is _____ .

10. _____ is a food-borne illness
    caused by eating raw eggs, poultry, or
    shellfish.

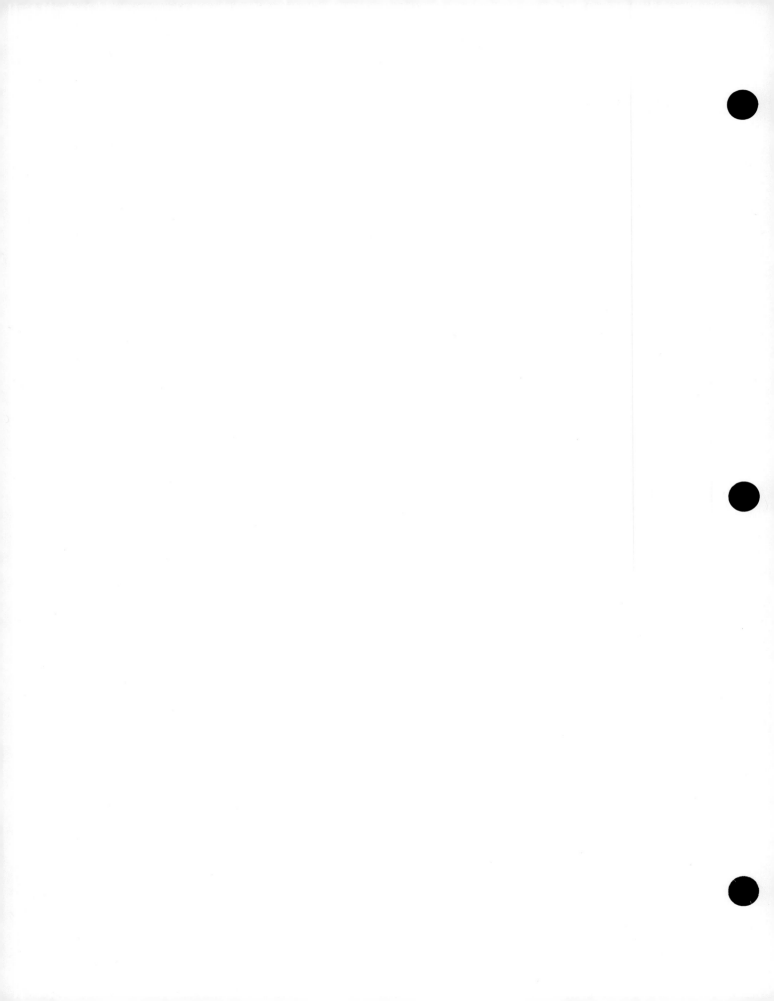

CHAPTER **15**

Assisting in Urology and Male Reproduction

Part I. Medical Terminology

Directions: Define the following terms.

1. albuminuria

_____

_____

2. azotemia

_____

_____

3. casts

_____

_____

4. copulation

_____

_____

5. erythropoietin

_____

_____

6. urgency

_____

_____

7. urology

_____

_____

Part II. Spelling

Directions: Supply the correct spelling for four types of urinary tract infections.

1. _____ inflammation of the urethra.

2. _____ infection of the urinary bladder.

3. _____ an inflammation of the renal pelvis and kidney.

4. _____ degenerative inflammation of the glomeruli.

Part III. Anatomy and Physiology

Directions: Label the structures of the scrotum on the figure below.

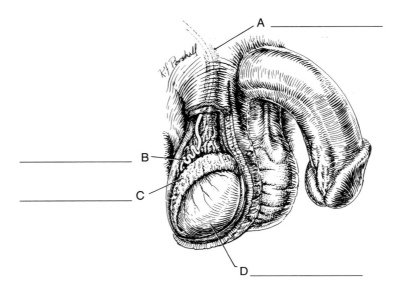

Part IV. Theory/Triage

List five reasons for performing a catheterization.

1. _____

2. _____

3. _____

4. _____

5. _____

Part V. Documentation _____

You performed a catheterization on a male patient for collection of a sterile urine specimen. The urine is dark orange but clear. The amount of urine was 460 cc. The patient appeared to be comfortable during the procedure. Document your findings on p. 129. Use appropriate abbreviations. Be sure to include the date and your signature. Correct mistakes by drawing one line. Use black ink.

Documentation

Part VI. Drugs to Know

A. **Directions:** Use a drug reference book or the Internet to make drug cards for the following.

1. Keflex

2. Bactrim

3. Viagra

4. Flomax

5. Hytrin

6. Detrol

7. Ditropan

8. Xylocaine

130 ASSISTING IN UROLOGY AND MALE REPRODUCTION

B. **Directions:** Review drugs that are used to treat sexually transmitted diseases and complete the table below.

Disease (Causative Organism)	Treatment
Chlamydia (*Chlamydia trachomatis*)	
Genital herpes simplex virus (HSV-2)	
Genital warts (human papillomavirus)	
Gonorrhea (*Neisseria gonorrhoeae* [bacteria])	
Syphilis (*Treponema pallidum* [spirochete bacteria])	
Trichomoniasis (*Trichomonas vaginalis* [protozoa])	

Part VII. Laboratory Tests and Diagnostic Tools to Know

A. **Directions:** Complete the table of common urinary system diagnostic tests.

Test	Description	Patient Preparation
Kidney-ureter-bladder x-ray examination (KUB)		

Test	Description	Patient Preparation
Renal scanning		
Cystography and voiding cystourethrogram		
Intravenous pyelography (IVP)		
Arteriography (angiography)		
Renal computed tomography		
Renal ultrasonography		
Cystoscopy		
Retrograde pyelography		

B. **Directions:** Describe the following.

1. Creatinine

_____

_____

2. BUN

_____

_____

3. UA

_____

_____

Part VIII. Transdisciplinary Skills

ICD-9 Coding

You have looked up *prostatitis* in the index of diseases, and you are confirming codes in the tabular index.

○ **600 Hyperplasia of prostate**
   Use additional code to identify urinary incontinence (788.30–788.39)

   600.0 Hypertrophy (benign) of prostate
   Benign prostatic hypertrophy
   Enlargement of prostate
   Smooth enlarged prostate
   Soft enlarged prostate

   600.1 Nodular prostate
   Hard, firm prostate
   Multinodular prostate
   [Excludes] *malignant neoplasm of prostate (185)*

   600.2 Benign localized hyperplasia of prostate
   Adenofibromatous hypertrophy of prostate
   Adenoma of prostate
   Fibroadenoma of prostate
   Fibroma of prostate
   Myoma of prostate
   Polyp of prostate
   [Excludes] *benign neoplasms of prostate (222.2)*
   hypertrophy of prostate (600.0)
   malignant neoplasm of prostate (185)

   600.3 Cyst of prostate

❏ **600.9 Hyperplasia of prostate, unspecified**
   Median bar
   Prostatic obstruction NOS

○ **601 Inflammatory diseases of prostate**
   Use additional code to identify organism, such as Staphylococcus (041.1), or Streptococcus (041.0)

   601.0 Acute prostatitis

   601.1 Chronic prostatitis

   601.2 Abscess of prostate

   601.3 Prostatocystitis

● ***601.4 Prostatitis in diseases classified elsewhere***
   Code first underlying disease, as:
   actinomycosis (039.8)
   blastomycosis (116.0)
   syphilis (095.8)
   tuberculosis (016.5)
   [Excludes] *prostatitis:*
   gonococcal (098.12, 098.32)
   monilial (112.2)
   trichomonal (131.03)

❏ **601.8 Other specified inflammatory diseases of prostate**
   Prostatitis:
   cavitary
   diverticular
   granulomatous

❏ **601.9 Prostatitis, unspecified**
   Prostatitis NOS

◄ **New**   ◄▥ **Revised Code**   ● **Not a Principle Diagnosis**   ○ **Use Additional Digit(s)**   ❏ **Nonspecific Code**

Code the following diagnoses.

1. Stricture of prostate _____

2. BPH _____

3. Cyst of prostate _____

4. Acute prostatitis _____

5. Chronic prostatitis _____

Part IX. Certification Review

A. **Directions:** Define the following terms.

1. Epididymitis

_____

_____

2. Balanitis

_____

_____

3. Impotence

_____

_____

4. Infertility

_____

_____

5. Prostatitis

_____

_____

6. BPH

_____

_____

7. Cryptorchidism

_____

_____

8. Hydrocele

_____

_____

9. Enuresis

_____

_____

10. Renal calculi

_____

_____

B. In the figure below, the physician is examining the male patient for presence of a hernia. What region of the abdomen is he examining? _____

Why are males at risk for developing a hernia in this area?

_____

_____

_____

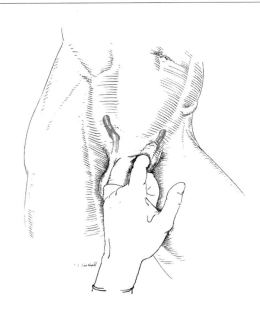

Chapter 15 Quiz

Name: _____

1. Renin regulates _____

   _____ .

2. Erythropoietin controls the formation of

   _____ .

3. Cryptorchidism means _____

   _____ .

4. KUB stands for

   _____ .

5. List two drugs used to treat UTIs.

   a. _____

   b. _____

6. True or False: The urethra connects the
   kidneys to the bladder.

7. Enuresis means _____

   _____ .

8. List two types of dialysis.

   a. _____

   b. _____

9. IVP stands for _____

   _____ .

10. _____ is the functional unit
    of the kidney.

CHAPTER 16

Assisting in Obstetrics and Gynecology

Part I. Medical Terminology

Directions: Define the following terms.

1. rectocele

_____

_____

2. uterine prolapse

_____

_____

3. cystocele

_____

_____

4. PID

_____

_____

5. endometriosis

_____

_____

6. dilation and curettage

_____

_____

7. abruptio placenta

_____

_____

8. placenta previa

_____

_____

9. hysterectomy

_____

_____

Part II. Spelling

Directions: Read each definition and supply the term with correct spelling.

1. Pertaining to women who have had two or more pregnancies _____

2. Thin, yellow, milky fluid secreted by the mammary glands a few days before and after delivery

   _____

3. An x-ray procedure to guide the insertion of a needle into a specific area of the breast

   _____

4. Spotting or bleeding between menstrual cycles _____

5. Excessive menstrual blood loss, such as a menses lasting longer than 7 days _____

6. The absence of menstruation for a minimum of 6 months _____

7. A woman who has not menstruated for a period of 35 days to 6 months is experiencing

   _____

Part III. Anatomy and Physiology _____

A. **Directions:** Fill in the blanks.

   The 28-day cycle is divided into three phases: _____ phase, _____

   phase, and _____ phase.

B. **Directions:** Label the structures in the figure below.

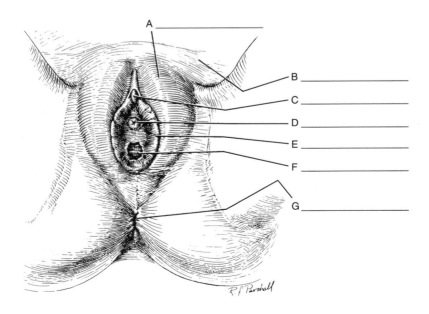

A _____

B _____

C _____

D _____

E _____

F _____

G _____

Part IV. Theory/Triage

A. You receive a telephone call from a female patient who is experiencing side effects from oral contraceptives. What symptoms will you ask about?

A _____

C _____

H _____

E _____

S _____

B. Name three bacterial STDs.

1. _____

2. _____

3. _____

C. Name an STD that is caused by protozoa.

_____

D. Name two viral STDs.

1. _____

2. _____

E. Name three benign gynecological tumors.

1. _____

2. _____

3. _____

F. Name four gynecological cancers.

1. _____

2. _____

3. _____

4. _____

G. **Directions:** Labor is the physiologic process by which the uterus expels the fetus and the placenta. It is divided into three stages. Complete the following definitions:

1. Stage I: From onset of labor through complete _____ and _____ of the cervix

2. Stage II: From complete dilation and effacement of the cervix through the _____

3. Stage III: From the birth of the fetus through the expulsion of the _____

Part V. Documentation

Directions: List five types of naturally occurring abortions.

1. _____

2. _____

3. _____

4. _____

5. _____

Part VI. Drugs to Know

A. **Directions:** Complete the table of various methods of contraception.

Type	Failure Rate	Contraindications	Side Effects
Condom (barrier method)			
Diaphragm or cervical cap (barrier method)			
Intrauterine device (IUD)			
Depo Provera (DMPA)			
Norplant			
Oral contraceptives (OCPs)			

B. **Directions:** Use a drug reference book or the Internet to make drug cards for the following.

   1. Tamoxifen

   2. Premarin

   3. Prempro

   4. Methotrexate (for use in ectopic pregnancies)

Part VII. Laboratory Tests and Diagnostic Tools to Know

Directions: Define the following terms.

1. Ultrasonography

_____

_____

2. Chorionic villus sampling

_____

_____

3. Amniocentesis

_____

_____

4. Alpha-fetoprotein (AFP)

_____

_____

5. Mammography

_____

_____

6. Colposcopy

_____

_____

7. Cryosurgery

_____

_____

Part VIII. Transdisciplinary Skills

ICD-9 Coding

You have looked up *menorrhagia* in the index of diseases, and you are confirming codes in the tabular index.

○ **626 Disorders of menstruation and other abnormal bleeding from female genital tract**

Excludes *menopausal and premenopausal bleeding (627.0)*
pain and other symptoms associated with menstrual cycle (625.2–625.4)
postmenopausal bleeding (627.1)

626.0 Absence of menstruation
Amenorrhea (primary) (secondary)

626.1 Scanty or infrequent menstruation
Hypomenorrhea
Oligomenorrhea

626.2 Excessive or frequent menstruation
Heavy periods
Menometrorrhagia
Menorrhagia
Polymenorrhea

Excludes *premenopausal (627.0)*
that in puberty (626.3)

626.3 Puberty bleeding
Excessive bleeding associated with onset of menstrual periods
Pubertal menorrhagia

626.4 Irregular menstrual cycle
Irregular:
bleeding NOS
menstruation
periods

626.5 Ovulation bleeding
Regular intermenstrual bleeding

626.6 Metrorrhagia
Bleeding unrelated to menstrual cycle
Irregular intermenstrual bleeding

626.7 Postcoital bleeding

❑ **626.8 Other**
Dysfunctional or functional uterine hemorrhage NOS
Menstruation:
retained
suppression of

❑ **626.9 Unspecified**

◀ **New**   ◀▥ **Revised Code**   ● **Not a Principle Diagnosis**   ○ **Use Additional Digit(s)**   ❑ **Nonspecific Code**

Code the following diagnoses.

1. amenorrhea _____

2. metrorrhagia _____

3. oligomenorrhea _____

4. menorrhagia _____

5. postcoital bleeding _____

Part IX. Certification Review

A. Name the position used for female pelvic examinations that is pictured below.

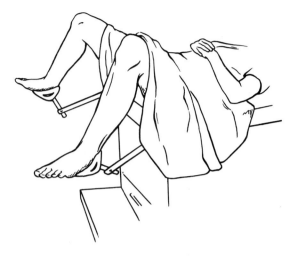

B. Name the instrument that is being used in the figure below.

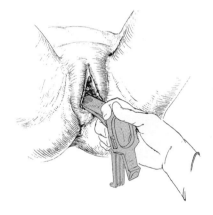

C. Name two supplies that will be needed to complete the bimanual exam illustrated below.

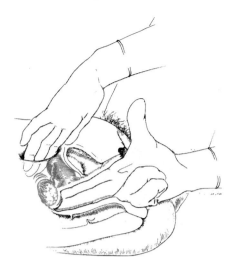

1. _____

2. _____

Chapter 16 Quiz

Name: _____

1. *Candida albicans* causes _____

   _____.

2. Menorrhagia means _____.

3. Multiparous means _____

   _____.

4. PID stands for:

   _____.

5. List two common causes of PID.

   a. _____

   b. _____

6. True or False: AZT is used to help treat HIV.

7. Amenorrhea means

   _____.

8. List two ways to screen for breast cancer.

   a. _____

   b. _____

9. A Papanicolaou smear helps detect

   _____ _____.

10. One in _____ women are at risk for breast cancer.

CHAPTER 17

Assisting in Pediatrics

Part I. Medical Terminology

Directions: Match the following terms and definitions.

1. _____ Weakened virulence or change in virulence of a pathogenic microorganism.

2. _____ Enlargement of the cranium caused by abnormal accumulation of cerebrospinal fluid within the cerebral system.

3. _____ Visual examination of the voice box area through an endoscope equipped with a light and mirrors for illumination.

4. _____ Small size of the head in relationship to the rest of the body.

5. _____ Continuous dry rattling in the throat or bronchial tube caused by partial obstruction.

6. _____ Thin, watery, serum-like drainage.

7. _____ Shrill, harsh respiratory sound heard during inhalation in laryngeal obstruction.

8. _____ Formation and/or discharge of pus.

A. microcephaly

B. serous

C. hydrocephaly

D. stridor

E. rhonchi

F. attenuated

G. suppurative

H. laryngoscopy

Part II. Spelling

Directions: Correct and define the following misspelled words.

1. Colick _____

_____

_____

2. Diareah _____

_____

_____

3. Rhinnitis _____

_____

_____

4. Azthma _____

_____

_____

5. Bronchialitus _____

_____

_____

6. Influensa _____

_____

_____

7. Diptherea _____

_____

_____

8. Tetnus _____

_____

_____

9. Mennengitis _____

_____

_____

10. Hepetitus B _____

_____

_____

11. Rye's Syndrone _____

_____

_____

12. Systic Fibrosis _____

_____

_____

13. Muscular Distrophy _____

_____

_____

14. Rubellia _____

_____

_____

15. Poleo _____

_____

_____

Part III. Anatomy and Physiology

Directions: Fill in the blanks.

1. An infant's birth weight doubles by _____.

2. By age _____, the child has reached approximately 50% of his or her adult height.

3. Growth in height is fairly well complete by age _____.

Part IV. Theory/Triage

A. **Directions:** Complete the following statements about developmental patterns.

1. By the age of 3 years, a child can:

_____

_____

_____

_____

2. During the preschool stage:

_____

_____

_____

_____

3. The school-aged child has perfected:

_____

_____

_____

_____

4. The adolescent, or transition, stage is when the individual attempts to:

_____

_____

_____

_____

B. **Directions:** Complete the table of action principles for telephone triage.

Complaint	Triage Questions
Pain	
Gastrointestinal	
Respiratory	

Part V. Documentation

Directions: A child weighs 20 pounds. You are asked to record the weight in kilograms. There are 2.2 pounds per kilogram. Show your work. Chart the weight below.

Part VI. Drugs to Know

Directions: Use a drug reference book or the Internet to make drug cards for the following.

1. Amoxicillin

2. Ceclor

3. Cipro

4. Augmentin

5. EryPed

6. Septra

Part VII. Laboratory Tests and Diagnostic Tools to Know _____

Directions: Give examples of how each of the following is assessed in children.

1. Gross motor skills: _____

_____

_____

2. Language skills:_____

_____

_____

3. Fine motor–adaptive skills: _____

_____

_____

4. Personal skills: _____

_____

_____

Part VIII. Transdisciplinary Skills

Teaching Injury Prevention

A. **Directions:** List 10 safety guidelines for parents with small children.

1. _____

2. _____

3. _____

4. _____

5. _____

6. _____

7. _____

8. _____

9. _____

10. _____

B. **Directions:** Complete the following statement.

The Federal Child Abuse Prevention and Treatment Act states that

_____

_____

_____

Part IX. Certification Review _____

1. What is a BRAT diet?

_____

_____

2. What is an MMR?

_____

_____

3. What is DPT?

_____

_____

4. Can you name the defect in the spine shown below?

_____

_____

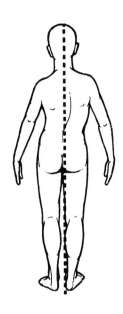

CHAPTER 18

Assisting in Orthopedic Medicine

Part I. Medical Terminology

Directions: Define the following terms.

1. kyphosis

_____

_____

2. lordosis

_____

_____

3. luxation

_____

_____

4. subluxation

_____

_____

5. thoracic

_____

_____

6. tendon

_____

_____

7. ligament

_____

_____

Part II. Spelling

Directions: Correct and define the misspelled words.

1. crepatation _____

_____

_____

2. epiphisis _____

_____

_____

3. cortisosteroeids _____

_____

_____

4. gonometer _____

_____

_____

5. ligiment _____

_____

_____

Part III. Anatomy and Physiology

A. **Directions:** In the figure below, label the bones of the extremities.

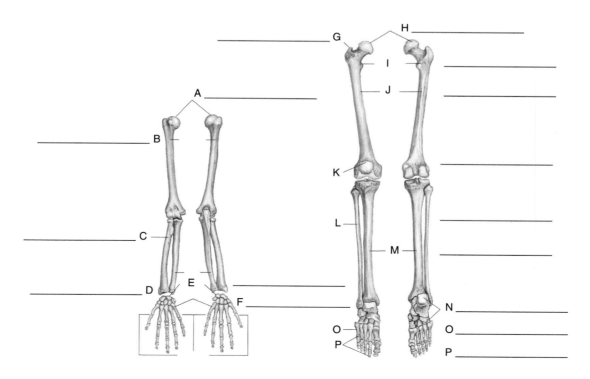

B. **Directions:** Label the drawing below with muscle, tendons, insertion, and origin.

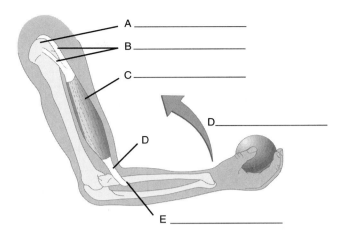

A _____

B _____

C _____

D _____

D

E _____

C. **Directions:** Label the three types of muscles shown in the figure below.

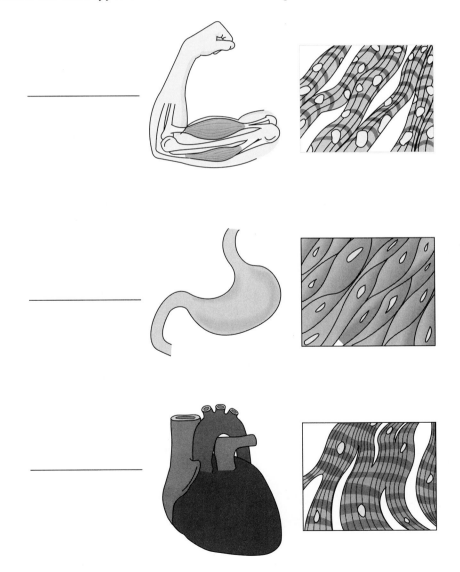

_____

_____

_____

D. **Directions:** Indicate which statements are true (T) and which statements are false (F).

1. _____ The tibia is distal to the femur.

2. _____ The patella is superior to meta carpals.

3. _____ The radius is lateral to the ulna.

4. _____ The tibia is medial to the fibula.

5. _____ The metatarsals are inferior to the tarsals.

Part IV. Theory/Triage

A. **Directions:** Label each type of range of motion.

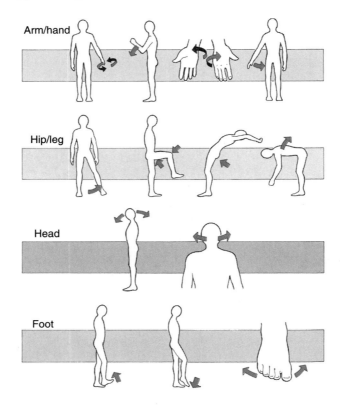

B. **Directions:** Differentiate among gout, osteoarthritis, and rheumatoid arthritis.

_____

_____

_____

_____

Part V. Documentation

Directions: A patient comes in with pain, tenderness, and deformity of fingers. What questions should you ask? What medications will you ask about?

_____

_____

_____

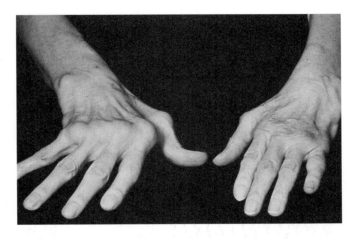

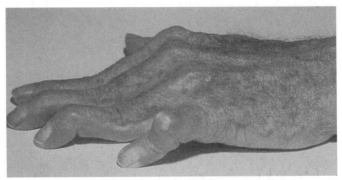

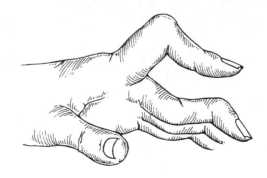

Part VI. Drugs to Know

Directions: Use a drug reference book or the Internet to make drug cards for the following.

1. Aspirin

2. Motrin

3. Prednisone

4. Zyloprim

5. Colchicine

6. Anaprox

7. Cataflam

8. Relafen

9. Toradol

10. Voltaren

11. Naprosyn

12. Orudis

13. Vioxx

14. Celebrex

15. Acetaminophen

Part VII. Laboratory Tests and Diagnostic Tools to Know

Directions: Discuss and record your responses to the following questions.

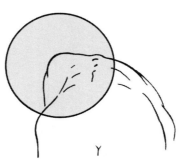

A. Discuss the procedure and findings for scoliosis assessment.

_____

_____

_____

_____

B. Define ESR.

_____

Part VIII. Transdisciplinary Skills

ICD-9 Coding

You have looked up *backache* in the index of diseases, and you are confirming codes in the tabular index.

○ **724 Other and unspecified disorders of back**
    Excludes *collapsed vertebra (code to*
              cause, e.g., osteoporosis,
              733.00–733.09)
          conditions due to:
           intervertebral disc disorders
             (722.0–722.9)
           spondylosis (721.0–721.9)

  ○ **724.0 Spinal stenosis, other than cervical**
    ❏ **724.00 Spinal stenosis, unspecified region**
      724.01 Thoracic region
      724.02 Lumbar region
    ❏ **724.09 Other**
  724.1 Pain in thoracic spine
  724.2 Lumbago
    Low back pain
    Low back syndrome
    Lumbalgia
  724.3 Sciatica
    Neuralgia or neuritis of sciatic nerve
    Excludes *specified lesion of sciatic nerve*
             (355.0)

❏ **724.4 Thoracic or lumbosacral neuritis or radiculitis, unspecified**
    Radicular syndrome of lower limbs
❏ **724.5 Backache, unspecified**
    Vertebrogenic (pain) syndrome NOS
  724.6 Disorders of sacrum
    Ankylosis, lumbosacral or sacroiliac (joint)
    Instability, lumbosacral or sacroiliac (joint)
○ **724.7 Disorders of coccyx**
    ❏ **724.70 Unspecified disorder of coccyx**
      724.71 Hypermobility of coccyx
    ❏ **724.79 Other**
      Coccygodynia
❏ **724.8 Other symptoms referable to back**
    Ossification of posterior longitudinal ligament NOS
    Panniculitis specified as sacral or affecting back
❏ **724.9 Other unspecified back disorders**
    Ankylosis of spine NOS
    Compression of spinal nerve root NEC
    Spinal disorder NOS
    Excludes *sacroiliitis (720.2)*

◀ **New** ⬅ **Revised Code** ● **Not a Principle Diagnosis** ○ **Use Additional Digit(s)** ❏ **Nonspecific Code**

Code the following diagnoses.

1. Sciatica _____

2. Lumbar spinal stenosis _____

3. Lumbago _____

4. Thoracic pain _____

5. Unspecific disorder of coccyx _____

Part IX. Certification Review

Directions: Review and label the fractures shown in the figure below. Match the name of the fracture with the letter corresponding to the illustration of the fracture in the figure below.

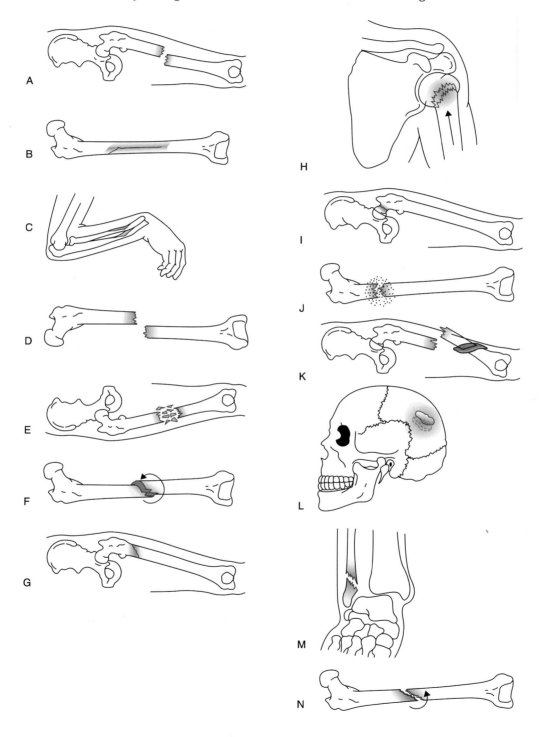

1. _____ transverse

2. _____ spiral

3. _____ simple

4. _____ pathologic

5. _____ oblique

6. _____ longitudinal

7. _____ intracapsular

8. _____ impacted

9. _____ greenstick

10. _____ extracapsular

11. _____ fracture/dislocation

12. _____ depressed

13. _____ compound

14. _____ comminuted

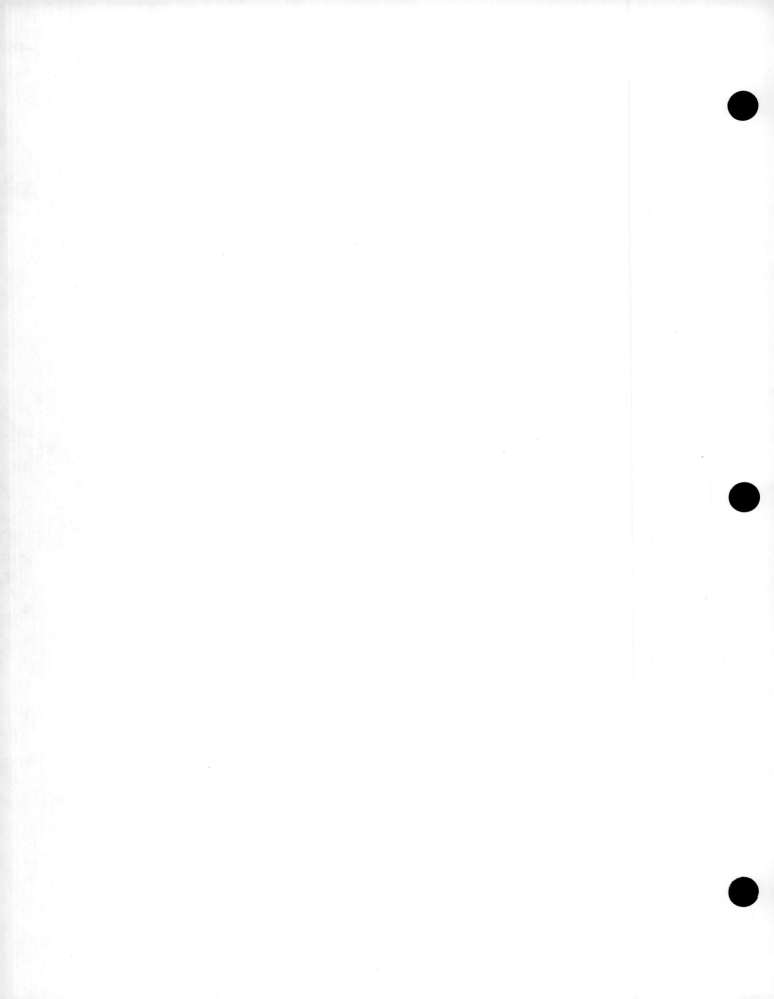

CHAPTER 19

Assisting in Neurology and Mental Health

Part I. Medical Terminology

Directions: Define the following terms.

1. anoxia

_____

_____

2. ataxia

_____

_____

3. atrophy

_____

_____

4. coma

_____

_____

5. diplopia

_____

_____

6. gait

_____

_____

Part II. Spelling

Directions: Correct and define the misspelled words.

Ideopathic _____

_____

_____

Ipselateral _____

_____

_____

Controlateral _____

_____

_____

Part III. Anatomy and Physiology

A. **Directions:** Label the functional structures and lobes of the brain on the figure below.

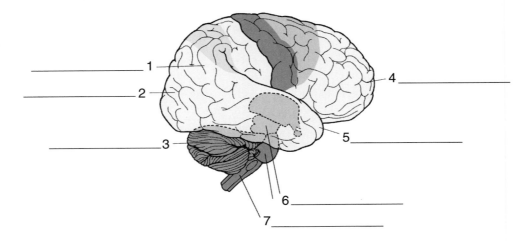

B. **Directions:** List the functions of each of the following.

1. CSF

_____

_____

2. cerebellum

_____

_____

3. brain stem

_____

_____

4. hypothalamus

_____

_____

5. cerebrum

_____

_____

6. spinal nerves

_____

_____

7. cranial nerves

_____

_____

8. autonomic nerves

_____

_____

C. **Directions:** Label the cranial nerves on the figure below.

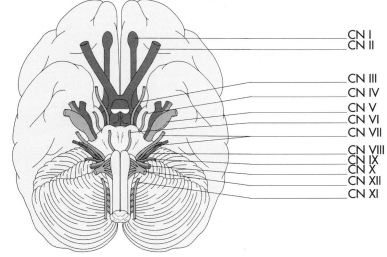

CN I _____

CN II _____

CN III _____

CN IV _____

CN V _____

CN VI _____

CN VII _____

CN VIII _____

CN IX _____

CN X _____

CN XI _____

Part IV. Theory/Triage

Directions: Fill in the blanks or indicate whether statements are true or false.

A. Differentiate between a thrombus and an embolus.

_____

_____

B. True or False: The cause of Alzheimer's disease remains unknown and there is no known cure.

_____

C. CVA is commonly referred to as _____ or brain attack.

D. True or False: Transient ischemic attacks (TIAs) are also called *mini strokes*. _____

E. This _____ often consists of some form of visual disturbance, such as dark lines across or spots within the visual field.

F. Absence or _____ _____ seizures are a less serious form of seizure consisting of momentary clouding of consciousness and loss of contact with reality.

G. The typical presentation of _____ includes muscular rigidity, unilateral pill-rolling tremor of the hand, high-pitched monotone voice, and a _____-like facial expression. The patient has a bent-forward posture with the head bowed. Muscular tremors and _____ increase. The cause is unknown, but some research indicates that it sometimes occurs after a remote earlier _____ infection. There is a deficiency of the neurotransmitter _____ in the brain.

H. _____ _____ results from the progressive inflammation and deterioration of these myelin sheaths, leaving the nerve fibers uncovered.

I. _____, or Lou Gehrig's disease, is a progressive, destructive neurologic disease that results in muscle atrophy.

J. _____ _____ affects the seventh cranial nerve of the face. It occurs suddenly and usually subsides spontaneously over several weeks to several months.

K. Carpal tunnel syndrome results from a compression or entrapment of the _____ nerve as it courses past the carpal bones of the _____ toward the hand.

Part V. Documentation _____

PSS stands for _____.

ADD stands for _____.

LD stands for _____.

List six symptoms of depression.

a. _____

b. _____

c. _____

d. _____

e. _____

f. _____

Part VI. Drugs to Know

Directions: Use a drug reference book or the Internet to make drug cards for the following.

1. Coumadin

2. Plavix

3. Aspirin

4. Heparin

5. methysergide maleate

6. sumatriptan succinate

7. L-dopa

8. Dilantin

9. phenobarbital

10. valproic acid

11. Prozac

12. Paxil

Part VII. Laboratory Tests and Diagnostic Tools to Know

Directions: Define the following.

1. MRI

_____

_____

2. CT

_____

_____

3. EEG

_____

_____

4. Lumbar puncture

_____

_____

Part VIII. Transdisciplinary Skills

A. **Direction:** If you have a *CPT* coding book in your classroom or library, try to code the four diagnostic tests in the previous exercise.

1. MRI of wrist _____

2. CT of head without contrast _____

3. EEG (standard) _____

4. Lumbar puncture _____

B. *ICD-9* Coding

Directions: You have looked up *hemiplegia* in the index of diseases, and you are confirming codes in the tabular index.

○ **342 Hemiplegia and hemiparesis**

Note: This category is to be used when hemiplegia (complete) (incomplete) is reported without further specification, or is stated to be old or long-standing but of unspecified cause. The category is also for use in multiple coding to identify these types of hemiplegia resulting from any cause.

Excludes *congenital (343.1)*
hemiplegia due to late effect of cerebrovascular accident (438.20–438.22)
infantile NOS (343.4)

The following fifth digits are for use with codes 342.0–342.9

❏ **0 affecting unspecified side**
1 affecting dominant side
2 affecting nondominant side

○ **342.0 Flaccid hemiplegia**
○ **342.1 Spastic hemiplegia**
❏ ○ **342.8 Other specified hemiplegia**
❏ ○ **342.9 Hemiplegia, unspecified**

○ **343 Infantile cerebral palsy**

Includes: cerebral:
palsy NOS
spastic infantile paralysis
congenital spastic paralysis (cerebral)
Little's disease
paralysis (spastic) due to birth injury:
intracranial
spinal

Excludes *hereditary cerebral paralysis, such as:*
hereditary spastic paraplegia (334.1)
Vogt's disease (333.7)
spastic paralysis specified as noncongenital or non-infantile (344.0–344.9)

343.0 Diplegic
Congenital diplegia
Congenital paraplegia

343.1 Hemiplegic
Congenital hemiplegia
Excludes *infantile hemiplegia NOS (343.4)*

343.2 Quadriplegic
Tetraplegic

343.3 Monoplegic

343.4 Infantile hemiplegia
Infantile hemiplegia (postnatal) NOS

❏ **343.8 Other specified infantile cerebral palsy**

❏ **343.9 Infantile cerebral palsy, unspecified**
Cerebral palsy NOS

◀ **New**   ◀▥ **Revised Code**   ● **Not a Principle Diagnosis**   ○ **Use Additional Digit(s)**   ❏ **Nonspecific Code**

Code the following diagnoses with all five digits.

1. spastic hemiplegia, unspecified _____

2. flaccid hemiplegia, dominant side _____

3. hemiplegia _____

4. spastic hemiplegia, nondominant side _____

5. flaccid hemiplegia, nondominant side _____

Part IX. Certification Review

Directions: Define the following.

1. CVA

_____

_____

2. ALS

_____

_____

3. MS

_____

_____

4. PTSD

_____

_____

5. ADD

_____

_____

6. TIA

_____

_____

CHAPTER 20

Assisting in Endocrinology

Part I. Medical Terminology

Directions: Match the following terms and definitions.

1. _____ a hormone produced by the alpha cells of the pancreatic islets; it stimulates the liver to convert glycogen into glucose.

2. _____ the abnormal presence of glucose in the urine.

3. _____ the sugar (starch) formed from glucose and stored mainly in the liver.

A. glucosuria

B. glycogen

C. glucagon

Part II. Spelling

Phone-etics Game

Directions: Use the telephone keypad on p. 174 to spell out the missing words.

1. 7-6-5-4 is excessive thirst. _____

2. 2-2-8-4 is a hormone that stimulates the production and secretion of glucocorticoids; it is released by the anterior pituitary gland. _____

3. 4-6-7-8-5-4-6 is a hormone secreted by the beta cells of the pancreatic islets in response to increased levels of glucose in the blood. _____

4. 5-3-8-6-7-4-7 means abnormal production of ketone bodies in the blood and tissues, resulting from fat catabolism in cells. Ketones accumulate in large quantities when fat, instead of, sugar is used as fuel for energy in cells. _____

5. 8-7-4 is a hormone secreted by the anterior lobe of the pituitary gland that stimulates the secretion of hormones produced by the thyroid gland. _____

6. 7-6-5-4-7-4-2-4-4-2 means increased appetite. _____

7. 2-3-4 is a hormone secreted by the posterior pituitary gland; it causes water retention in the kidneys and an elevation in blood pressure. It is also known as *vasopressin.* _____

8. 7-6-5-4-8-7-4-2 is excessive urine production.

1	ABC 2	DEF 3
GHI 4	JKL 5	MNO 6
PRS 7	TUV 8	WXY 9
*	0	#

Part III. Anatomy and Physiology

Directions: Fill in the blanks.

1. The posterior pituitary gland secretes _____ and _____.

2. The hormones released by the anterior pituitary gland are:

   a. _____
   b. _____
   c. _____
   d. _____
   e. _____
   f. _____

3. Three conditions related to alterations in growth hormone are:

   a. _____
   b. _____
   c. _____

Part IV. Theory/Triage

A. **Directions:** Complete the chart of endocrine diseases by writing in common signs and symptoms.

Location	Disease	Common Signs/Symptoms
Adrenal gland	Addison's disease	
	Cushing's disease	
	Pheochromocytoma	
Pancreas	Diabetes mellitus	
	Hyperinsulinism	
Pituitary gland (anterior lobe)	Acromegaly	
	Gigantism	
	Dwarfism	
Pituitary gland (posterior lobe)	Diabetes insipidus	
Thyroid gland	Hyperthyroidism	
	Hypothyroidism	

B. **Directions:** Differentiate between type 1 and type 2 diabetes.

_____

_____

_____

_____

C. **Directions:** Differentiate between diabetic coma and insulin shock.

_____

_____

_____

_____

D. **Directions:** Name and define the three "poly" conditions of diabetes.

1. _____

_____

_____

2. _____

_____

_____

3. _____

_____

_____

Directions: Fill in the blanks.

E. People with diabetes are _____ times more likely to have heart disease or

_____. The destruction of the blood vessels is from atherosclerosis.

_____ _____ _____ (CAD) occurs at a quicker rate in both

patients with type 1 and those with type 2 diabetes. It affects women as often as men and is

often fatal. In individuals with diabetes, _____ _____ is strongly

associated with an increased risk of CAD.

F. Diabetes is a leading cause of _____ _____ in people 20 to 74 years of

age, which is often a result of 8 to 10 years of poorly controlled diabetes.

G. _____ disease is present in 10% to 21% of all patients with diabetes.

Part V. Documentation _____

A. A patient with diabetes has come to your office because of a sore on the right big toe. He states
that he was trimming a corn a week ago and the area has become painful. You notice that the
area is red and warm to the touch. Pedal pulses are weak. The patient is wearing beach sandals.
The patient's fasting blood sugar (FBS) is 348. Oral temperature is 100.9. The blood pressure is
182/110 and pulse is 88.

Directions: Use the correct medical terminology to chart your findings. Use appropriate abbreviations. Be sure to include the date and your signature. Correct mistakes by drawing one line. Use black ink.

Documentation

Part VI. Drugs to Know

Directions: Describe a use for each of the following drugs.

Synthroid	
Hydrocortisone	
DDAVP	
DiaBeta	
Glucophage	
Glynase	
Micronase	
Glucovance	
Avandia	
Actos	

Part VII. Laboratory Tests and Diagnostic Tools to Know

A. **Directions:** Describe each of the following laboratory tests.

1. Thyroid stimulating hormone (TSH)

_____

_____

_____

2. Sodium

_____

_____

_____

3. Potassium

_____

_____

_____

4. Fasting blood sugar (FBS)

_____

_____

_____

5. Glucose tolerance test (GTT)

_____

_____

_____

6. Glycohemoglobin or hemoglobin A_{1c}

_____

_____

_____

○ **250 Diabetes mellitus**

Excludes *gestational diabetes (648.8)*
hyperglycemia NOS (790.6)
neonatal diabetes mellitus
(775.1)
nonclinical diabetes (790.2)

The following fifth-digit subclassification is
for use with category 250:

0 type II [non-insulin dependent type]
[NIDDM type] [adult-onset type] or
unspecified type, not stated as
uncontrolled
Fifth-digit 0 is for use for type II,
adult-onset, diabetic patients, even
if the patient requires insulin

1 type I [insulin dependent type]
[IDDM] [juvenile type], not stated as
uncontrolled

2 type II [non-insulin dependent type]
[NIDDM type] [adult-onset type] or
unspecified type, uncontrolled
Fifth-digit 2 is for use for type II,
adult-onset, diabetic patients, even
if the patient requires insulin

3 type I [insulin dependent type]
[IDDM] [juvenile type], uncontrolled

○ **250.0 Diabetes mellitus without mention**
of complication
Diabetes mellitus without mention
of complication or manifestation classifiable to 250.1–250.9
Diabetes (mellitus) NOS

○ **250.1 Diabetes with ketoacidosis**
Diabetic:
acidosis without mention of coma
ketosis without mention of coma

○ **250.2 Diabetes with hyperosmolarity**
Hyperosmolar (nonketotic) coma

○ **250.3 Diabetes with other coma**
Diabetic coma (with ketoacidosis)
Diabetic hypoglycemic coma
Insulin coma NOS

Excludes *diabetes with hyperosmolar*
coma (250.2)

○ **250.4 Diabetes with renal manifestations**
Use additional code to identify
manifestation, as:
diabetic:
nephropathy NOS (583.81)
nephrosis (581.81)

intercapillary glomerulosclerosis
(581.81)
Kimmelstiel-Wilson syndrome
(581.81)

○ **250.5 Diabetes with ophthalmic**
manifestations
Use additional code to identify
manifestation, as:
diabetic:
blindness (369.00–369.9)
cataract (366.41)
glaucoma (365.44)
retinal edema (362.83)
retinopathy (362.01–362.02)

○ **250.6 Diabetes with neurological**
manifestations
Use additional code to identify
manifestation, as:
diabetic:
amyotrophy (358.1)
mononeuropathy (354.0–355.9)
neurogenic arthropathy (713.5)
peripheral autonomic neuropathy
(337.1)
polyneuropathy (357.2)

○ **250.7 Diabetes with peripheral circulatory**
disorders
Use additional code to identify
manifestation, as:
diabetic:
gangrene (785.4)
peripheral angiopathy (443.81)

❑ ○ **250.8 Diabetes with other specified**
manifestations
Diabetic hypoglycemia
Hypoglycemic shock
Use additional code to identify
manifestation, as:
any associated ulceration
(707.10–707.9)
diabetic bone changes (731.8)
Use additional E code to identify cause,
if drug-induced

❑ ○ **250.9 Diabetes with unspecified complication**

◀ **New**   ◀▥ **Revised Code**   ● **Not a Principle Diagnosis**   ○ **Use Additional Digit(s)**   ❑ **Nonspecific Code**

Part VIII. Transdisciplinary Skills

ICD-9 Coding

Directions: You have looked up *diabetes* in the index of diseases, and you are confirming codes in the tabular index.

Code the following diagnoses with five digits.

1. Hypoglycemia, insulin, juvenile, shock (uncontrolled) _____

2. Ketoacidosis, NIDDM (uncontrolled) _____

3. Hyperosmolar nonketotic coma, insulin dependent (uncontrolled) _____

4. Controlled juvenile diabetes _____

5. Uncontrolled noninsulin-dependent diabetes _____

6. Diabetes type 2 _____

7. Controlled adult-onset diabetes _____

8. Uncontrolled IDDM _____

9. Diabetic cataract, controlled, juvenile onset _____ _____

10. Diabetic renal failure, NIDDM (uncontrolled) _____

Part IX. Certification Review

Directions: Fill in the blanks or indicate whether statements are true or false.

1. True or False: Type 1 diabetes is insulin dependent. _____

2. True or False: Ketoacidosis can occur if blood sugar gets too low. _____

3. Cushing's disease in an _____ in cortisol.

4. Graves' disease is an excess of _____ hormones.

5. True or False: A simple goiter is any thyroid enlargement that has not been caused by an infection or neoplasm. _____

Part X. Class Project

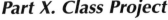

Directions: Evaluate the sample daily food plan for a patient with diabetes. With a partner, see whether you can follow the diet for 24 hours. Read labels to determine calories. Be careful to monitor serving sizes. If you need to estimate, allow 100 calories for one serving of fruit, bread, cereal, and egg. At the end of 24 hours, evaluate the experience. Note: **Any dietary changes should be approved by your doctor.**

Breakfast
   one piece of fruit
   small bowl of unsweetened cereal
   one slice of whole wheat bread or toast
   one egg
   coffee or tea with skim milk

Snack
  one piece of fruit
  coffee or tea with skim milk

Lunch
  one slice of whole wheat bread
  one medium serving of fish, lean meat, or low-fat cheese
  small salad
  one piece of fruit
  coffee or tea with skim milk

Snack
  one piece of fruit
  coffee or tea with skim milk

Dinner
  small serving of vegetable or clear soup
  medium serving of fish, lean meat, or chicken
  one potato or one serving of corn or rice
  three servings of vegetables
  coffee or tea with skim milk

Snack
  one piece of fruit or three plain crackers

Food Choice	Calories	Personal Thoughts
Breakfast		
Snack		
Lunch		
Snack		
Dinner		
Snack		
No. of glasses of water =	Total calories	

Ideas to share with the class about the diabetic diet experience.

_____

_____

_____

_____

Chapter 20 Quiz

Name: _____

1. The posterior pituitary gland secretes:

    a. _____

    b. _____

2. Too much growth hormone causes

    _____.

3. Another term for hyperthyroidism is

    _____ *disease*.

4. Cortisol _____ blood sugar
   levels.

5. List two types of diabetes mellitus.

    a. _____

    b. _____

6. True or False: Insulin shock occurs when
   the blood sugar level is too low.

    _____

7. Diabetic coma occurs with a very

    _____ blood glucose level.

8. Older adults are at risk for:

    a. type 1 diabetes

    b. type 2 diabetes

9. A hemoglobin A_{1c} test can detect

    _____.

10. True or False: Iodine deficiency is related to
    simple goiter formation. _____

183

Assisting in Pulmonary Medicine

Part I. Medical Terminology

A. **Directions:** Define the following terms.

Medical Term	Definition
Apnea	
Atelectasis	
Dyspnea	
Empyema	
Hemoptysis	
Hemothorax	
Hypercapnia	
Hyperpnea	
Hypoxemia	
Orthopnea	
Pleurisy	
Pneumothorax	
Pyothorax	
Rhinoplasty	
Rhinorrhea	
Tachypnea	
Thoracotomy	

Part II. Spelling

Phone-etics Game

Directions: Use the telephone keypad on p. 186 to spell out the missing words.

1. 5-8-6-4 cancer is the leading cause of cancer-related deaths for both men and women in the

   United States. _____

2. A positive 6-2-6-8-6-8-9 reaction indicates the possibility of active or dormant tuberculosis or

   exposure to the disease. _____

3. Pulse 6-9-4-6-3-8-7-9 is a noninvasive method of evaluating the oxygen saturation of hemoglobin in arterial blood, as well as the pulse rate. _____

4. Bronchoscopy provides an 3-6-3-6-7-2-6-7-4-2 view of the larynx, trachea, and bronchi.

_____

1	ABC 2	DEF 3
GHI 4	JKL 5	MNO 6
PRS 7	TUV 8	WXY 9
*	0	#

Part III. Anatomy and Physiology _____

A. **Directions:** Label the drawing below with the anatomical landmarks: anterior, posterior, and mid-axillary lines.

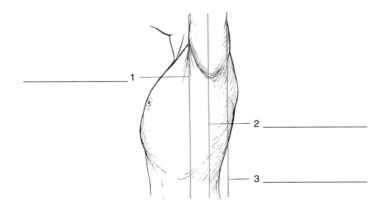

B. **Directions:** On the figure below, label the structures of the respiratory system, head, and chest.

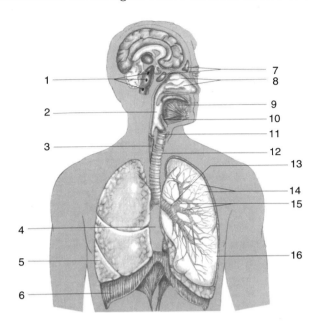

1. _____

2. _____

3. _____

4. _____

5. _____

6. _____

7. _____

8. _____

9. _____

10. _____

11. _____

12. _____

13. _____

14. _____

15. _____

16. _____

C. **Directions:** Label the lobes of the lungs on the figure below.

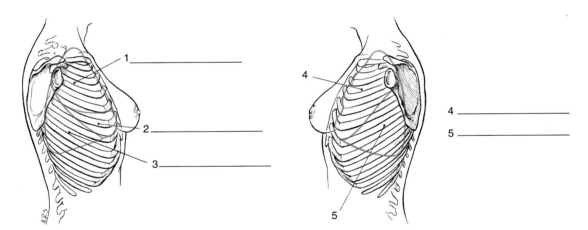

1 _____

2 _____

3 _____

4 _____

5 _____

Part IV. Theory/Triage

Directions: Indicate whether each statement is true (T) or false (F).

1. _____ In asthma and/or emphysema, the individual has difficulty in getting the air out of the lungs, and accessory muscles in the chest are needed to assist the intercostal and diaphragm muscles for complete exhalation.

2. _____ Cigarette smoking is the primary contributing factor to emphysema; however, patients in whom emphysema develops at an early age may have a genetic predisposition to the disease.

Directions: Match the following occupations with the associated lung diseases.

1. _____ stone cutting or sand blasting

2. _____ insulation and shipbuilding

3. _____ coal mining

A. anthracosis

B. silicosis

C. asbestosis

Part V. Documentation

A. Your patient has had a fever and cough for four days. Oral temperature is 102.4°F. You hear a high-pitched, musical sound on expiration when you auscultate the posterior chest near the left side of the neck.

Directions: Use the correct medical terminology to chart your findings. Use appropriate abbreviations. Be sure to include the date and your signature. Correct mistakes by drawing one line. Use black ink.

Documentation

Part VI. Drugs to Know

A. **Directions:** Complete the chart below.

Drug	Use
Oxygen	
INH	
Allergra	
Rifampin	
Zyrtec	
Prednisone	
Ventolin	
Azmacort	

B. Identify the oxygen delivery devices shown in the figure below as simple face mask, non-rebreathing mask, or nasal cannula.

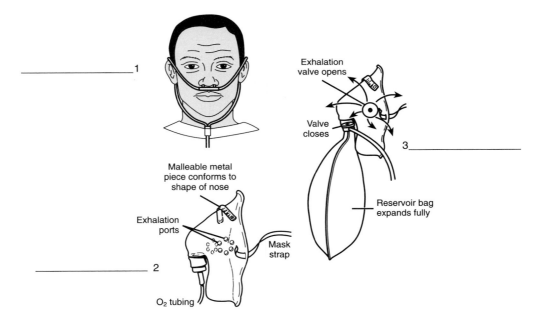

Part VII. Laboratory Tests and Diagnostic Tools to Know _____

A. **Directions:** Describe the condition shown in the figure below.

_____

_____

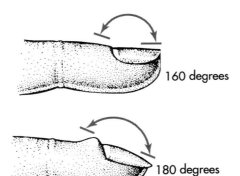

160 degrees

180 degrees

B. **Directions:** Describe the following.

1. Complete blood cell count

_____

_____

2. Chest radiographs

_____

_____

3. Spirometric evaluation

_____

_____

Part VIII. Transdisciplinary Skills

ICD-9 Coding

You have looked up *COPD* in the index of diseases, and you are confirming codes in the tabular index.

❏ **490 Bronchitis, not specified as acute or chronic**
Bronchitis NOS:
catarrhal
with tracheitis NOS
Tracheobronchitis NOS
Excludes *bronchitis:*
allergic NOS (493.9)
asthmatic NOS (493.9)
due to fumes and vapors
(506.0)

○ **491 Chronic bronchitis**
Excludes *chronic obstructive asthma*
(493.2)

491.0 Simple chronic bronchitis
Catarrhal bronchitis, chronic
Smokers' cough

491.1 Mucopurulent chronic bronchitis
Bronchitis (chronic) (recurrent):
fetid
mucopurulent
purulent

○ **491.2 Obstructive chronic bronchitis**
Bronchitis:
asthmatic, chronic
emphysematous
obstructive (chronic) (diffuse)
Bronchitis with:
chronic airway obstruction
emphysema
Excludes *asthmatic bronchitis (acute)*
(NOS) 493.9
chronic obstructive asthma 493.2

491.20 Without mention of acute exacerbation
Chronic asthmatic bronchitis
Emphysema with chronic bronchitis

491.21 With acute exacerbation
Acute bronchitis with chronic obstructive pulmonary disease [COPD]
Acute and chronic obstructive bronchitis
Acute exacerbation of chronic obstructive pulmonary disease [COPD]
Chronic asthmatic bronchitis with acute exacerbation
Emphysema with acute and chronic bronchitis

Excludes *chronic obstructive asthma with*
acute exacerbation (493.22) ◀

❏ **491.8 Other chronic bronchitis**
Chronic:
tracheitis
tracheobronchitis

❏ **491.9 Unspecified chronic bronchitis**

○ **492 Emphysema**
492.0 Emphysematous bleb
Giant bullous emphysema
Ruptured emphysematous bleb
Tension pneumatocele
Vanishing lung

❏ **492.8 Other emphysema**
Emphysema (lung or pulmonary):

NOS	panacinar
centriacinar	panlobular
centrilobular	unilateral
obstructive	vesicular

MacLeod's syndrome
Unilateral hyperlucent lung
Excludes *emphysema:*
with both acute and chronic
bronchitis (491.21)
with chronic bronchitis
(491.20)
compensatory (518.2)
due to fumes and vapors
(506.4)
interstitial (518.1)
newborn (770.2)
mediastinal (518.1)
surgical (subcutaneous)
(998.81)
traumatic (958.7)
with chronic bronchitis
(491.20)

○ **493 Asthma**   ◀▥
The following fifth-digit subclassification is for use with catergory 493:
0 without mention of status asthmaticus or acute exacerbation or unspecified
1 with status asthmaticus
2 with acute exacerbation
Excludes *wheezing NOS (786.07)*

○ **493.0 Extrinsic asthma**
Asthma:
allergic with stated cause
atopic
childhood
hay
platinum
Hay fever with asthma

◀ **New**   ◀▥ **Revised Code**   ● **Not a Principle Diagnosis**   ○ **Use Additional Digit(s)**   ❏ **Nonspecific Code**

Excludes *asthma:*
  allergic:
  allergic NOS (493.9)
  detergent (507.8)
  miners' (500)
  wood (495.8)
○ **493.1 Intrinsic asthma**
  Late-onset asthma
○ **493.2 Chronic obstructive asthma**
  Asthma with chronic obstructive
   pulmonary disease (COPD)
 Excludes *acute bronchitis (466.0)* ◀
  chronic asthmatic bronchitis
   (491.2)
  chronic obstructive
   bronchitis (491.2)

❏ ○ **493.9 Asthma, unspecified**
  Asthma (bronchial) (allergic NOS)
  Bronchitis:
   allergic   asthmatic
○ **494 Bronchiectasis**
  Bronchiectasis (fusiform) (postinfectious)
   (recurrent)
  Bronchiolectasis
  Excludes *congenital (748.61)*
   tuberculous bronchiectasis
    (current disease) (011.5)
 494.0 Bronchiectasis without acute
  exacerbation
 494.1 Bronchiectasis with acute
  exacerbation
   Acute bronchitis with bronchiectasis

◀ **New** ◀■■ **Revised Code** ● **Not a Principle Diagnosis** ○ **Use Additional Digit(s)** ❏ **Nonspecific Code**

Code the following diagnoses.

1. Emphysema _____

2. Chronic bronchitis (smoker's cough) _____

3. Chronic tracheitis _____

4. Asthma (unspecified) _____

5. Intrinsic asthma _____

6. Bronchitis _____

7. Hay fever with asthma (extrinsic) _____

8. Bronchiectasis with exacerbation _____

Part IX. Certification Review

Directions: Fill in the blanks or indicate whether statements are true or false.

1. True or False: *Mycobacterium tuberculosis* is the bacterium that causes tuberculosis (TB). _____

2. Name three ways to screen for TB.

 a. _____

 b. _____

 c. _____

3. The lungs are part of the _____ airway.

4. The upper respiratory tract transports air from the atmosphere to the lungs and includes the:

 a. _____

 b. _____

 c. _____

Chapter 21 Quiz

Name: _____

1. COPD includes:

   a. _____

   b. _____

2. Apnea means _____

   _____ .

3. Another term for sore throat is

   _____ .

4. The _____ are part of the
   lower airway.

5. List two types upper respiratory infections.

   a. _____

   b. _____

6. True or False: Allegra and Zyrtec are used

   to treat allergies and hay fever. _____

7. Laryngitis means _____ .

8. Coughing up blood is:

   a. hemothorax

   b. hemoptysis

   c. atelectasis

9. Rhinorrhea means _____

   _____ .

10. Another name for the windpipe is the

    _____ .

CHAPTER 22

Assisting in Cardiology

Part I. Medical Terminology

Directions: Fill in the blanks:

1. _____ Abnormal sound or murmur heard on auscultation of an organ, vessel, or gland.

2. _____ claudication. Recurring cramping in the calves caused by poor circulation of blood to the muscles of the lower leg.

3. _____ Autoimmune disorder that affects the blood vessels and connective tissue, causing fibrous degeneration of the major organs.

Part II. Spelling

Phone-etics Game

Directions: Use the telephone keypad on p. 196 to spell out the missing words.

1. The heart is enclosed in a double-membrane sac called the *7-3-7-4-cardium*. _____

2. The outer layer of the pericardial sac is a tough protective membrane that connects the heart to the diaphragm, and the inner layer, the visceral membrane or *3-7-4-cardium*, forms the first layer of the heart. _____

3. The middle layer of the heart is the *6-9-6-cardium*, which is the muscle layer that comprises the largest percentage of the heart wall. _____

4. The inner layer of the heart is the *3-6-3-6-cardium*, which forms the heart valves that separate the chambers of the heart and provides a means of blocking the flow of blood from major blood vessels entering and exiting the heart. _____

1	ABC 2	DEF 3
GHI 4	JKL 5	MNO 6
PRS 7	TUV 8	WXY 9
*	0	#

Part III. Anatomy and Physiology

Directions: Label the parts of the heart on the figure below.

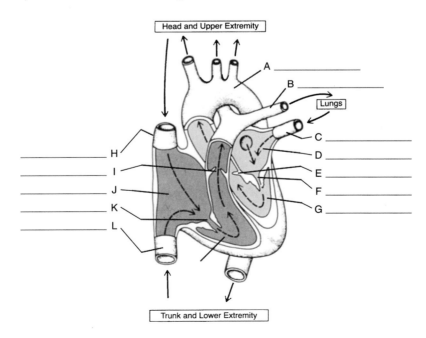

Part IV. Theory/Triage

A. CAD stands for _____ _____ _____ .

B. List five symptoms of myocardial infarction in women:

1. _____

2. _____

3. _____

4. _____

5. _____

C. Telephone screening for chest pain

List five situations in which the medical assistant should activate emergency medical services.

1. _____

2. _____

3. _____

4. _____

5. _____

D. List five conditions that can result from hypertension.

1. _____

2. _____

3. _____

4. _____

5. _____

E. A myocardial infarction is

_____

_____

_____

F. Identify the causes of the various types of shock.

Type	Causes
Cardiogenic	
Hypovolemic	
Neurogenic	

Type	Causes
Anaphylactic	
Septic (septicemia)	

Part V. Documentation

A. Your patient has congestive heart failure and complains of swelling of both legs. When you press on the pre-tibia area of the leg, you notice that your finger leaves a 6-mm indention.

Directions: Use the correct medical terminology to chart your findings. Use appropriate abbreviations. Be sure to include the date and your signature. Correct mistakes by drawing one line. Use black ink.

Documentation

Part VI. Drugs to Know

Directions: Look up the generic names of these drugs. Make a drug card for each one. What do you notice about the generic names within each category?

1. beta blockers (Tenormin, Lopressor, or Inderal)

   generic names _____ _____ _____

2. angiotensin-converting enzyme (ACE) inhibitors (Lotensin, Capoten, or Vasotec)

   generic names _____ _____ _____

3. anticholesterol agents (Lipitor, Mevacor, or Zocor)

   generic names _____ _____ _____

4. anticoagulants (Coumadin)

   generic name _____

5. cardiac glycosides (Lanoxin)

   generic name _____

6. diuretics (HCTZ, Lasix, or Dyazide)

   generic names _____ _____ _____

Part VII. Laboratory Tests and Diagnostic Tools to Know _____

Directions: Research and describe the following.

1. ECG

   _____

   _____

2. CPK and LDH

   _____

   _____

3. ESR

   _____

   _____

Part VIII. Transdisciplinary Skills

ICD-9 Coding

You have looked up *rheumatic fever* in the index of diseases, and you are confirming codes in the tabular index.

---

390 Rheumatic fever without mention of heart involvement
Arthritis, rheumatic, acute or subacute
Rheumatic fever (active) (acute)
Rheumatism, articular, acute or subacute
Excludes *that with heart involvement (391.0–391.9)*

○ **391 Rheumatic fever with heart involvement**
Excludes *chronic heart diseases of rheumatic origin(393.0–398.9) unless rheumatic fever is also present or there is evidence of recrudescence or activity of the rheumatic process*

391.0 Acute rheumatic pericarditis
Rheumatic:
fever (active) (acute) with pericarditis
pericarditis (acute)
Any condition classifiable to 390 with pericarditis
Excludes *that not specified as rheumatic (420.0–420.9)*

391.1 Acute rheumatic endocarditis
Rheumatic:
endocarditis, acute
fever (active) (acute) with endocarditis or valvulitis
valvulitis, acute
Any condition classifiable to 390 with endocarditis or valvulitis

391.2 Acute rheumatic myocarditis
Rheumatic fever (active) (acute) with myocarditis
Any condition classifiable to 390 with myocarditis

❑ **391.8 Other acute rheumatic heart disease**
Rheumatic:
fever (active) (acute) with other or multiple types of heart involvement
pancarditis, acute
Any condition classifiable to 390 with other or multiple types of heart involvement

❑ **391.9 Acute rheumatic heart disease, unspecified**
Rheumatic:
carditis, acute
fever (active) (acute) with unspecified type of heart involvement
heart disease, active or acute
Any condition classifiable to 390 with unspecified type of heart involvement

◄ New   ◄▪ Revised Code   ● Not a Principle Diagnosis   ○ Use Additional Digit(s)   ❑ Nonspecific Code

---

Code the following diagnoses.

1. Acute rheumatic myocarditis _____

2. Acute rheumatic endocarditis _____

3. Acute rheumatic pericarditis _____

4. Rheumatic fever, active _____

5. Rheumatic valvulitis _____

Part IX. Certification Review

Directions: Fill in the blanks or indicate whether statement is true or false.

1. The heart is divided into four chambers. The _____, the top chambers, receive

   blood, and the _____, the bottom chambers, pump the blood out.

2. The cardiac impulse originates in specialized muscle tissue called the _____ node.

3. _____ _____ _____ occurs when the myocardium is

   unable to pump an adequate amount of blood to meet the needs of the body.

4. _____ heart failure, when the left ventricle cannot completely empty, causes a

   backup of blood in the lungs resulting in pulmonary edema, a collection of fluid in the lungs.

5. _____-sided heart failure, when the ventricle cannot maintain complete output,

   causes a backup of blood in the _____ atrium, which prevents complete emptying

   of the vena cava and results in systemic edema, especially in the legs and feet.

6. True or False: The most common valve defect is mitral valve prolapse (MVP), an incompetence in

   the mitral valve. _____

Chapter 22 Quiz

Name: _____

1. Name two diuretics.

   a. _____

   b. _____

2. A common name for MI is a

   _____ .

3. What generic names end in "pril"?

   a. ACE inhibitors

   b. beta blockers

   c. calcium channel blockers

4. What does MVP mean? _____

   _____ _____

5. Describe two types of valve disorders.

   a. _____

   b. _____

6. What is another name for right-sided heart

   failure? _____

   _____

7. _____-sided heart failure
   causes lung congestion.

8. What generic names end in "lol"?

   a. ACE inhibitors

   b. beta blockers

   c. calcium channel blockers

9. Lasix, KCL, and _____ are the
   drugs that are used commonly for CHF.

10. Describe four different types of shock.

    a. _____

    b. _____

    c. _____

    d. _____

CHAPTER 23

Assisting in Geriatrics

Part I. Theory/Triage

Directions: List five myths and stereotypes about aging.

1. _____
2. _____
3. _____
4. _____
5. _____

Part II.

Directions: Complete the table of health promotion and body system changes associated with aging.

Body System	Age-Related Changes	Health Promotion
Cardiovascular		
Central nervous system		
Endocrine		
Gastrointestinal		

Body System	Age-Related Changes	Health Promotion
Musculoskeletal		
Pulmonary		
Sensory organs		
Urinary		
Sexuality		

Part III.

List six suggestions for helping the elderly prevent and treat dry skin.

1. _____
2. _____
3. _____
4. _____
5. _____
6. _____

Part IV.

List six suggestions for helping the older adult with mobility, dexterity, and balance.

1. _____
2. _____
3. _____
4. _____

5. _____

6. _____

Part V.

List eight suggestions for preventing falls.

1. _____
2. _____
3. _____
4. _____
5. _____
6. _____
7. _____
8. _____

Part VI.

List seven risk factors for cognitive decline.

1. _____
2. _____
3. _____
4. _____
5. _____
6. _____
7. _____

Part VII.

Describe the stages of Alzheimer's disease.

First Stage:

_____

_____

Second Stage:

_____

_____

Terminal Stage:

_____

_____

Part VIII.

Describe the guidelines for effective patient education with older adults.

_____

_____

_____

_____

_____

_____

_____

_____

Part IX. _____

Describe the patient's stooped posture and possible causes. Who is at risk for this condition? What can be done to prevent this condition?

_____

_____

_____

_____

Chapter 23 Quiz

Name: _____

1. Describe two skin changes in the elderly:

    a. _____

    b. _____

2. Alopecia means _____

    _____ .

3. Older adults frequently have problems with:

    a. diarrhea

    b. constipation

    c. vomiting

4. Presbycusis means _____

    _____ .

5. Describe glaucoma.

    _____

6. What is a cataract? _____

    _____ .

7. _____ cause the greatest number of injuries in the elderly.

8. DNR stands for _____

    _____ _____ .

9. _____ is used to treat impotence.

10. PLMD stands for _____

    _____ _____

    _____ .

CHAPTER 24

Principles of Electrocardiography

Part I. Medical Terminology

Directions: Match the following terms and definitions.

1. _____ bradycardia
2. _____ bundle of His
3. _____ cardiac arrest
4. _____ cardioversion
5. _____ defibrillator
6. _____ dyspnea
7. _____ hypertension
8. _____ infarction
9. _____ ischemic
10. _____ myocardial
11. _____ myocardium
12. _____ orthopnea
13. _____ sinoatrial (SA) node
14. _____ tachycardia

A. Complete cessation of cardiac contractions

B. Use of an electroshock to convert an abnormal cardiac rhythm to a normal one

C. Heart muscle

D. Heart rate of less than 60 beats per minute

E. Fibers that conduct electrical impulses from AV node to ventricular myocardium

F. Heart rate greater than 100 beats per minute

G. Area of tissue that has died because of lack of blood supply

H. Temporary interruption in blood supply to a tissue or organ

I. Pertaining to the heart muscle

J. Difficulty breathing when in supine position

K. Pacemaker of the heart located in the right atrium

L. Machine used to deliver an electroshock to the heart through electrodes placed on the chest wall

M. difficulty breathing

N. High blood pressure in which the diastolic pressure is greater than 90 mm Hg

Part II. Spelling

Phone-etics Game

Directions: Use the telephone keypad below to spell out the missing words. Write the corresponding numbers in the blanks provided.

_____ The two upper chambers of the heart

_____ The two lower chambers of the heart

_____ Dizziness

_____ Divide from one into two branches

	ABC	DEF
1	2	3
GHI 4	JKL 5	MNO 6
PRS 7	TUV 8	WXY 9
*	0	#

Part III. Visual Aids

Directions: Use the figures on p. 213 to answer the following questions.

1. Describe the conduction pathways of the heart and label the structures of the heart on the following figure.

_____

_____

_____

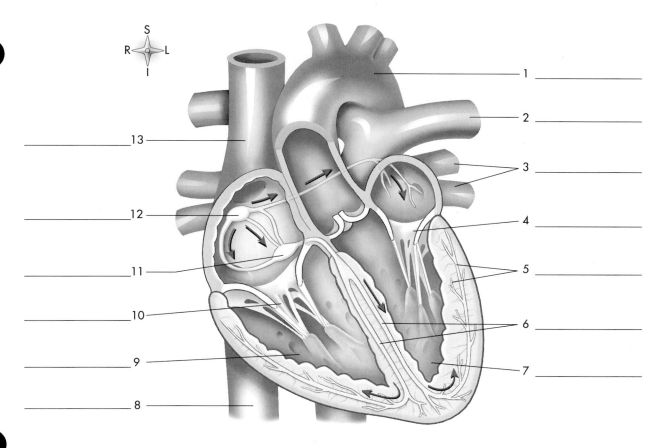

1 _____

2 _____

3 _____

4 _____

5 _____

6 _____

7 _____

13 _____

12 _____

11 _____

10 _____

9 _____

8 _____

2. Label the precordial leads on the drawing below.

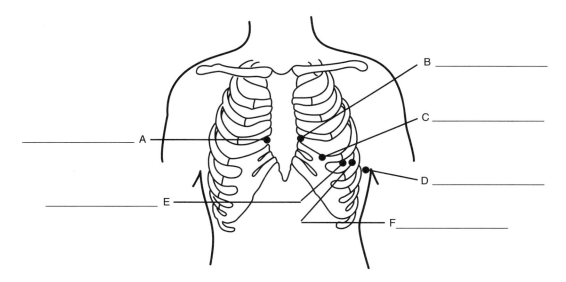

A _____

B _____

C _____

D _____

E _____

F _____

3. Draw in correct placement of leads for a 12-lead electrocardiogram (ECG). _____

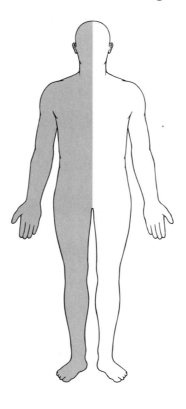

4. Name the rhythm shown below. _____

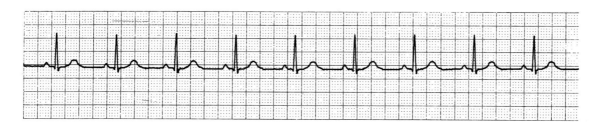

5. Name the rhythm shown below. _____

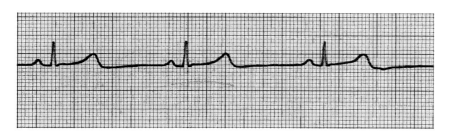

6. Name the rhythm shown below. _____

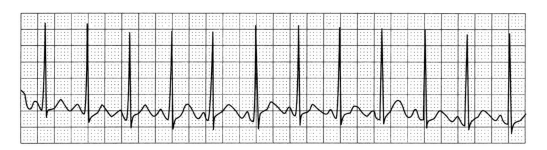

7. Name the rhythm shown below. _____

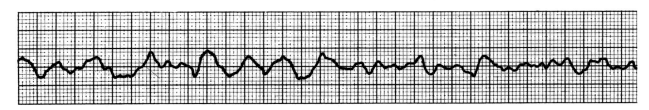

8. Name the rhythm shown below. _____

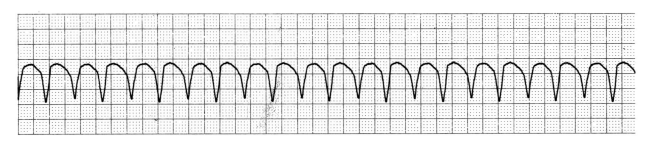

9. Name the rhythm shown below. _____

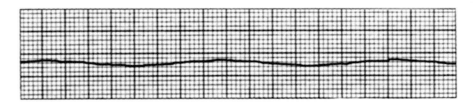

10. Describe the procedure shown in the drawing below.

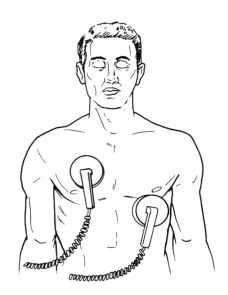

_____

_____

_____

_____

Part IV. Theory

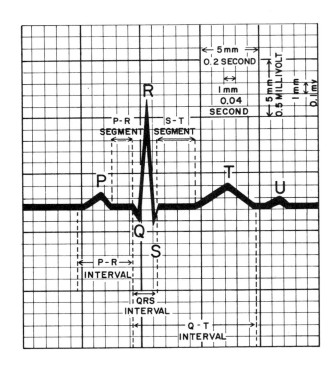

1. The _____ wave occurs during the contraction of the atria and shows the beginning of cardiac depolarization.

2. The _____ complex shows the contraction of both ventricles and also reflects the completion of cardiac depolarization.

3. The _____ interval is the time from the beginning of atrial contraction to the beginning of ventricular contraction.

4. The T wave indicates ventricular recovery or _____ of the ventricles.

5. ECG paper has horizontal and vertical lines at _____ mm intervals.

6. When running at normal speed, one small, 1-mm square passes the stylus every

   _____ seconds.

7. One large 5-mm square passes the stylus every _____ seconds.

8. Lead I records the electrical activity between the _____ arm and the

   _____ arm.

9. Lead _____ records the electrical activity between the right arm and the left leg.

10. Lead III records the electrical activity between the _____ arm and the left leg.

11. _____ records the activity from midway between the left leg and the left arm to the right arm.

12. _____ records the activity from midway between the right arm and the left leg to the left arm.

13. _____ records the activity from midway between the right arm and the left arm to the left leg.

14. The standardization button should cause the stylus to make a _____ mm deflection or two large squares when the sensitivity is set at 1.

15. With the _____ baseline, the stylus gradually shifts away from the center of the paper.

16. _____ _____ shows up on the recording as jagged peaks of irregular height and spacing and a shifting baseline.

17. _____ _____ occurs when the electric connection has been interrupted.

18. _____ interference appears as a series of uniform small spikes on the paper.

19. Cardiac _____ testing is conducted to observe and record the patient's cardiovascular response to measured exercise challenges.

20. A _____ monitor is a portable system for recording the cardiac activity of a patient over a 24-hour period or longer.

Part V. Documentation

Refer to Table 24-2 in the text and complete the following statements.

A. On some older machines, standard marking codes for limb leads are indicated by:

_____

B. Augmented leads are indicated by:

_____

C. Precordial leads are indicated by:

_____

Part VI. Transdisciplinary Skills

Procedural Coding

You have looked up ECG in the index, and you are confirming codes in the Medicine Section below. Answer the questions for the Cardiography subsection.

Cardiography

93000   Electrocardiography, routine ECG with at least 12 leads: with interpretation and report

93005   tracing only without interpretation and report

93010   interpretation only

93230   Electrocardiographic monitoring for 24 hours by continuous waveform recoding and storage....

93225   recording (includes hook-up, recording and disconnection)

93226   scanning analysis with report

93227   physician review and interpretation

1. You work for a cardiologist that reads 12 Lead ECGs for the local hospital. How would you code for the interpretation? _____

2. A patient comes in with chest pain, and the physician orders a 12-lead ECG and makes a diagnosis of acute MI. What procedure code would you use? _____

3. You are placing a Holter monitor on a patient. What *CPT* code would you choose?

    _____

4. When the Holter is taken off the next day and interpreted by the physician, which code would be placed on the HCFA 1500 form? _____

Part VII. Certification Review _____

1. Limb leads are

    a. unipolar

    b. bipolar

2. Precordial leads are placed on the _____.

3. Precordial leads are

    a. unipolar

    b. bipolar

4. What is the standard speed of ECG paper? _____

5. Which leads are recorded from a midpoint? _____

6. Name the limb leads.

    a. _____

    b. _____

    c. _____

7. Name the augmented leads.

    a. _____

    b. _____

    c. _____

8. Name the precordial leads.

    a. _____

    b. _____

    c. _____

    d. _____

    e. _____

    f. _____

9. What does a p-wave represent? _____

10. PVC stands for _____ _____ _____.

CHAPTER 25

Assisting in Diagnostic Imaging

Part I. Medical Terminology

Directions: Fill in the blanks with the correct terms.

1. _____ refers to the making of x-ray images called *radiographs*.

2. X-rays can penetrate most substances to some degree, but some substances, such as metals and bones, are more difficult to penetrate and are said to be _____.

3. _____ is a technique performed with special equipment that permits the radiologist to view x-ray images in motion.

4. The _____ scanner consists of a movable table with remote control, a circular gantry structure that supports the x-ray tube and detectors, an operator console with a monitor, and the supporting computer system.

5. _____ medicine scans do not provide clear images of anatomical structures. They are used to obtain information about the function of organs and tissues.

Anatomical Position Matching

Directions: Match the following terms and definitions.

1. _____ Forward or front portion of the body or body part

2. _____ Pertaining to the head; toward the head

3. _____ Away from the head; the opposite of cephalad

4. _____ Away from the source or point of origin; for example, the wrist is distal to the elbow; being farther from the point of origin of the arm, which is the shoulder

5. _____ To the outside, at or near the surface of the body or a body part

6. _____ Below, farther from the head

7. _____ Deep, near the center of the body or a part; the opposite of external

8. _____ Referring to the side; away from the center to the left or right

9. _____ Toward the center of the body or of a body part; the opposite of lateral

10. _____ Referring to the palm (anterior surface) of the hand

A. distal

B. internal

C. plantar

D. medial or mesial

E. palmar

F. external

G. anterior

H. inferior

I. lateral

J. posterior

K. cephalic, cephalad

L. caudal, caudad

M. anterior

N. proximal

O. superior

11. _____ Referring to the sole of the foot

12. _____ Backward or back portion of the body or body part; the opposite of anterior

13. _____ Toward the source or point of origin; the opposite of distal

14. _____ Above, toward the head; the opposite of inferior

Part II. Spelling

Phone-etics Game

Directions: Use the telephone keypad below to spell out the missing words. Write the corresponding numbers in the blanks provided.

1. The _____ gantry houses the magnet and the main radiographic/fluoroscopic (R/F) coil.

2. Ultrasound or _____ uses high-frequency sound waves to produce echoes within the body.

3. _____ projections are those in which the sagittal plane of the body or body part is parallel to the film. Lateral projections are always named for the side of the patient that is nearest the film.

4. _____ projections are those in which the body or part is rotated so that the projection is neither frontal nor lateral.

5. _____ projections are radiographs taken with a longitudinal angulation of the x-ray beam.

	ABC	DEF
1	2	3
GHI 4	JKL 5	MNO 6
PRS 7	TUV 8	WXY 9
*	0	#

Part III. Visual Aids

Directions: Name the directions and planes of the body shown in the figure below.

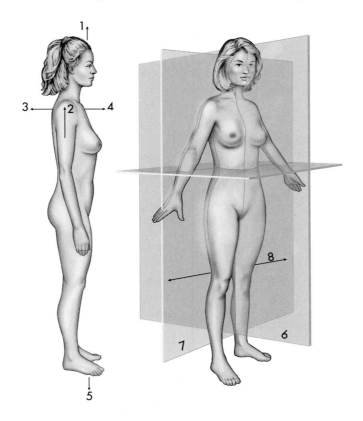

1. _____

2. _____

3. _____

4. _____

5. _____

6. _____

7. _____

8. _____

Part IV. Theory

Directions: Indicate which statements are true and which statements are false. For other statements, fill in the blanks.

1. True or False: Cardiac pacemakers are a particular hazard, and patients with pacemakers cannot

   have MRI examinations. _____

2. True or False: Radiation control regulations do not require that female patients of childbearing age be advised of potential radiation hazards before x-ray examination. _____

3. True or False: If the patient is supine, or facing the x-ray tube, the projection is said to be anteroposterior (AP). _____

4. The radiographer then selects the correct cassette and places a _____ _____ marker on it to identify the patient's right or left side.

5. The _____ (R) is the conventional unit of radiation exposure that represents a measurement of radiation intensity and is determined by the interaction of the x-ray beam with air.

6. To measure both therapeutic radiation doses and specific tissue doses received in diagnostic applications, the conventional unit is the _____, which stands for "radiation absorbed dose."

7. To measure occupational dose or other exposure that may involve more than one type of radiation, the dose equivalent unit used is the _____, which stands for "roentgen equivalent in man."

8. True or False: X-rays do not linger in the room after the exposure, and they are not capable of making the objects in the room radioactive. _____

Part V. Workplace Applications

Directions: Identify each type of x-ray in the pictures below.

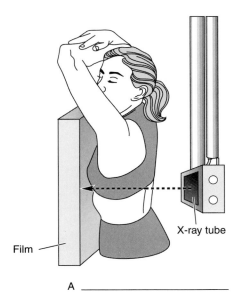

Film

X-ray tube

A _____

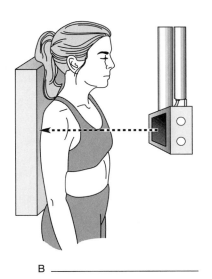

B _____

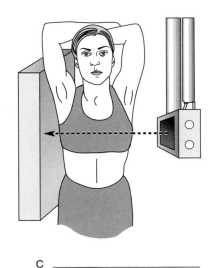

C _____

Part VI. Transdisciplinary Skills

Procedural Coding

You have looked up *chest x-ray* in the *CPT* index, and you are confirming codes in the Radiology Section below. Answer the questions for the diagnostic studies.

Radiology

71010	Radiologic examination, chest, single view, frontal
71015	stereo, frontal
71020	Radiologic examination, chest, two views, frontal and lateral
71021	with apical lordotic posture
71022	with oblique view
71023	with fluoroscopy
71250	Computerized axial tomography, thorax, with contrast material
71260	with contrast material
71550	Magnetic Resonance Imaging, chest, without contrast material
71551	with contrast material

1. What is the *CPT* code for chest CT with contrast? _____

2. What code do you use for anteroposterior (AP) and lateral chest x-ray? _____

3. What is the *CPT* code for magnetic resonance imaging of the chest without contrast?

_____

4. A portable chest x-ray examination that only has one view would need which *CPT* code?

_____

Part VII. Certification Review

Directions: Fill in the blanks by choosing the correct terms from the list below.

recumbent

upright

prone

lateral recumbent

supine

dorsal recumbent

ventral recumbent

1. Lying face down is known as the _____ position.

2. Lying down is referred to as _____.

3. Lying on the back, supine is called _____ _____.

4. Lying on the side would be _____.

5. Lying face down, prone is called _____ _____.

6. Lying face up is known as the _____ position.

7. Having an x-ray examination while standing or seated would be called an _____ view.

CHAPTER 26

Assisting in the Clinical Laboratory

Part I. Medical Terminology

Directions: Write the correct term in the space provided.

1. _____ A portion of a well-mixed sample removed for testing.

2. _____ A chemical added to the blood after collection to prevent clotting.

3. _____ The substance or chemical being analyzed or detected in a specimen.

4. _____ A substance that is known to cause cancer.

5. _____ A substance that burns or destroys tissue by chemical action.

6. _____ _____ Fluid within the subarachnoid space, the central canal of the spinal cord, and the four ventricles of the brain.

7. _____ A liquid used to dilute a specimen or reagent.

8. _____ Fluids with a high concentration of protein and cellular debris that have escaped from the blood vessels and been deposited in tissues or on tissue surfaces.

9. _____ A sac filled with blood that may be the result of trauma.

10. _____ A term used to describe a blood sample in which the red blood cells have ruptured.

11. _____ A cylindrical glass or plastic tube used to deliver fluids.

12. _____ Substances added to a specimen to prevent deterioration of cells or chemicals.

13. _____ _____ Private or hospital-based laboratories that perform a wide variety of tests, many of them specialized. Physicians often send specimens collected in the office to one of these for testing.

14. _____ The ability of the eye to distinguish two objects that are very close together; the sharpness of an image.

15. _____ A sample of body fluid, waste product, or tissue that is collected for analysis.

16. _____ An order found on a laboratory requisition indicating that the test must be done immediately (from the Latin word statin, meaning "at once").

17. _____ A substance that is known to cause birth defects.

Part II. Spell It Out

Phone-etics Game

Directions: Use the telephone keypad to spell out the acronyms for the following agencies beside their laboratory certifications. Write the corresponding letters in the blanks provided.

1. (2-7-2-7) MT, MLT _____

2. (2-6-8) MT, MLT _____

3. (2-2-6-2) CMA _____

4. (2-2-4-3-7) RMA _____

	ABC	DEF
1	2	3
GHI	JKL	MNO
4	5	6
PRS	TUV	WXY
7	8	9
*	0	#

Part III. Visual Aids

Accuracy and Precision

Directions: Read the following scenario and answer the questions in the space provided.

1. One blood glucose meter always reads 10% too high. Another meter reads anywhere between 5% and 9% too high. Which one is the most precise? Which one is the most accurate? How is accuracy different from precision?

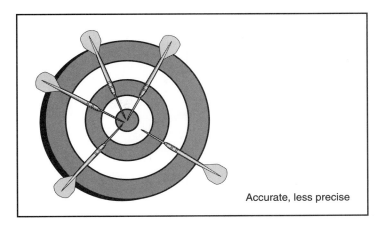

Accurate, less precise

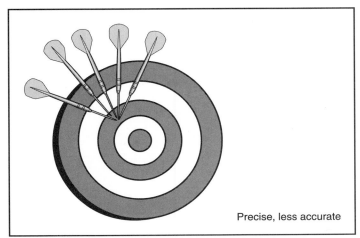

Precise, less accurate

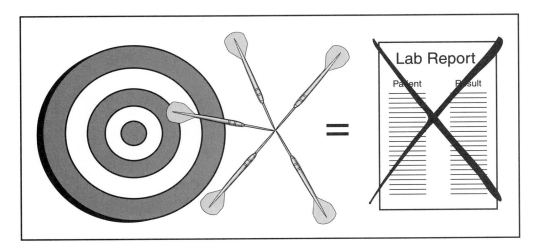

2. Look at the clock below and write the military time for both afternoon and morning for the time shown.

    a. PM _____

    b. AM _____

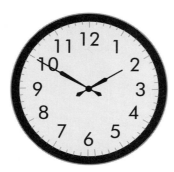

3. Label the parts of a microscope in the figure below.

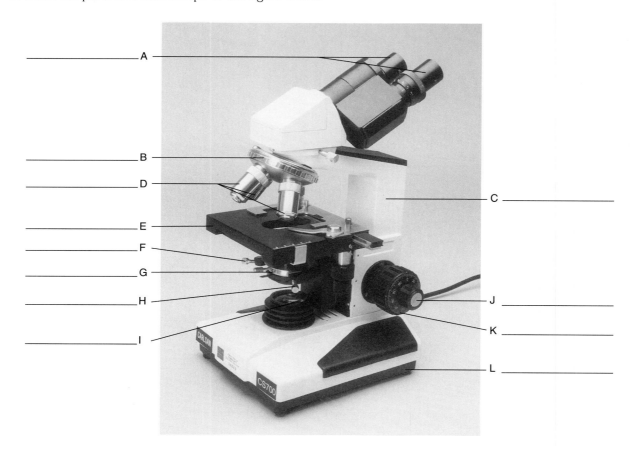

Part IV. Theory

1. List five reasons when it is absolutely required to wash your hands in the laboratory area.

   A. _____

   B. _____

   C. _____

   D. _____

   E. _____

2. Name three types of hazards in the lab setting:

   A. _____

   B. _____

   C. _____

3. Differentiate between qualitative and quantitative results. Give an example of each.

   _____

   _____

4. Name the four major divisions of the clinical lab.

   A. _____

   B. _____

   C. _____

   D. _____

5. Label each of the following according to its division.

   A. Hemoglobin _____

   B. Urine specific gravity _____

   C. Urine culture _____

   D. Blood glucose _____

   E. Throat culture _____

   F. White blood cell count _____

   G. Cholesterol _____

   H. Complete blood count _____

6. What is an MSDS?

   _____

   _____

   _____

7. What is the role of OSHA?

_____

_____

_____

8. What is CLIA and what are the levels of laboratory testing?

_____

_____

_____

_____

_____

9. List the items that must be present on the label of a collected specimen.

_____

_____

_____

_____

_____

Part V. Workplace Applications

1. On the thermometer drawings provided, mark the range of common laboratory temperatures for:

   a. Body and incubator temperature

   b. Room temperature

   c. Freezer temperature

   d. Refrigerator temperature

A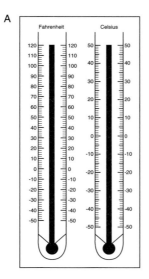

B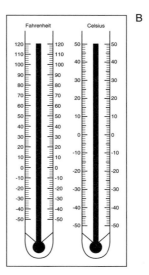

C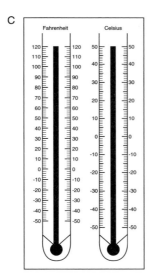

D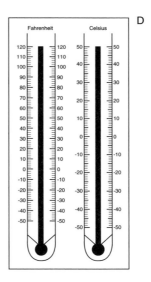

2. Record the volume in milliliters for the two cylinders pictured.

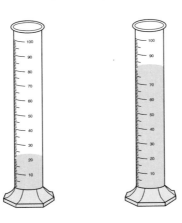

a. How much diluent do you have to add to a 1 ml sample to make a 1:10 dilution?

_____ ml

b. How much diluent do you have to add to a 2 ml sample to make a 1:10 dilution?

_____ ml

c. How much diluent do you have to add to a 1 ml sample to make a 1:20 dilution?

_____ ml

d. How much diluent do you have to add to a 2 ml sample to make a 1:10 dilution?

_____ ml

e. Your centrifuge starts to vibrate markedly while you are spinning a specimen. What should you check?

Part VI. Transdisciplinary Skills

Directions: Proofread and make corrections to the following transcription.

4-14-20XX The patient arrived complaining of disuria and fever x 3 days. A urinalisis was performed. The microscopic results show presence of bacteria. CBC shows an elevated WBC.

Part VII. Certification Review

1. True or False: Mouth-pipetting is forbidden in the laboratory setting. _____

2. If the eyepiece of the microscope is 10x and the high power is 40x, what is the total magnification?

   _____

3. True or False: The coarse adjustment should always be used with the oil emersion lens. _____

4. Always carry the microscope by the _____ with one hand under the

   _____.

CHAPTER 27

Assisting in the Analysis of Urine

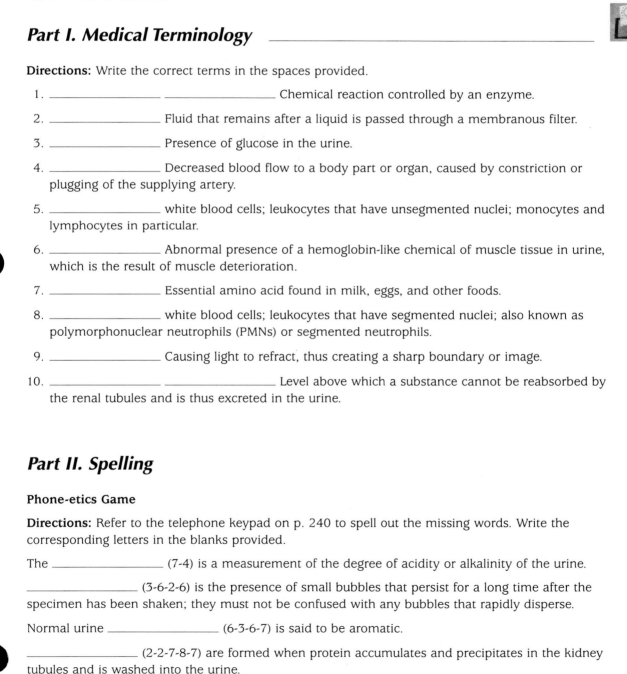

Part I. Medical Terminology

Directions: Write the correct terms in the spaces provided.

1. _____ _____ Chemical reaction controlled by an enzyme.

2. _____ Fluid that remains after a liquid is passed through a membranous filter.

3. _____ Presence of glucose in the urine.

4. _____ Decreased blood flow to a body part or organ, caused by constriction or plugging of the supplying artery.

5. _____ white blood cells; leukocytes that have unsegmented nuclei; monocytes and lymphocytes in particular.

6. _____ Abnormal presence of a hemoglobin-like chemical of muscle tissue in urine, which is the result of muscle deterioration.

7. _____ Essential amino acid found in milk, eggs, and other foods.

8. _____ white blood cells; leukocytes that have segmented nuclei; also known as polymorphonuclear neutrophils (PMNs) or segmented neutrophils.

9. _____ Causing light to refract, thus creating a sharp boundary or image.

10. _____ _____ Level above which a substance cannot be reabsorbed by the renal tubules and is thus excreted in the urine.

Part II. Spelling

Phone-etics Game

Directions: Refer to the telephone keypad on p. 240 to spell out the missing words. Write the corresponding letters in the blanks provided.

The _____ (7-4) is a measurement of the degree of acidity or alkalinity of the urine.

_____ (3-6-2-6) is the presence of small bubbles that persist for a long time after the specimen has been shaken; they must not be confused with any bubbles that rapidly disperse.

Normal urine _____ (6-3-6-7) is said to be aromatic.

_____ (2-2-7-8-7) are formed when protein accumulates and precipitates in the kidney tubules and is washed into the urine.

	ABC	DEF
1	2	3
GHI	JKL	MNO
4	5	6
PRS	TUV	WXY
7	8	9
*	0	#

Part III. Visual Aids

Directions: Identify the structures of the urinary system shown in the figure below.

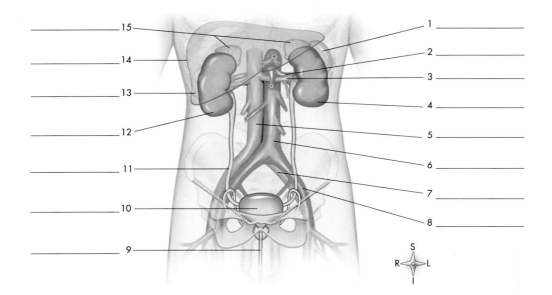

1. _____

2. _____

3. _____

4. _____

5. _____

6. _____

7. _____

8. _____

9. _____

10. _____

11. _____

12. _____

13. _____

14. _____

15. _____

Directions: Label the structures of the kidney shown in the figure below.

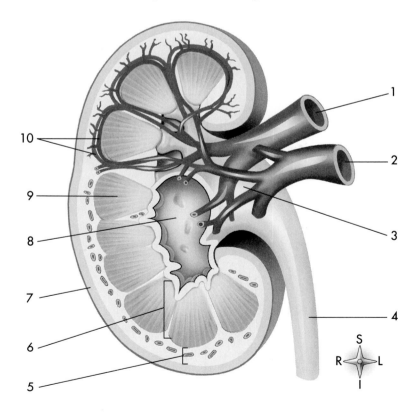

1. _____

2. _____

3. _____

4. _____

5. _____

6. _____

7. _____

8. _____

9. _____

10. _____

Part IV. Theory

A. List eight types of urine specimens.

1. _____

2. _____

3. _____

4. _____

5. _____

6. _____

7. _____

8. _____

B. Name three examinations in a routine urinalysis and give some examples of information determined from each examination.

1. _____

_____

2. _____

_____

3. _____

_____

C. Describe a urinometer.

_____

_____

D. Describe a refractometer.

_____

_____

E. Differentiate between a Clinitest and a Acetest.

_____

_____

F. What is a sulfosalicylic acid test used for?

_____

_____

G. How does a urine pregnancy test work?

_____

_____

Part V. Workplace Applications

1. You are performing a microscopic examination of urine and you notice the blood cells shown in the figure below. What type are they?

   A. _____

   B. _____

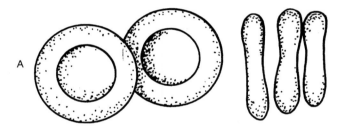

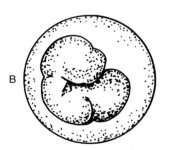

2. You are performing a microscopic examination of urine and you notice the pathogens shown in the figure below. What type are they?

A. _____

B. _____

C. _____

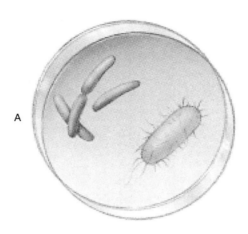

A

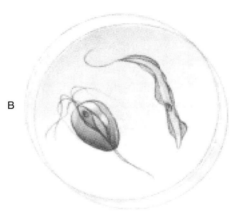

B

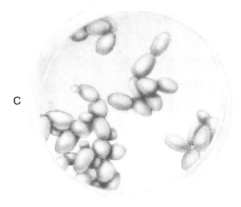

C

Part VI. Transdisciplinary Skills

Procedural Coding

You have looked up *urinalysis* in the *CPT* index, and you are confirming codes in the Pathology and Laboratory Section below. Answer the questions for these diagnostic studies.

Urinalysis

81000	Urinalysis by dipstick or tablet reagent for bilirubin, glucose, hemoglobin, ketones, leukocytes, nitrate, pH, protein, specific gravity, urobilinogen, any number of constituents: non-automated, with microscopy
81001	automated, with microscopy
81002	non-automated, without microscopy
81003	automated, without microscopy

1. What is the *CPT* code for a manual routine UA without microscopy? _____

2. What code do you use for automated, without microscopy? _____

3. What is the *CPT* manual routine UA with microscopy? _____

4. An automated UA with a microscopic exam would need which *CPT* code? _____

Part VII. Certification Review _____

Draw the following urine crystals.

1. Calcium oxalate (shaped like kites)

2. Triple phosphates (shaped like envelopes)

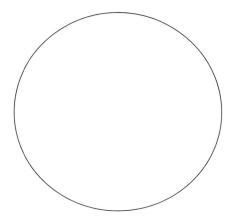 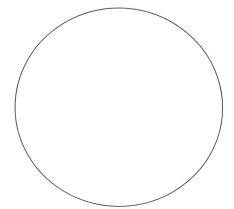

CHAPTER 28

Assisting in Phlebotomy

Part I. Medical Terminology

Directions: Fill in the blanks with the correct terms.

1. _____ An agent that inhibits bacterial growth that can be used on human tissue.

2. _____ The point of forking or separating into two branches.

3. _____ a situation in which the concentration of blood cells is increased in proportion to the plasma.

4. _____ The destruction or dissolution of red blood cells, with subsequent release of hemoglobin.

5. _____ The percentage by volume of packed red blood cells in a given sample of blood after centrifugation.

6. _____ Liquid portion of whole blood that contains active clotting agents.

7. _____ The liquid portion of whole blood that remains after the blood has clotted.

8. _____ Fainting.

9. _____ A material that appears to be a solid and appears as such until subjected to a disturbance such as centrifugation, upon which it becomes a liquid.

Part II. Spelling

Phone-etics Game

Directions: Use the telephone keypad on p. 248 to spell out the missing words and write the words in the blanks provided.

1. Found in the lavender-topped tube, _____ (3-3-8-2) prevents platelet clumping and preserves the appearance of blood cells for microscopic examination.

2. If blood is allowed to clot and then centrifuged, the liquid portion is referred to as

   _____ (7-3-7-8-6).

3. With no delay; at once _____ (7-8-2-8)

4. Some patients are allergic to _____ (5-2-8-3-9) tourniquets.

	ABC	DEF
1	2	3
GHI	JKL	MNO
4	5	6
PRS	TUV	WXY
7	8	9
*	0	#

Part III. Visual Aids

1. **Directions:** On the figure below, identify the parts of a Vacutainer (evacuated tube) system.

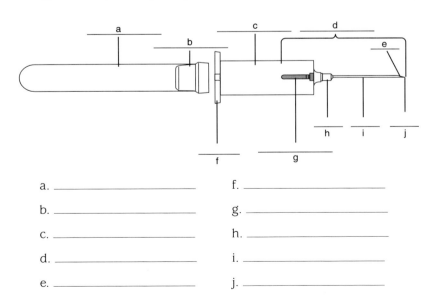

a. _____   f. _____

b. _____   g. _____

c. _____   h. _____

d. _____   i. _____

e. _____   j. _____

2. **Directions:** On the figure below, label the veins that are used for venipuncture:

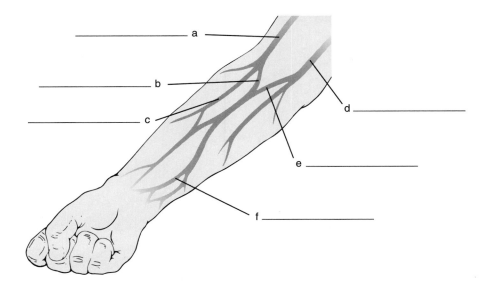

a _____

b _____

c _____

d _____

e _____

f _____

Part IV. Theory

A. **Directions:** List seven reasons that the laboratory may reject a specimen.

1. _____

2. _____

3. _____

4. _____

5. _____

6. _____

7. _____

B. The National Committee for Clinical Laboratory Standards has developed a set of standards outlining the order of draw for a multi-tube draw. The same order applies to the filling of tubes when the blood is collected in a syringe. A mnemonic device that is useful for remembering the order of the draw is **ST**OP, **R**ED **L**IGHT, **G**REEN **L**IGHT, **R**EADY, **G**O.

Directions: Use the mnemonic device and fill in the blanks.

1. _____ _____ tubes are collected first because they are sterile.

2. _____-topped tubes are second because they have no additive and thus nothing to transfer to another tube.

3. _____ blue-topped tubes are next because other anticoagulants might contaminate the sample that is collected for coagulation studies.

4. _____-topped tubes are next because heparin is less likely to interfere with EDTA than vice versa.

5. _____-topped tubes follow. EDTA binds with calcium, so this tube is drawn near the end.

6. _____/_____ marble-topped tubes are next. They contain clot activator that could interfere with specimens if passed into another tube.

7. The _____-topped tube is last because the contents can elevate electrolyte levels or damage cells if passed into another tube.

Part V. Workplace Applications

A. Identify the venipuncture supplies pictured below.

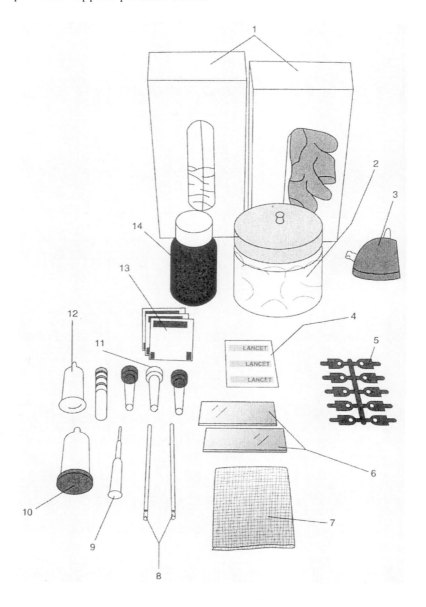

1. _____
2. _____
3. _____
4. _____
5. _____
6. _____
7. _____
8. _____
9. _____
10. _____
11. _____
12. _____
13. _____
14. _____

B. Capillary puncture may be warranted in:

1. _____
2. _____
3. _____
4. _____
5. _____
6. _____
7. _____

Directions: Fill in the blanks.

C. _____ tubes, also known as *microhematocrit tubes,* are small glass or plastic tubes, open on each end, that will hold a volume of 75 microliters.

D. Microcollection, or _____, tubes hold up to 750 microliters of blood and are available with a variety of anticoagulants and additives.

E. For children younger than 1 year, dermal puncture is performed on the medial and lateral surfaces of the _____ (bottom) of the heel.

F. True or False: After puncturing the dermis, it is important to wipe away the first drop of blood because this drop contains tissue fluid that could interfere with test results. _____

G. The most commonly used skin preparation is _____ % _____ _____, also known as *rubbing alcohol.*

H. If a blood culture is ordered, additional preparation is needed at the venipuncture site to eliminate contaminating bacteria. _____-iodine solution (_____) is commonly used.

CHAPTER **29**

Assisting in the Analysis of Blood

Part I. Medical Terminology

Matching:

1. _____ A condition marked by deficiency of red blood cells

2. _____ An apparatus consisting essentially of a compartment spun about a central axis to separate contained materials of different specific gravities, or to separate colloidal particles suspended in a liquid.

3. _____ Any of several complex proteins that are produced by cells and act as catalysts in specific biochemical reactions

4. _____ A substance, usually a peptide or steroid, produced by one tissue and conveyed by the bloodstream to another to effect physiological activity, such as growth or metabolism

5. _____ A substance produced by metabolism.

6. _____ An instrument for measuring the intensity of light, or, more especially, for comparing the relative intensities of different lights, or their relative illuminating power.

7. _____ A condition marked by an abnormally large number of red blood cells in the circulatory system

8. _____ An abnormal condition of pregnancy characterized by hypertension, edema, and protein in the urine

9. _____ Tests performed to assess the compatibility of blood to be transfused

10. _____ The major nitrogenous end product of protein metabolism and the chief nitrogenous component of the urine

11. _____ An enzyme that catalyzes the hydrolysis of urea to form ammonium carbonate

A. anemia

B. enzyme

C. urea

D. hormone

E. polycythemia vera

F. toxemia

G. metabolite

H. photometer

I. centrifuge

J. urease

K. type and cross match

Part II. Spell It Out

Phone-etics Game

Directions: Use the telephone keypad below to spell out the missing words. Write the corresponding words in the blanks provided.

1. The _____ (2-2-2) is the most frequent laboratory procedure ordered on blood.

2. The _____ (4-2-8) is a measurement of the percentage of packed red blood cells in a volume of blood.

3. The _____ (4-4-2) determination is a rough measure of the oxygen-carrying capacity of the blood.

4. Increases in _____ (7-2-2) are found in people with dehydration and polycythemia vera.

5. The _____ (3-7-7) is a laboratory test that measures the rate at which erythrocytes gradually separate from plasma and settle to the bottom of a specially calibrated tube in an hour, and it is used as a general indication of inflammation.

	ABC	DEF
1	2	3
GHI	JKL	MNO
4	5	6
PRS	TUV	WXY
7	8	9
*	0	#

Part III. Visual Aids

A. **Directions:** Identify the blood cells shown in the figure below.

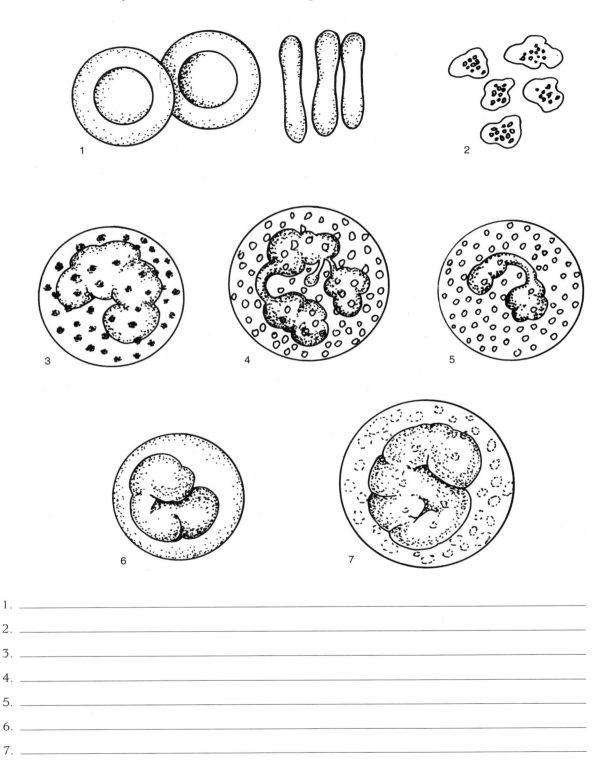

1. _____

2. _____

3. _____

4. _____

5. _____

6. _____

7. _____

B. Practice counting manual differentials in the lab by using a Neubauer-type hemacytometer.

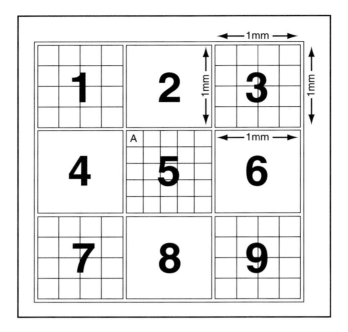

Part IV. Theory

Directions: Fill in the blanks.

A. Whole blood is composed of formed elements suspended in a clear yellow liquid portion called

_____. It makes up about 55% of the blood by volume. The remaining 45%

consists of the formed cellular elements, which are the _____ (red blood cells),

_____ (white blood cells), and _____ (platelets).

B. _____ actually carries the oxygen and carbon dioxide throughout the body. The life

span of an erythrocyte is about _____ days.

C. The granular leukocytes are called *polymorphonuclear leukocytes* and include the (hint "phils")

_____, _____, and _____.

D. The agranular leukocytes are the (hint "cytes") _____ and _____, both
of which have clear cytoplasm and a solid nucleus.

E. _____ are the smallest formed elements of the blood.

F. The platelets produce a substance that combines with _____ ions in the blood to

form _____, which in turn converts the protein _____ into thrombin in
a complex series of reactions. Thrombin, an enzyme, converts fibrinogen, a protein substance,

into _____, an insoluble protein that forms an intricate network of minute thread-
like structures called *fibrils* and causes the blood plasma to gel.

G. The _____ test is also used to monitor the condition of patients who are taking warfarin (Coumadin).

H. Complete the following statements.

1. One person in _____ is O positive.

2. One person in 15 is O _____.

3. One person in _____ is A positive.

4. One person in 16 is _____ negative.

5. One person in 12 is B _____.

6. One person in _____ is B negative.

7. One person in 29 is _____ positive.

8. One person in _____ is AB negative.

I. List several commonly used blood chemistry tests.

1. _____

2. _____

3. _____

Part V. Workplace Applications _____

Directions: Identify the cells in the picture below. _____

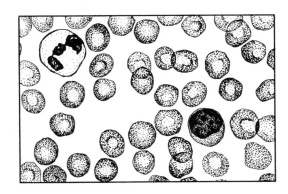

Part VI. Transdisciplinary Skills

Procedural Coding

You have looked up *blood count* in the *CPT* index, and you are confirming codes in the Pathology and Laboratory Section below. Answer the questions for the diagnostic studies.

Hematology and Coagulation

85007   Blood count, manual differential WBC count (includes RBC morphology and platelet estimation

85008   manual blood smear examination without differential parameters

85009   differential WBC count, buffy coat

85013   spun microhematocrit

85014   other than spun hematocrit

85014   hemoglobin

1. What is the *CPT* code for HCT? _____

2. What code do you use for microhematocrit? _____

3. What is the *CPT* code for Hgb? _____

4. A CBC with manual diff would need which *CPT* code? _____

CHAPTER 30

Assisting in Microbiology

Part I. Medical Terminology

Directions: Fill in the blanks with the correct terms.

1. _____ _____ A drug that is used to treat infection.

2. _____ The process of removing pathogenic microorganisms or protecting against infection by such organisms.

3. _____-_____ _____ _____ A drug used to treat a broad range of infections.

4. _____ A small capsule-like sac that encloses certain organisms in their dormant or larval stage.

5. _____ A single-celled or multicellular organism in which each cell contains a distinct membrane-bound nucleus.

6. _____ Requiring specialized media or growth factors to grow.

7. _____ _____ Refers to conditions outside of a living body.

8. _____ The molecules needed for metabolism: carbohydrates, lipids, proteins, and nucleic acids.

9. _____ A group of like or different atoms held together by chemical forces.

10. _____ An organism of microscopic or submicroscopic size.

11. _____ One billionth (10^{-9}) of a meter.

12. _____ Pertaining to or originating in the hospital; said of an infection not present or incubating before admission to the hospital.

13. _____ A differentiated structure within a cell, such as a mitochondrion, vacuole, or chloroplast, that performs a specific function.

14. _____ An agent that causes disease, especially a living microorganism such as a bacterium or fungus.

15. _____ A unicellular organism that lacks a membrane-bound nucleus.

16. _____ _____ A bacterial or fungal culture that contains a single organism.

17. _____ A sample, as of tissue, blood, or urine, used for analysis and diagnosis.

18. _____ _____ The technique or process of keeping tissue alive and growing in a culture medium.

19. _____ _____ A medium used to keep an organism alive during transport to the laboratory.

20. _____ Capable of living, developing, or germinating under favorable conditions.

21. _____ _____ A slide preparation in which a drop of liquid specimen or the like is covered with a coverslip and observed with a microscope.

Part II. Spell It Out

Phone-etics Game

Directions: Use the telephone keypad below to spell out the missing words. Write the words in the blanks provided.

1. Helminths go through the same life cycle as other worms. The adult worm lays eggs or

_____ (6-8-2).

2. Liquid media is called _____ (2-7-6-8-4).

3. The addition of a powdered extract of seaweed to media is called _____ (2-4-2-7).

	ABC	DEF
1	2	3
GHI 4	JKL 5	MNO 6
PRS 7	TUV 8	WXY 9
*	0	#

Part III. Visual Aids

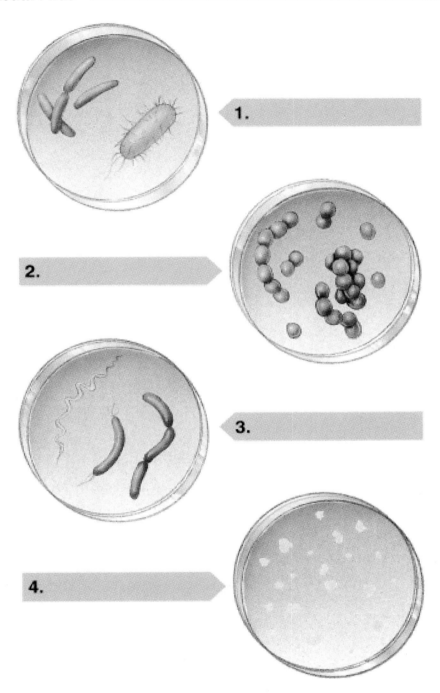

A. **Directions:** Identify the four shapes of bacteria shown in the figure above.

1. _____

2. _____

3. _____

4. _____

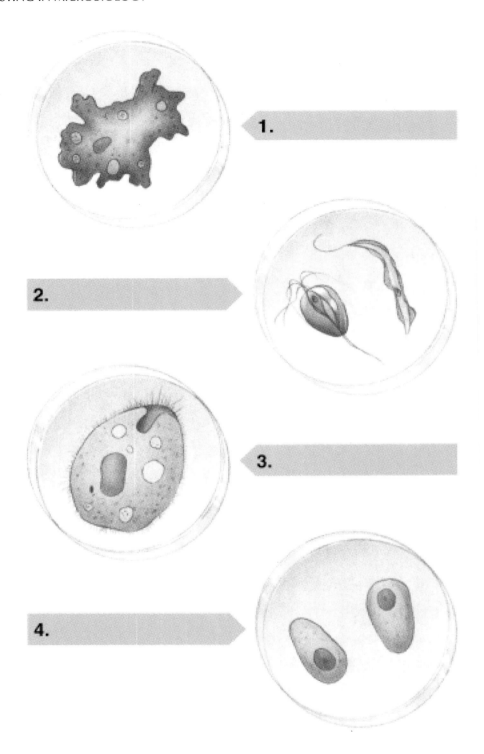

B. **Directions:** Identify the four types of disease-causing protozoa shown in the figure above.

1. _____

2. _____

3. _____

4. _____

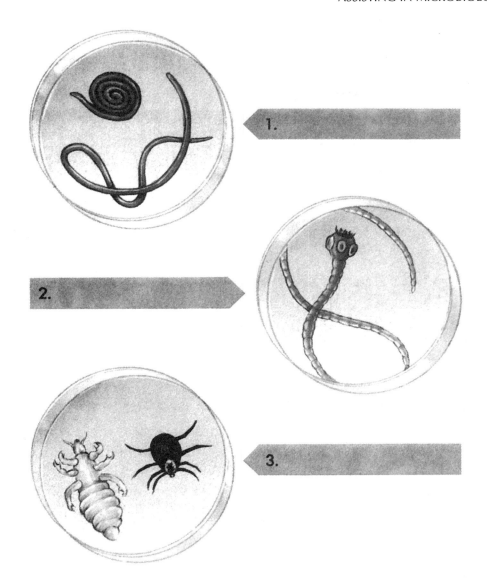

C. Identify the three pathogenic animals shown in the figure above.

1. _____

2. _____

3. _____

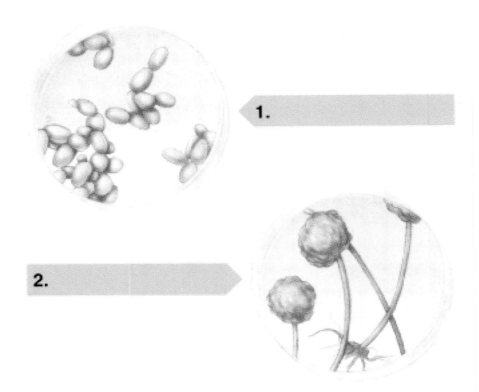

D. Identify the two fungi shown in the figure above.

1. _____

2. _____

Part IV. Theory _____

A. Bacteria are also classified according to oxygen requirements. Those that require oxygen to live

are called _____; those that will die in the presence of oxygen are called

_____.

B. _____ is the study of fungi and the diseases they cause.

C. _____ are transmitted through contaminated feces, food, or drink and are present in
moist environments and in bodies of water such as lakes and ponds.

D. Differentiate between Gram stain and acid fast stain.

_____

_____

_____

_____

E. Describe the four different classifications of media.

All-purpose or nutritive:

_____

_____

_____

_____

Selective:

_____

_____

_____

_____

Differential:

_____

_____

_____

_____

Enriched:

_____

_____

_____

_____

F. Complete the chart for transporting and processing of microbiology specimens.

Collection, Transport, and Processing of Specimens Commonly Submitted to the Physician's Office Laboratory

Specimen	Container	Patient Preparation	Special Instructions	Storage Before Processing
Blood		Disinfect venipuncture site with alcohol swab and Betadine.	Draw blood during febrile episodes; draw two sets from right and left arms.	
Body fluids (peritoneal, synovial. pleural, etc.)		Disinfect aspiration site with alcohol swab and Betadine.	Needle aspirations are preferable to swab collections.	
Eye			Moisten swab with Amie's or Stuart's medium before collection.	
Stool			Transport to lab within 24 hours if storing at 4°C.	

Specimen	Container	Patient Preparation	Special Instructions	Storage Before Processing
Rectal swab			Insert swav approx. 2.5 cm past anal sphincter.	
Gonorrhea culture		Wipe away exudate before culture; obtain culture with swab.	Do not refrigerate.	
Chlamydia culture		Urogenital swabs are preferred; epithelial cells, not exudate, must be obtained.	Transport immediately on ice to lab.	
Skin scraping (fungal culture)		Wipe skin with alcohol prep pad.	Scrape skin at leading edge of lesion.	
Sputum		Patient should rinse or gargle with mouthwash before collection.	Have patient collect from deep cough; do not collect saliva.	
Throat		Moisten swab with Stuart's or Amie's transport medium.	Swab pharynx and tonsils, not mouth, tongue, or teeth.	
Ova and parasites		A minimum of 3 specimens should be collected every other day for outpatients.	Wait 7 to 10 days if patient has been taking Pepto-Bismol, Kaopectate, or milk of magnesia.	
Urine		Instruct patient on clean-catch midstream collection.	Hold at 4°C and deliver to lab within 24 hours.	
Superficial wound		Wipe area with sterile saline solution or alcohol prep pad before collection.	Moisten swab with Amie's or Stuart's medium before collection.	
Deep wound or abscess		Wipe area with sterile saline solution or alcohol prep pad before collection.	Aspirate material, excise tissue,or insert swab deep into wound.	

Part V. Workplace Applications

A. What two questions should the medical assistant ask himself or herself before collecting specimens for microbiological analysis?

_____

_____

B. Draw the pattern that you should make when you prepare a culture on an agar plate.

Part VI. Transdisciplinary Skills

Procedural Coding

You have looked up *culture* in the *CPT* Index, and you are confirming codes in the Pathology and Laboratory section below. Answer the questions for the diagnostic studies.

Microbiology

87040	Culture, bacterial; blood with isolation and presumptive identification of isolates (includes anaerobic)
87045	stool, with isolation and preliminary examination (e.g., KIA, LIA) *Salmonella* and *Shigella* species
87046	stool, additional pathogens (includes Campylobacter, Yersinia, Vibro, and E. coli), each plate
87070	any source, except urine, blood, stool

1. What is the *CPT* code for a stool culture for salmonella? _____

2. What code do you use for a blood culture? _____

3. What is the *CPT* code for a throat culture? _____

4. A wound culture would need which *CPT* code? _____

5. What is the *CPT* code for an extra stool culture for *Escherichia coli*? _____

CHAPTER 31

Surgical Supplies and Instruments

Part I. Medical Terminology

Directions: Fill in the blanks with the appropriate terms.

1. Act of scraping a body cavity with a surgical instrument, such as a curette _____.

2. Opening or widening the circumference of a body orifice with a dilating instrument

   _____.

3. Sheet or band of fibrous tissue located deep in the skin that covers muscles and body organs

   _____.

4. Abnormal, tube-like passage between internal organs or from an internal organ to the body

   surface _____.

5. Open space, such as within a blood vessel, the intestine, the inside of a needle, or an examining

   instrument _____.

6. Rigid tube that surrounds a blunt trocar or a sharp, pointed trocar inserted into the body; when
   withdrawn, fluid may escape from the body through it, depending on where it is inserted

   _____.

7. Metal rod with a smooth rounded tip that is placed into hollow instruments to decrease

   destruction of the body tissues during insertion _____.

8. Localized collection of pus that may be under the skin or deep within the body that causes

   tissue destruction _____.

9. Open condition of a body cavity or canal _____.

10. Tumors with stems, frequently found on mucous membranes _____.

11. Metal probe that is inserted into or passed through a catheter, needle, or tube used for clearing

    purposes or to facilitate passage into a body orifice _____.

12. To cut or separate tissue with a cutting instrument or scissors _____.

Part II.

A. List some of the features of a minor surgery room.

1. _____

2. _____

3. _____

4. _____

5. _____

B. List four surgical solutions.

1. _____

2. _____

3. _____

4. _____

C. List three local anesthetics.

1. _____

2. _____

3. _____

D. List two medications that help control bleeding.

1. _____

2. _____

E. List four groups of surgical instruments and give an example of each.

1. _____

2. _____

3. _____

4. _____

Part III. Visual Aids

1. **Directions:** Name the instruments pictured below.

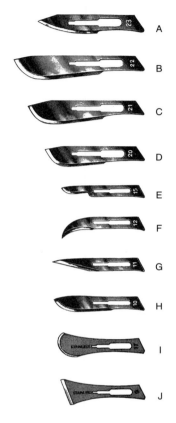

A. _____

B. _____

C. _____

D. _____

E. _____

F. _____

G. _____

H. _____

I. _____

J. _____

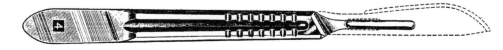

2. _____

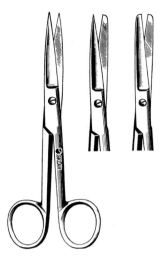

3. _____

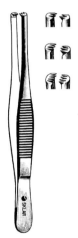

4. _____

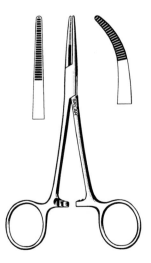

5. _____

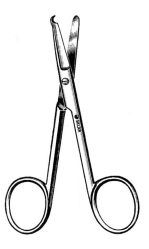

6. _____

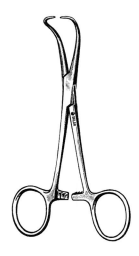

7. _____

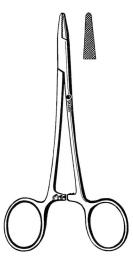

8. _____

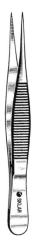

9. _____

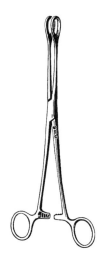

10. _____

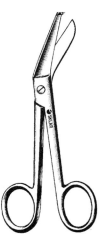

11. _____

Part IV.

A. **Directions:** Indicate which statements are true (T) and which statements are false (F).

1. _____ Each instrument should always be unlocked before immersion in the chemical decontaminate to permit cleansing of the entire surface area.

2. _____ Instruments are always named after the person who designed them.

3. _____ Scissors have ratchets.

4. _____ *A mosquito* and *Kelly* are names of hemostats.

B. **Directions:** Match the following descriptions and instruments.

1. _____ Blade has beak or hook to slide under sutures.

2. _____ Jaws are shorter and look stronger than hemostat jaws.

3. _____ Design and construction vary; has fine tip for foreign object retrieval.

4. _____ Have very sharp hooks.

5. _____ Valves can be spread to facilitate viewing.

6. _____ Bandage scissors.

7. _____ Manufactured in different lengths; smooth-tipped; used to insert packing into or remove objects from nose and ear.

A. Bayonet forceps

B. Towel forceps (towel clamp)

C. Littauer stitch or suture scissors

D. Needle holders

E. Splinter forceps

F. Nasal specula

G. Probe tip is blunt

C. Search the Internet for surgical instruments. Review the names of instruments that you find on the Internet.

_____   _____

_____   _____

_____   _____

_____   _____

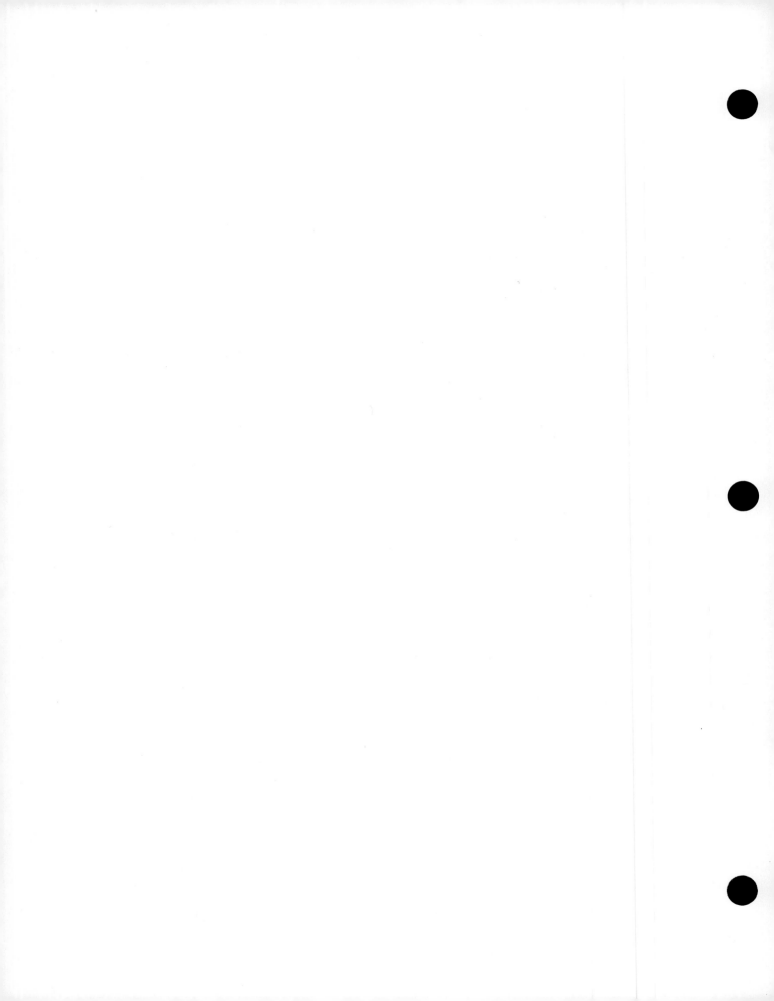

CHAPTER 32

Surgical Asepsis and Assisting with Surgical Procedures

Part I. Vocabulary

Directions: Match the following terms and definitions.

1. _____ Invasion of body tissues by microorganisms, which then proliferate and damage tissues

2. _____ Living organisms that can only be seen with a light microscope

3. _____ Disease-causing microorganisms

4. _____ Allowing a substance to pass or soak through

5. _____ Presence of pus-forming organisms in the blood

6. _____ Reducing the number of microorganisms to a relatively safe level

7. _____ Thick-walled dormant form of bacteria, very resistant to disinfection measures

8. _____ Complete destruction of all forms of microbial life

9. _____ Chemical agents that kill pathogens

10. _____ Having a rapid onset and severe symptoms

11. _____ Substance that kills microorganisms

12. _____ Being free from infection or infectious materials

13. _____ Persisting for a prolonged period

14. _____ Becoming unsterile by contact with any nonsterile material

15. _____ Pathologic process having a descriptive set of signs and symptoms

16. _____ Destruction of pathogens by physical or chemical means

17. _____ Swelling between layers of tissue

A. permeable

B. contamination

C. asepsis

D. disease

E. chronic

F. infection

G. antiseptic

H. edema

I. spores

J. pathogens

K. germicides

L. pyemia

M. acute

N. sterilization

O. disinfection

P. microorganisms

Q. sanitization

Part II.

Directions: Rate yourself on the knowledge of the following procedures, with 1 being the lowest score and 5 being the highest score.

1. Demonstrate proper hand washing technique for surgical asepsis.   1 2 3 4 5

2. Clean and wrap instruments and equipment for autoclaving.   1 2 3 4 5

3. Load, run, and unload the autoclave properly.   1 2 3 4 5

4. Open a sterile pack to create a sterile field.   1 2 3 4 5

5. Open and add the contents of a sterile pack to a sterile field.   1 2 3 4 5

6. Transfer sterile instruments.   1 2 3 4 5

7. Assist with a minor surgical procedure.   1 2 3 4 5

8. Assist with suturing.   1 2 3 4 5

9. Remove sutures.   1 2 3 4 5

10. Properly apply dressing and bandage to surgical site.   1 2 3 4 5

Part III.

Directions: Fill in the blanks.

1. The physician must have the patient's written, _____ consent before doing any surgical procedure. To sign an informed consent form, permitting the physician to legally perform

the surgery, the patient must understand _____ procedure will be done,

_____ it should be done, the potential _____ and _____ of the surgery, alternative treatments (including no treatment), and the possible risks of any alternative treatment. This legal requirement is not simply met by having the patient

_____ the operative permit. A _____ must occur during which the physician provides the patient or the patient's legal representative with enough information to decide whether to proceed with the proposed surgical treatment. After this discussion, the patient

either _____ or _____ to consent to the surgery.
The patient then signs or refuses to sign the consent form. If the patient signs with an X, the medical assistant should write "patient's mark" beside the X, and in addition, have a

_____ _____ witness the signature. The discussion must be fully

_____ in the patient's medical record. A copy of the _____ form must also be included in the patient's record. Treatment may not exceed the scope of the permit.

NOTE: The patient must not be under the influence of any _____ medication at the

time he or she is signing the consent form. This condition must _____ be violated.

Part IV.

A. List five reasons a postoperative patient should call the office.

1. _____

2. _____

3. _____

4. _____

5. _____

B. **Directions:** Indicate which statements are true (T) and which statements are false (F).

1. _____ Air currents carry bacteria, so body motions over a sterile field and talking should be kept to a minimum.

2. _____ Infection can cause death in some circumstances.

3. _____ A sterile field can get wet.

4. _____ Sterile team members should always face each other.

5. _____ You should always keep the sterile field in your view.

6. _____ You should never turn your back on a sterile field or wander away from it.

7. _____ When autoclaving, you should place a gauze sponge around the tips of sharp instruments to prevent them from piercing the wrapping material.

8. _____ Nonsterile persons should never reach over a sterile field.

9. _____ All hinged instruments are wrapped in the closed position to allow full steam penetration of the joint.

10. _____ When using sterilizing bags, you should insert the grasping end of the instruments first.

CHAPTER 33

Career Development and Life Skills

Part I. Vocabulary

Directions: Match the following terms and definitions.

1. _____ To give an expert judgment of the value or merit of; in this chapter, the evaluation of work performance.

2. _____ A return offer made by one who has rejected an offer or job.

3. _____ A failure to pay financial debts, especially a student loan.

4. _____ A postponement, especially of repayment of a student loan.

5. _____ Expressing sincerity and honest feeling.

6. _____ Not tolerable or bearable.

7. _____ To imitate or practice.

8. _____ The exchange of information or services among individuals, groups, or institutions; in this chapter, it involves meeting and getting to know individuals in the same or similar career fields and sharing information about available opportunities.

9. _____ Having a clear decisive relevance to the matter in hand.

10. _____ To read and mark corrections.

11. _____ Something produced by a cause or necessarily following from a set of conditions.

12. _____ To correct by removing errors.

13. _____ Having or marked by keen insight and ability to penetrate deeply and thoroughly.

14. _____ Marked by compact, precise expression without wasted words.

15. _____ A condensed statement or outline.

16. _____ The work in which a person is regularly employed.

A. succinct

B. counteroffer

C. synopsis

D. appraisals

E. rectify

F. proofread

G. intolerable

H. default

I. pertinent

J. ramification

K. networking

L. vocation

M. subtle

N. genuineness

O. mock

P. deferment

Part II.

A. **Directions:** List nine methods of job searching.

1. _____
2. _____
3. _____
4. _____
5. _____
6. _____
7. _____
8. _____
9. _____

B. **Directions:** Complete the job application that is included in this workbook. Use factual information. Remember: Neatness counts.

C. **Directions:** Prepare a draft resume using the blank pages included in this chapter.

APPLICATION FOR EMPLOYMENT

This application is not a contract. It is intended to provide information for evaluating your suitability for employment. Please read each question carefully and give an honest and complete answer. Qualified applicants receive consideration for employment without unlawful discrimination because of sex, religion, race, color, national origin, age, disability, or other classification protected by law. Applications will remain active for three months.

PLEASE TYPE OR PRINT ALL INFORMATION

Date: _____

Position(s) applying for: _____

How did you learn about us? ☐ Walk-in ☐ Friend ☐ Relative ☐ Job hotline ☐ Employee ☐ Other
☐ Advertisement (Please state name of publication) _____ Referred by: _____

Name: _____
　　　　　　Last　　　　　　　　　　　First　　　　　　　　　Middle initial

Mailing address: _____
　　　　　　　　　　City　　　　　　　　State　　　　　　　　Zip code

Phone: (____)_____ (____)_____ Social Security #: _____
　　　　Home　　　　　　　　　Message

If related to anyone in our employ, state name and department: _____

If you have been employed under another name, please list here: _____

Are you under 18 years of age?---------------------------------- ☐Yes　☐No

Are you currently employed?------------------------------------- ☐Yes　☐No

May we contact your present employer?-------------------------- ☐Yes　☐No

Do you have legal rights to work in this country?
　(Proof of legal rights to work in this country will be required upon employment)--- ☐Yes　☐No

Have you ever been employed with us before?------------------- ☐Yes　☐No If "yes," give date(s): _____

Are you available to work: --------------------------------------- ☐Full-time ☐Part-time ☐ Shift work ☐ Temporary

Are you available to work overtime if required?----------------- ☐Yes　☐No

How flexible are you in accepting varying scheduled hours?----------- ☐Very flexible ☐Somewhat flexible
　　　　　　　　　　　　　　　　　　　　　　　　　　　　　　　　☐Need set schedule

Minimum salary desired: _____

Have you ever been discharged from a job or forced to resign? -------- ☐Yes　☐No
　Explain:_____

Have you ever been convicted of a felony?
　If "yes," please explain: -- ☐Yes　☐No
　Criminal convictions are not an absolute bar to _____
　employment but will be considered with respect _____
　to the specific requirements of the job for which _____
　you are applying.

EDUCATION

High school: _____ High school graduate/GED: ☐Yes ☐No
_____ Date: _____

College: _____ Graduated: ☐Yes ☐No
Major/field(s) of study: _____ Degree: _____
Date: _____

College: _____ Graduated: ☐Yes ☐No
Major/field(s) of study: _____ Degree: _____
Date: _____

Technical, business, or correspondence school: _____ Graduated: ☐Yes ☐No
Major/field(s) of study: _____ Degree: _____
Date: _____

Describe any specialized training, apprenticeship, and skills such as computer, office equipment, etc. _____
_____
_____
_____
_____

LICENSES AND CERTIFICATIONS

Type of license(s)/certification(s): _____ Expiration date: _____
Type of license(s)/certification(s): _____ Expiration date: _____
Type of license(s)/certification(s): _____ Expiration date: _____
Verified by: _____
Date: _____

REFERENCES

(Give name, address, and telephone number of three references that you have known for at least one year who are not related to you.)

Name: _____ Phone: _____ Years acquainted: _____
Address: _____ Business: _____

Name: _____ Phone: _____ Years acquainted: _____
Address: _____ Business: _____

Name: _____ Phone: _____ Years acquainted: _____
Address: _____ Business: _____

EMPLOYMENT EXPERIENCE

(Please list all employment experience, with most recent employment first. If more space is needed, please use the Additional Employment form.)

Employer: _____ Duties and skills performed: _____

Address: _____ _____

Phone number(s) _____ _____

Job title: _____ _____

Supervisor's name/title: _____ _____

Reason for leaving: _____ _____

Salary received: _____ *hourly / weekly / monthly* _____

Employed from: _____ to _____ _____
           month / year   *month / year*

Employer: _____ Duties and skills performed: _____

Address: _____ _____

Phone number(s) _____ _____

Job title: _____ _____

Supervisor's name/title: _____ _____

Reason for leaving: _____ _____

Salary received: _____ *hourly / weekly / monthly* _____

Employed from: _____ to _____ _____
           month / year   *month / year*

Employer: _____ Duties and skills performed: _____

Address: _____ _____

Phone number(s) _____ _____

Job title: _____ _____

Supervisor's name/title: _____ _____

Reason for leaving: _____ _____

Salary received: _____ *hourly / weekly / monthly* _____

Employed from: _____ to _____ _____
           month / year   *month / year*

Do you expect any of the employers listed above to give you a poor reference? ☐ *Yes* ☐ *No*

If yes, explain: _____

_____

APPLICANT'S STATEMENT

I hereby certify that the statements and information provided are true, and I understand that any false statements or omissions are cause for termination. I agree to submit to a drug test and physical following any conditional offer of employment, and I grant permission to Diamonte Hospital to investigate my criminal history, education, prior employment history, and references, and hereby release all persons or agencies from all liability or any damage for issuing this information.

I understand that this application is current for only **three months**. At the end of that time, if I do not hear from Diamonte Hospital and still wish to be considered for employment, it will be necessary to update my application.

_____   _____
Signature of Applicant   *Date*

_____
Print Name

DIAMONTE
HOSPITAL

Draft Resumé

Draft Resumé

Part III.

Directions: Evaluate Teresa O'Sullivan's cover letter. Describe what you like about the letter and make notes of additional information that you would include in your own cover letter.

Theresa O'Sullivan
233 Wentworth Street, San Diego, CA 92100
Telephone (619) 222-3333

June 15, 20xx

Arthur M. Blackburn, MD
2200 Broadway
Any Town, US 98765

Dear Doctor Blackburn:

In a few weeks, I will complete my formal training in medical assisting with an Associate in Science degree from Ola Vista Community College.

The medical assisting program at Ola Vista includes theory and practical application in both administrative and clinical skills. My six-week supervised externship gave me additional practical experience in two specialty practices.

While studying at Ola Vista, I also worked part-time for a physician in family practice, while maintaining a 3.5 grade point average. My experience as Dr. Madden's employee is outlined on the enclosed resumé. I have enjoyed my work in Dr. Madden's office and am now seeking full-time employment.

If you will require a replacement or addition to your staff in the near future, may I be considered as an applicant? I will follow up with a telephone call within a week.

Sincerely yours,

Theresa O'Sullivan

Enc. Resumé

Part IV.

A. **Directions:** Set some realistic goals for your career in medical assisting by answering the following questions.

1. Where am I today?

_____

_____

_____

_____

_____

_____

2. Where will I be in five years?

_____

_____

_____

_____

_____

_____

3. Where will I be in ten years?

_____

_____

_____

_____

_____

_____

4. What additional skills do I need to get where I want to be?

_____

_____

_____

_____

_____

_____

B. **Directions:** Plan a budget for yourself using your actual living expenses.

The Guideline Budget

MONTHLY INCOME	AMOUNT
Net Income	
Spouse Net Income	
Child Support	
Other Income	

MONTHLY EXPENSES	AMOUNT
Rent	
Gas	
Electric	
Home/Renters Insurance	
Water/Sewage	
Trash	
Home Telephone	
Cell Telephone	
Pager	
Cable TV/Satellite	
Internet/DSL	
Child Care	
Lawn Care	
Clothing	
Food-Home	
Food-Work or School	
Food-Eating Out	
Laundry/Dry Cleaning	
Medical Expenses	
Dental Expenses	
Life Insurance	
Medical Insurance	
Dental Insurance	
Eyeglasses	
Prescriptions	
Automobile Payment	
Automobile Insurance	
Repairs	
Gas/Oil	
Furniture	
Beauty/Barber Shop	
Pet Expenses	
Student Loan	
Others Loans	
Credit Cards	
Church/charities	
Birthdays	
Anniversaries	
Christmas	
Vacation Planning	
Entertainment	

PROCEDURE CHECKLISTS

Procedure 2-1 Performing Medical Aseptic Hand Washing

Task: To minimize the number of pathogens on your hands, thus reducing the risk of pathogenic transmission.

Equipment and Supplies:
• Sink with running water
• Anti-microbial liquid soap in a dispenser (bar soap is not acceptable)
• Nail brush or orange stick
• Paper towels in a dispenser
• Water-based antimicrobial lotion

Standards: Complete the procedure and all critical steps in _____ minutes with a minimum

score of _____ % within three attempts.

Scoring: Divide points earned by total possible points. Failure to perform a critical step that is indicated with an asterisk (*), will result in an unsatisfactory overall score.

Time began _____ **Time ended** _____

Steps	Possible Points	First Attempt	Second Attempt	Third Attempt
1. Remove all jewelry except your wristwatch, which should be pulled up above your wrist or removed, and a plain gold wedding ring.	10			
2. Turn on the faucet and regulate the water temperature to lukewarm.	10			
3. Allow your hands to become wet, apply soap, and lather using a circular motion with friction while holding your fingertips downward. Rub well between your fingers.	10			
4. Rinse well, holding your hands so that the water flows from your wrists downward to your fingertips.	10			
5. Wet your hands again and repeat the scrubbing procedure using vigorous, circular motion over wrists and hands for at least 1 to 2 minutes.	10			
6. Rinse your hands a second time, keeping fingers lower than your wrists.	10			
7. Dry your hands with paper towels. Do not touch the paper towel dispenser as you are obtaining towels.	10			
8. If faucets are not foot operated, turn off the water faucet with the paper towel.*	10			

Steps	Possible Points	First Attempt	Second Attempt	Third Attempt
9. After completion of drying your hands and turning off faucets (if necessary) place used towels into waste container	**10**			
10. Apply a water-based antibacterial hand lotion to prevent chapped or dry skin.	**10**			

Comments:

Total Points Earned _____ Divided by _____ Total Possible Points = _____ % Score

Instructor's Signature _____

Procedure 2-2 Sanitization of Instruments

Task: To remove all contaminated matter from instruments in preparation for disinfection or sterilization.

Equipment and Supplies:
- Sink with hot running water
- Sanitizing agent or low-sudsing soap with enzymatic action
- Utility gloves
- Brush
- Towels
- Appropriate waste container

Standards: Complete the procedure and all critical steps in _____ minutes with a minimum score of _____ % within three attempts.

Scoring: Divide points earned by total possible points. Failure to perform a critical step that is indicated with an asterisk (*), will result in an unsatisfactory overall score.

Time began _____ **Time ended** _____

Steps	Possible Points	First Attempt	Second Attempt	Third Attempt
1. Put on utility gloves.*	20			
2. Separate sharp instruments from other instruments to be sanitized.	10			
3. Rinse the instruments under cold running water.	10			
4. Open hinged instruments and scrub all grooves, crevices, and serrations with a brush.*	20			
5. Rinse well with hot water.	10			
6. Towel dry all instruments thoroughly.	10			
7. Remove utility gloves and wash hands thoroughly.	10			
8. Place sanitized instruments in designated area for disinfection or sterilization.	10			

Comments:

Total Points Earned _____ Divided by _____ Total Possible Points = _____ % Score

Instructor's Signature _____

Procedure 2-3 Removing Contaminated Latex Gloves

Task: To minimize pathogen exposure by aseptically removing and discarding contaminated gloves.

Equipment and Supplies:
• Latex examination gloves
• Biohazard waste container

Standards: Complete the procedure and all critical steps in _____ minutes with a minimum

score of _____ % within three attempts.

Scoring: Divide points earned by total possible points. Failure to perform a critical step that is indicated with an asterisk (*), will result in an unsatisfactory overall score.

Time began _____   **Time ended** _____

Steps	Possible Points	First Attempt	Second Attempt	Third Attempt
1. With the dominant hand, grasp the glove of the opposite hand near the palm and begin removing the first glove. Arms should be extended from the body and hands pointed down.	20			
2. Pull the glove inside out until you reach the fingers, holding the contaminated glove in the dominant gloved hand.	20			
3. Insert the thumb of the non-gloved hand inside the cuff of the remaining contaminated glove.	20			
4. Pull the glove down the hand inside out over the contaminated glove being held leaving the contaminated side of both gloves on the inside.	20			
5. Properly dispose of the inside out contaminated gloves in a biohazard waste container. Perform a medical aseptic hand wash as described in Procedure 2-1.	20			

Documentation in the Medical Record

_____

_____

_____

_____

Comments:

Total Points Earned _____ Divided by _____ Total Possible Points = _____ % Score

Instructor's Signature _____

Procedure 3-1 Obtaining a Medical History

Task: To obtain an acceptable written background from the patient to help the physician determine the cause and effects of the present illness. This includes the chief complaint (CC), present illness (PI), past history (PH). family history (FH), and social history (SH).

Equipment and Supplies:
- A history form
- Two pens, a red pen for recording patient allergies and a black pen to meet legal documentation guidelines
- A quiet, private area

Standards: Complete the procedure and all critical steps in _____ minutes with a minimum score of _____ % within three attempts.

Scoring: Divide points earned by total possible points. Failure to perform a critical step that is indicated with an asterisk (*), will result in an unsatisfactory overall score.

Time began _____ Time ended _____

Steps	Possible Points	First Attempt	Second Attempt	Third Attempt
1. Greet and identify the patient in a pleasant manner. Introduce yourself and explain your role.	10			
2. Take patient to a quiet, private area for the interview and explain to the patient why the information is needed.	10			
3. Complete the history form by utilizing therapeutic communication techniques. Make sure that all medical terminology is adequately explained. A self-history may have been mailed to the patient before the visit. If so, review the self-history for completeness.	10			
4. Speak in a pleasant, distinct manner, remembering to keep eye contact with your patient.	10			
5. Record the following statistical information on the patient information form: • Patient's full name, including middle initial • Address, including apartment number and ZIP code • Marital status • Sex (gender) • Age and date of birth • Telephone number for home and work • Insurance information if not already available • Employer's name, address, telephone number	10			

Steps	Possible Points	First Attempt	Second Attempt	Third Attempt
6. Record the following medical history on the patient history (PH) form: Chief complaint Present illness Past history Family history Social history	10			
7. Ask about allergies to drugs and any other substances, and record any allergies in red ink on every page of the history form, on the front of the chart, and on each progress note page. Some practices apply allergy alert labels to the front of each chart.	10			
8. Record all information legibly and neatly, and spell words correctly. Print rather than write in longhand. Do not erase, scribble or use white-out. If you make an error, draw a single line through the error, write error above it, add the correction, and initial and date the entry.	10			
9. Thank the patient for cooperating, and direct him or her back to the reception area.	10			
10. Review the record for errors before you pass it to the physician. Use the information on the record to complete the patient's chart. Keep the information confidential.	10			

Documentation:

Your patient's CC is dizziness for 2 weeks. She denies headaches, history (Hx) of ear infections, or Hx of hypertension. Her BP is 172/94, T – 97.6, P – 88, R – 22. Document pertinent patient findings using the SOAPE method.

S: _____

O: _____

A: _____

P: _____

E: _____

Total Points Earned _____ Divided by _____ Total Possible Points = _____ % Score

Instructor's Signature _____

Procedure 5-1 Determining Fat-Fold Measurement

Task: To accurately determine and record a measurement of body fat.

Equipment and Supplies:
- Fat-fold body calipers
- Pencil and paper

Standards: Complete the procedure and all critical steps in _____ minutes with a minimum

score of _____ % within three attempts.

Scoring: Divide points earned by total possible points. Failure to perform a critical step that is indicated with an asterisk (*), will result in an unsatisfactory overall score.

Time began _____ **Time ended** _____

Steps	Possible Points	First Attempt	Second Attempt	Third Attempt
1. Read the directions for the caliper before you begin.	5			
2. Gather the equipment and supplies needed to complete the procedure and wash hands.	5			
3. Identify the patient.	5			
4. Explain the procedure to the patient.	5			
5. Using the triceps of the upper arm, grasp the skinfold with thumb and index finger. Make sure that the fold is in a parallel angle by keeping the thumb and index finger in line with one another. Be sure you do not grasp muscle tissue or pinch too tightly.	5			
6. Place calipers over the fold and measure.	10			
7. Record the measurement.	10			
8. Grasp the subscapular region located beneath the shoulder blade and obtain your second measurement.	10			
9. Record the measurement.	5			
10. Using the suprailiac area located posteriorly and immediately superior to the fanning of the hip bone, obtain your third measurement.	10			
11. Record the measurement.	5			

Steps	Possible Points	First Attempt	Second Attempt	Third Attempt
12. Determine total percent of body fat using Table 27-4.	10			
13. Record the calculations in the patient's medical record.	5			
14. Disinfect equipment and return to its proper place.	5			
15. Wash your hands.	5			

Documentation in the Medical Record

_____

_____

_____

_____

Comments:

Total Points Earned _____ Divided by _____ Total Possible Points = _____ % Score

Instructor's Signature _____

Procedure 5-2 Teaching the Patient to Read Food Labels

Task: To accurately explain the nutritional labeling of food products to the patient.

Equipment and Supplies:
• One each of four bars: Snickers, Twix, Healthy Choice, Fat Free Fruit Bar
• Pencil and Paper

Standards: Complete the procedure and all critical steps in _____ minutes with a minimum

score of _____ % within three attempts.

Scoring: Divide points earned by total possible points. Failure to perform a critical step that is indicated with an asterisk (*), will result in an unsatisfactory overall score.

Time began _____ **Time ended** _____

Steps		Possible Points	First Attempt	Second Attempt	Third Attempt
1.	Explain what you are going to talk about to the patient. Be sure to include reasons why food labels are a valuable source of nutritional information in diet planning.	10			
2.	Using the labels on each bar, point out the nutritional information according to the guidelines in the text.	10			
3.	Give the patient pencil and paper to write down the serving size of each type of candy bar.	10			
4.	Together compare similarities and differences.	10			
5.	Next have the patient write down the total caloric amount for each product serving.	10			
6.	Compare similarities and differences.	10			
7.	Write down the percentage of total, saturated, and unsaturated fats.	10			
8.	Compare similarities and differences.	10			
9.	Together analyze the nutritional level of each.	10			
10.	Discuss any new information that was learned and ask the patient if he or she will use this information when shopping and how it will be implemented into nutritional planning.	10			

Comments:

Total Points Earned _____ Divided by _____ Total Possible Points = _____ % Score

Instructor's Signature _____

Procedure 6-1 Obtaining an Oral Temperature Using a Digital Thermometer

Task: To accurately determine and record a patient's temperature using a digital thermometer.

Equipment and Supplies:
- Digital thermometer
- Probe covers
- Biohazard waste container

Standards: Complete the procedure and all critical steps in _____ minutes with a minimum score of _____ % within three attempts.

Scoring: Divide points earned by total possible points. Failure to perform a critical step that is indicated with an asterisk (*), will result in an unsatisfactory overall score.

Time began _____ **Time ended** _____

Steps	Possible Points	First Attempt	Second Attempt	Third Attempt
1. Wash hands and assemble equipment and supplies.*	10			
2. Identify your patient and explain the procedure. Be sure that the patient has not eaten, drunk fluids, smoked, or exercised for 30 minutes before taking the temperature.*	20			
3. Prepare the probe for use as described in package directions. Make sure probe covers are *always* used.	10			
4. Place the probe under the patient's tongue, and instruct the patient to close the mouth tightly. Assist the patient by holding the probe end.	10			
5. When the "beep" is heard, remove the probe from the patient's mouth and immediately eject the probe cover into the appropriate waste container.	10			
6. Note the reading in the LED window of the processing unit you are holding.	10			
7. Record the reading on the patient's medical record as T = 97.7°.	20			
8. Wash hands and disinfect equipment as indicated.	10			

Documentation in the Medical Record

_____

_____

_____

_____

Comments:

Total Points Earned _____ Divided by _____ Total Possible Points = _____ % Score

Instructor's Signature _____

Procedure 6-2 Obtaining an Aural Temperature Using the Tympanic Thermometer

Task: To accurately determine and record a patient's temperature using the tympanic thermometer.

Equipment and Supplies:
- Tympanic thermometer
- Disposable probe covers
- Biohazard waste container

Standards: Complete the procedure and all critical steps in _____ minutes with a minimum

score of _____ % within three attempts.

Scoring: Divide points earned by total possible points. Failure to perform a critical step that is indicated with an asterisk (*), will result in an unsatisfactory overall score.

Time began _____ **Time ended** _____

Steps	Possible Points	First Attempt	Second Attempt	Third Attempt
1. Wash hands.	10			
2. Gather the necessary equipment and supplies.	10			
3. Identify your patient and explain the procedure.	10			
4. Place disposable probe cover on probe.	10			
5. Follow the package directions to start the thermometer.	10			
6. Insert the probe into the ear canal far enough to seal the opening. Do not apply pressure.	10			
7. Press the button on the probe as directed. The temperature will be on the display screen in 1 to 2 seconds.	10			
8. Remove the probe, note the reading, and discard the probe cover without touching it.	10			
9. Wash your hands and disinfect the equipment if indicated.	10			
10. Record temperature results as T = 98.6° (T) on the patient's medical record.	10			

Documentation in the Medical Record

_____

_____

_____

_____

Comments:

Total Points Earned _____ Divided by _____ Total Possible Points = _____ % Score

Instructor's Signature _____

Student Name _____ Date _____ Score _____

Procedure 6-3 Obtaining an Axillary Temperature

Task: To accurately determine and record a patient's temperature using the axillary method.

Equipment and Supplies:
• Digital unit
• Thermometer sheath or probe cover
• Supply of tissues
• Biohazard waste container

Standards: Complete the procedure and all critical steps in _____ minutes with a minimum

score of _____ % within three attempts.

Scoring: Divide points earned by total possible points. Failure to perform a critical step that is indicated with an asterisk (*), will result in an unsatisfactory overall score.

Time began _____ **Time ended** _____

Steps	Possible Points	First Attempt	Second Attempt	Third Attempt
1. Wash your hands.	10			
2. Gather equipment and supplies.	5			
3. Introduce yourself, identify your patient, and explain the procedure.	10			
4. Prepare thermometer or digital unit in same manner as done for oral usage.	10			
5. Remove clothing and gown patient as needed to access axillary region.	5			
6. Pat the patient's axillary area dry if needed.	10			
7. Cover the thermometer or probe and place the tip into the center of the armpit, pointing the stem to the upper chest, making sure the thermometer is touching only skin, not clothing.	10			
8. Instruct the patient to hold the arm snugly across the chest or abdomen until the thermometer beeps.	10			
9. Remove the thermometer, note the digital reading, and dispose of the cover in the biohazard waste container.	10			
10. Disinfect the thermometer if indicated and Wash hands.	10			
11. Record the axillary temperature on the patient's medical record, for example, T = 97.6° (A)	10			

313

Documentation in the Medical Record

_____

_____

_____

_____

Comments:

Total Points Earned _____ Divided by _____ Total Possible Points = _____ % Score

Instructor's Signature _____

Procedure 6-4 Obtaining Rectal Temperature

Task: To accurately determine and record a patient's temperature using the rectal method.

Equipment and Supplies:
- Digital thermometer for rectal use
- Thermometer sheath or probe cover
- Lubricant
- A supply of tissues
- Nonsterile gloves
- Biohazard waste container

Standards: Complete the procedure and all critical steps in _____ minutes with a minimum

score of _____ % within three attempts.

Scoring: Divide points earned by total possible points. Failure to perform a critical step that is indicated with an asterisk (*), will result in an unsatisfactory overall score.

Time began _____ **Time ended** _____

Steps	Possible Points	First Attempt	Second Attempt	Third Attempt
1. Wash your hands.	10			
2. Introduce yourself, identify your patient, and explain the procedure.	5			
3. Remove patient clothing from waist down and drape as needed.	5			
4. Place adult patient in Sims' position.	5			
5. Prepare thermometer using a sheath or probe cover on the red probe in the digital unit.	10			
6. Put on gloves.*	10			
7. Lubricate the probe tip and insert into the rectum past the sphincter.*	10			
8. Hold the thermometer in place until a beep is heard.	10			
9. Remove the thermometer and note the reading on the LED window. Offer tissues to patient.	5			
10. Remove the sheath or probe cover as well as your gloves and discard into appropriate biohazard waste container.	15			
11. Wash hands.*	10			

Steps	Possible Points	First Attempt	Second Attempt	Third Attempt
12. Assist patient with positioning and dressing as needed.	5			
13. Record temperature with (R) which indicates a rectal temperature for example, T = 99.6° (R).	10			

Documentation in the Medical Record

_____

_____

_____

_____

Comments:

Total Points Earned _____ Divided by _____ Total Possible Points = _____ % Score

Instructor's Signature _____

Procedure 6-5 Obtaining an Apical Pulse

Task: To assess the patient's apical heart rate.

Equipment and Supplies:
- A watch with a second hand
- Stethoscope
- Alcohol wipes
- Patient gown

Standards: Complete the procedure and all critical steps in _____ minutes with a minimum

score of _____ % within three attempts.

Scoring: Divide points earned by total possible points. Failure to perform a critical step that is indicated with an asterisk (*), will result in an unsatisfactory overall score.

Time began _____ **Time ended** _____

Steps	Possible Points	First Attempt	Second Attempt	Third Attempt
1. Wash your hands and clean stethoscope earpieces with alcohol swabs.	10			
2. Introduce yourself, identify your patient, and explain the procedure.	10			
3. Assist patient in disrobing from waist up and provide patient gown open to the front.	10			
4. Patient should be either sitting or in supine position.	10			
5. Place the stethoscope just below the left nipple in the intercostal space between the 5th and 6th ribs.	10			
6. Listen carefully for the heartbeat.	10			
7. Count the pulse for one full minute.* Note any irregularities in rhythm and volume.	10			
8. Assist the patient to sit up and dress.	10			
9. Wash hands.	10			
10. Record the pulse in the patient chart as AP (e.g., AP = 96) and record any arrhythmias.	10			

Documentation in the Medical Record

_____

_____

_____

_____

Comments:

Total Points Earned _____ Divided by _____ Total Possible Points = _____ % Score

Instructor's Signature _____

Procedure 6-6 Assessing the Patient's Pulse

Task: To determine and record a patient's pulse rate, rhythm, volume, and elasticity.

Equipment and Supplies:
• A watch with a second hand

Standards: Complete the procedure and all critical steps in _____ minutes with a minimum

score of _____ % within three attempts.

Scoring: Divide points earned by total possible points. Failure to perform a critical step that is indicated
with an asterisk (*), will result in an unsatisfactory overall score.

Time began _____ **Time ended** _____

Steps	Possible Points	First Attempt	Second Attempt	Third Attempt
1. Wash your hands.	10	_____	_____	_____
2. Introduce yourself, identify your patient, and explain the procedure.	10	_____	_____	_____
3. Place the patient's arm in a relaxed position, palm downward.	10	_____	_____	_____
4. Gently grasp the palm side of the patient's wrist with your first three fingertips approximately 1 inch above the base of the thumb.	20	_____	_____	_____
5. Count the beats for 1 full minute, using a watch with a second hand. Note* if measured for 30 seconds, multiply by two.	20	_____	_____	_____
6. Wash your hands.	10	_____	_____	_____
7. Record the count and any irregularities on the patient's medical record. Record as P = 72. Pulse is usually recorded immediately after temperature.	20	_____	_____	_____

Documentation in the Medical Record

_____

_____

_____

_____

Comments:

Total Points Earned _____ Divided by _____ Total Possible Points = _____ % Score

Instructor's Signature _____

Procedure 6-7 Determining Respirations

Task: To determine and record a patient's respirations.

Equipment and Supplies:
• A watch with a second hand

Standards: Complete the procedure and all critical steps in _____ minutes with a minimum

score of _____ % within three attempts.

Scoring: Divide points earned by total possible points. Failure to perform a critical step that is indicated with an asterisk (*), will result in an unsatisfactory overall score.

Time began _____ **Time ended** _____

Steps	Possible Points	First Attempt	Second Attempt	Third Attempt
1. Wash your hands.	_____	_____	_____	_____
2. Identify your patient.	_____	_____	_____	_____
3. The patient's arm will be in the same positions when counting the pulse. If having difficulty noticing breathing, place the arm across the chest to pick up movement.	_____	_____	_____	_____
4. Count the respirations for 30 seconds, using a watch with a second hand, and multiply by 2.	_____	_____	_____	_____
5. Release the patient's wrist.	_____	_____	_____	_____
6. Record the respirations on the patient's medical record after the pulse recording. Record as R = 18.	_____	_____	_____	_____

Documentation in the Medical Record

_____

_____

_____

_____

Comments:

Total Points Earned _____ Divided by _____ Total Possible Points = _____ % Score

Instructor's Signature _____

Student Name _____ Date _____ Score _____

Procedure 6-8 Determining a Patient's Blood Pressure

Task: To perform a blood pressure measurement that is correct in technique, accurate, and comfortable for the patient.

Equipment and Supplies:
- Sphygmomanometer
- Stethoscope
- Antiseptic wipes

Standards: Complete the procedure and all critical steps in _____ minutes with a minimum

score of _____ % within three attempts.

Scoring: Divide points earned by total possible points. Failure to perform a critical step that is indicated with an asterisk (*), will result in an unsatisfactory overall score.

Time began _____ **Time ended** _____

Steps	Possible Points	First Attempt	Second Attempt	Third Attempt
1. Wash your hands.	5			
2. Assemble the equipment and supplies needed. Clean the earpieces of the stethoscope with alcohol swabs.	5			
3. Introduce yourself, identify the patient, and explain the procedure.	5			
4. Seat the patient in a comfortable position with legs uncrossed and arm resting at heart level on the lap or table.	5			
5. Determine the correct cuff size.	5			
6. Roll up the sleeve to about 5 inches above the elbow, or have the patient remove his or her arm from the sleeve.				
7. Palpate the brachial artery at the antecubital space in both arms. If one arm has a stronger pulse, use that arm. If the pulses are equal, select the right arm.	5			
8. Center the cuff bladder over the brachial artery, with the connecting tube away from the patient's body and the tube to the bulb close to the body.	5			
9. Place the lower edge of the cuff about 1 inch above the palpable brachial pulse, normally located in the natural crease of the inner elbow, and wrap it snugly and smoothly.	5			

Copyright © 2003, Elsevier Science (USA). All rights reserved.

323

Steps	Possible Points	First Attempt	Second Attempt	Third Attempt
10. Position the gauge of the sphygmomanometer so that it is at eye level.	5			
11. Take the patient's brachial pulse, and mentally add 40 mm to the reading.	5			
12. Insert the earpieces of the stethoscope turned down and forward into your ears.	5			
13. Place the stethoscope bell over the palpated brachial artery firmly enough to obtain a seal but not so tightly that you constrict the artery.	5			
14. Close the valve, and squeeze the bulb to inflate the cuff at a rapid but smooth rate to 20 mm above the palpated pulse level that was previously determined in step 12.	10			
15. Open the valve slightly and deflate the cuff at the constant rate of 2 mm Hg per second.	5			
16. Listen throughout the entire deflation until the sounds have stopped for at least 10 mm Hg.	10			
17. Remove the stethoscope from your ears, and record the systolic and diastolic readings as BP systolic/diastolic (e.g., BP 120/80).	10			
18. Note: If you are uncertain of your reading, release the air from the cuff, wait 1 to 2 minutes, then repeat the process. Wash your hands.*				

Documentation in the Medical Record

_____

_____

_____

_____

Comments:

Total Points Earned _____ Divided by _____ Total Possible Points = _____ % Score

Instructor's Signature _____

Procedure 6-9 Measuring a Patient's Height and Weight

Task: To accurately weigh and measure a patient as part of the physical assessment.

Equipment and Supplies:
• A balance scale with a measuring bar

Standards: Complete the procedure and all critical steps in _____ minutes with a minimum

score of _____ % within three attempts.

Scoring: Divide points earned by total possible points. Failure to perform a critical step that is indicated
with an asterisk (*), will result in an unsatisfactory overall score.

Time began _____ **Time ended** _____

Steps	Possible Points	First Attempt	Second Attempt	Third Attempt
1. Wash your hands.	5			
2. Identify your patient and explain the procedure.	5			
3. If the patient is to remove his or her shoes for weighing, place a paper towel on the scale platform.	5			
4. Check to see that the balance bar pointer floats in the middle of the balance frame when all weights are at zero.	5			
5. Help the patient onto the scale. Be sure that the female patient is not holding a purse and that the male patient has removed any heavy objects from pockets.	5			
6. Move the large weight into the groove closest to the estimated weight of the patient.	5			
7. While the patient is standing still, slide the small upper weight to the right along the pound markers until the pointer balances in the middle of the balance frame.	10			
8. Leave the weights in place.	5			
9. Ask the patient to stand up straight and to look straight ahead. On some scales the patient may need to turn with the back to the scale.	5			

Steps	Possible Points	First Attempt	Second Attempt	Third Attempt
10. Adjust the height bar so that it just touches the top of the patient's head	5			
11. Leave the elevation bar set but fold down the horizontal bar.	5			
12. Assist the patient off the scale. Be sure all items removed for weighing are given back to the patient.	5			
13. Read the weight scale. Add the numbers at the markers of the large and the small weights and record the total to the nearest pound on the patient's medical record.	15			
14. Record the height. Read the marker at the movable point of the ruler, and record the measurement to the nearest quarter inch on the patient's medical record.	15			
15. Return the weights and the measuring bar to zero. Wash hands.	5			

Documentation in the Medical Record

_____

_____

_____

_____

Comments:

Total Points Earned _____ Divided by _____ Total Possible Points = _____ % Score

Instructor's Signature _____

Student Name _____ Date _____ Score _____

Procedure 7-1 Preparing for and Assisting with the Physical Examination

Task: To help the physician examine patients by preparing the necessary equipment and ensuring patient safety and comfort during the examination.

Equipment and Supplies:

- Stethoscope
- Scale
- Cotton balls
- Examination light
- Lubricating gel
- Sphygmomanometer
- Tape measure
- Pen light
- Tuning fork
- Laboratory request forms
- Patient gown
- Thermometer

- Ophthalmoscope
- Tongue depressor
- Examination light
- Percussion hammer
- Latex gloves/finger cots
- Otoscope
- Gauze sponges
- Nasal speculum
- Biohazard container
- Specimen bottles/glass slides
- Drapes
- Cotton-tipped applicators

Standards: Complete the procedure and all critical steps in _____ minutes with a minimum

score of _____ % within three attempts.

Scoring: Divide points earned by total possible points. Failure to perform a critical step that is indicated with an asterisk (*), will result in an unsatisfactory overall score.

Time began _____ **Time ended** _____

Steps	Possible Points	First Attempt	Second Attempt	Third Attempt
1. Prepare the examining room according to acceptable medical aseptic rules.	5			
2. Wash hands.	6			
3. Locate the instruments for the procedure. Set them out in sequence.	5			
4. Identify the patient, and determine whether the patient understands the procedure.	6			
5. Review the medical history with the patient and investigate the purpose of the visit.	6			
6. Measure and record the patient's vital signs, height, and weight.	6			
7. Instruct the patient on how to collect the urine specimen, and hand the patient the properly labeled specimen container (see Chapter 27). Obtain any blood samples that are required (see Chapter 28). Obtain resting ECG if ordered (see Chapter 24).	6			

Steps	Possible Points	First Attempt	Second Attempt	Third Attempt
8. Hand the patient a gown and drape. Instruct the patient on how to put the gown on. Help patient with undressing as needed.	6			
9. Assist the patient in sitting on the narrow end of the examination table; place the drape over the patient's lap and legs. If the patient is elderly, confused, or feeling faint or dizzy, DO NOT leave him or her alone.	6			
10. Advise the physician that the patient is ready.	6			
11. Assist during the examination by handing the physician each instrument as it is needed and by positioning and draping the patient.	6			
12. When the physician has completed the examination, allow the patient to rest for a moment, then help the patient from the table. Assist with dressing, if necessary. Use proper body mechanics if assistance in transfer is needed.	6			
13. Record the necessary notes on the patient's chart and forward it to the physician for further notations.	6			
14. Return to the patient and ask him or her if there are any questions. Give the patient any final instructions, and schedule tests as ordered by the physician and/or the next appointment.	6			
15. Put on gloves and dispose of used supplies and linens in designated waste containers. Clean tabletop surfaces with disinfectant. Disinfect all equipment.	6			
16. Remove gloves and discard them in the bio-hazard waste container and wash hands.	6			
17. Replace used supplies and prepare room for next patient.	6			

2222222

Documentation in the Medical Record

_____
_____
_____
_____

Comments:

Total Points Earned _____ Divided by _____ Total Possible Points = _____ % Score

Instructor's Signature _____

Procedure 8-1 Preparing a Prescription for the Physician's Signature

Task: To accurately prepare a prescription for the physician's signature using appropriate abbreviations and prescription format.

Equipment and Supplies:
- Prescription pad
- Drug reference materials if needed
- Black pen
- Patient chart

Standards: Complete the procedure and all critical steps in _____ minutes with a minimum

score of _____ % within three attempts.

Scoring: Divide points earned by total possible points. Failure to perform a critical step that is indicated with an asterisk (*), will result in an unsatisfactory overall score.

Time began _____ Time ended _____

Steps	Possible Points	First Attempt	Second Attempt	Third Attempt
1. Refer to the physician's written order for the prescription. If the physician gives a verbal order to write a prescription, write down the order and review it with the physician for accuracy.	10			
2. If unfamiliar with the medication, look up the drug in a drug reference book (such as the PDR). recommended dose, storage guidelines, drug-to-drug interactions, and possible side effects to make sure the transcription is correct and to be prepared to answer patient questions about the medication.	10			
3. Ask the patient about drug allergies.	10			
4. Using a prescription pad that has the physician's name, address, telephone number, and DEA registration number pre-printed on the slip, begin to transcribe the physician order.	10			
5. Record the patient's name, address, and date on which the prescription is being written.	10			
6. Next to the Rx write in legible handwriting the name of the drug (correctly spelled), the dosage form (such as tablet, capsule, etc., using correct abbreviations), and the strength ordered. For example, if the physician orders Lipitor, 40 mg tablets, by mouth, one tablet at bedtime then the first line of the prescription should read: Lipitor 40 mg tabs. This is the *inscription*.	10			

Steps	Possible Points	First Attempt	Second Attempt	Third Attempt
7. On the next line write *Disp*. This is the subscription which includes directions to the pharmacist on the amount to be dispensed and the form of the drug. For the Lipitor order, the subscription would read: Disp: #30	__10__	_____	_____	_____
8. Next comes the *signature*. This includes directions for the patient, such as how and when to take the medicine, and is usually preceded by the symbol *Sig*. For the Lipitor order the signature would read: Sig: i tab po hs	__10__	_____	_____	_____
9. The physician tells you the patient can get 3 refills of the prescription so this information should be added at the bottom of the prescription.	__10__	_____	_____	_____
10. The physician must sign the prescription before it is given to the patient.	__10__	_____	_____	_____
11. Document on the patient's chart the medication order and any pertinent details including patient education and refill information.	__10__	_____	_____	_____

Documentation in the Medical Record

_____

_____

_____

_____

Comments:

Total Points Earned _____ Divided by _____ Total Possible Points = _____ % Score

Instructor's Signature _____

Procedure 9-1 Calculating the Correct Dosage for Administration

Task: To calculate the correct dosage amount and choose the correct equipment when the physician orders 2.4 million IU of penicillin G benzathine (Bicillin) administered to a patient.

Equipment and Supplies:
- Premixed syringes of Bicillin in the following two strengths are available:
  - 0.6 million IU/syringe
  - 1.2 million IU/syringe
- Paper and pencil

Standards: Complete the procedure and all critical steps in _____ minutes with a minimum score of _____ % within three attempts.

Scoring: Divide points earned by total possible points. Failure to perform a critical step that is indicated with an asterisk (*), will result in an unsatisfactory overall score.

Time began _____ **Time ended** _____

Steps	Possible Points	First Attempt	Second Attempt	Third Attempt
1. Read the order in quiet surroundings to make sure that you fully understand it.*	15			
2. Write out the order.	15			
3. Examine the drug labels to see what strengths and amounts are available.	15			
4. Write down the standard formula.	15			
5. Rewrite the formula, replacing the unknown values with the known quantities. The unknown x will be the amount of the drug to give.	10			
6. Work the proportion problem by cross-multiplying to solve for x.	10			
7. State your answer by filling in the blanks, as follows: To administer 2.4 million IU of Bicillin, I would select _____ of the premixed syringes labeled _____.	20			

Documentation in the Medical Record

_____

_____

_____

_____

Comments:

Total Points Earned _____ Divided by _____ Total Possible Points = _____ % Score

Instructor's Signature _____

Procedure 9-2 Calculating the Correct Dosage for Administration Using Two Systems of Measurement

Task: To choose the correct system of measurement and calculate the correct dosage amount when the physician orders 120 mg of a drug to be administered to a patient.

Equipment and Supplies
- Tablets labeled 1 gr (grain) each
- Standard mathematical formula:

$$\frac{\text{Available strength}}{\text{Ordered strength}} = \frac{\text{Available amount}}{\text{Amount to give}}$$

- Conversion equivalent: 1 gr = 60 mg
- Paper and pencil

Standards: Complete the procedure and all critical steps in _____ minutes with a minimum score of _____ % within three attempts.

Scoring: Divide points earned by total possible points. Failure to perform a critical step that is indicated with an asterisk (*), will result in an unsatisfactory overall score.

Time began _____ **Time ended** _____

Steps	Possible Points	First Attempt	Second Attempt	Third Attempt
1. Read the order in quiet surroundings to make sure that you fully understand it.*	15			
2. Write out the order.	10			
3. Examine the drug labels to see what strengths and amounts are available.	15			
4. Convert the ordered system of measurement to the system of measurement on the label using the conversion formula. $$\text{Have} \times \frac{\text{Wanted}}{\text{Have}} = \text{Unit Wanted in New System}$$ (conversion)	15			
5. Write down the standard formula.	10			
6. Rewrite the formula, replacing the unknown values with the known quantities and using the system of measurement on the label. The unknown x will be the amount of the drug to give (amount to give).	10			

Steps	Possible Points	First Attempt	Second Attempt	Third Attempt
7. Work the proportion problem by cross-multiplying to solve for x.	10			
8. By filling in the blank, as follows: State your answer To administer 120 mg of a drug from tablets labeled 1 gr (grain) each, give _____ tablet(s).	15			

Documentation in the Medical Record

_____

_____

_____

_____

Comments:

Total Points Earned _____ Divided by _____ Total Possible Points = _____ % Score

Instructor's Signature _____

Procedure 9-3 Calculating the Correct Dosage for a Child when only Adult Medication is Available

Task: To calculate the correct dosage amount for a 90-pound child using Clark's rule when the adult dosage is 250 mg.

Equipment and Supplies:
• Adult dosage 250 mg/ml
• Clark's rule:

$$\text{Pediatric dose} = \frac{\text{Child's weight in pounds}}{150}$$

• Standard mathematical formula:

$$\frac{\text{Available strength}}{\text{Ordered strength}} = \frac{\text{Available amount}}{\text{Amount to give}}$$

• Paper and pencil

Standards: Complete the procedure and all critical steps in _____ minutes with a minimum

score of _____ % within three attempts.

Scoring: Divide points earned by total possible points. Failure to perform a critical step that is indicated with an asterisk (*), will result in an unsatisfactory overall score.

Time began _____ **Time ended** _____

Steps	Possible Points	First Attempt	Second Attempt	Third Attempt
1. Read the order in quiet surroundings to make sure that you fully understand it.	10			
2. Write out the order.	10			
3. Examine the drug labels to see what strengths and amounts are available.	10			
4. Write down Clark's rule.	10			
5. Using Clark's rule, replace the unknown values with the known quantities. The unknown x will be the pediatric strength ordered (pediatric dose).	20			
6. Write down the standard formula.	10			
7. Rewrite the formula, replacing the unknown values with the available quantities and the pediatric strength just determined. The unknown x will be the amount of the drug to give (amount to give).	10			

Steps	Possible Points	First Attempt	Second Attempt	Third Attempt
8. Work the proportion problem by cross-multiplying to solve for x.	10			
9. State your answer by filling in the blank, as follows: To administer an adult medication labeled 250 mg/mL to a 90-pound child, give _____ ml.	20			

Documentation in the Medical Record

_____

_____

_____

_____

Comments:

Total Points Earned _____ Divided by _____ Total Possible Points = _____ % Score

Instructor's Signature _____

Procedure 9-4 Calculating the Correct Dosage for Administration Using Body Weight

Task: To calculate correct dosage by using body weight method. Ordered: Zovirax capsules 5 mg/kg every 8 hours for 7 days for a patient who has a diagnosis of herpes zoster. The patient weighs 176 pounds. The capsules are labeled 200 mg = 1 capsule.

Equipment and Supplies:
- Weight conversion: 2.5 lb = 1 kg
- Capsules labeled 200 mg/kg
- Balance scale
- Formula for conversion of pounds to kilograms
- Standard math formula:

$$\frac{\text{Available strength}}{\text{Ordered strength}} = \frac{\text{Available amount}}{\text{Amount to give}}$$

- Paper and pencil

Standards: Complete the procedure and all critical steps in _____ minutes with a minimum

score of _____ % within three attempts.

Scoring: Divide points earned by total possible points. Failure to perform a critical step that is indicated with an asterisk (*), will result in an unsatisfactory overall score.

Time began _____ **Time ended** _____

Steps	Possible Points	First Attempt	Second Attempt	Third Attempt
1. Read the order in quiet surroundings to make sure that you fully understand it.	10			
2. Write out the order.	10			
3. Examine the drug label to check the strength and amount.	10			
4. Convert the patient's weight from pounds to kilograms.	10			
5. Write down the standard formula.	10			
6. Rewrite the formula, replacing the unknown values with the known quantities. The unknown x will be the amount of the drug to give.	10			
7. Work the problem by cross-multiplying to solve for x.	10			
8. State your answer by filling in the blank as follows: To administer 5 mg/kg of body weight of Zovirax from capsules labeled 200 mg each, I would give _____ capsule(s).	30			

Documentation in the Medical Record

_____

_____

_____

_____

Comments:

Total Points Earned _____ Divided by _____ Total Possible Points = _____ % Score

Instructor's Signature _____

Procedure 10-1 Dispensing and Administering Oral Medications

Task: To safely dispense and administer an oral medication to a patient.

Equipment and Supplies:
- Container of ordered medication
- Medication cup
- A written physician order, including the drug name, strength, dose, and route

Standards: Complete the procedure and all critical steps in _____ minutes with a minimum

score of _____ % within three attempts.

Scoring: Divide points earned by total possible points. Failure to perform a critical step that is indicated with an asterisk (*), will result in an unsatisfactory overall score.

Time began _____ **Time ended** _____

Steps	Possible Points	First Attempt	Second Attempt	Third Attempt
1. Read the order and clarify any questions with the physician.	5			
2. If unfamiliar with the drug, refer to the *PDR* or the package insert to determine the purpose of the drug, common side effects, typical dose, and any pertinent precautions or contraindications. Use the "seven rights" to prevent errors.	5			
3. Perform calculations needed to match the physician order. Confirm the answer with the physician if there are any questions.	5			
4. Dispense medication in a well-lit, quiet area.	5			
5. Wash your hands.*	5			
6. Compare the order with the label on the container of medicine when you remove it from storage. Check the expiration date on the container and dispose of the medication if it has expired.*	5			
7. Compare the order with the label on the container of medicine just before dispensing the ordered dose. Make sure that the strength on the label matches the order or that you dispense the correctly calculated dose.	5			
8. Gently tap the prescribed dose into the lid of the medication container. Avoid touching the inside of the lid, as well as the medication.	5			
9. Empty the medication in the container lid into a medicine cup.	5			

Steps	Possible Points	First Attempt	Second Attempt	Third Attempt

To Dispense Liquid Oral Preparations

1. Shake medication well if required. — 2

2. When you pour liquid medications, hold the labeled side of the container toward the palm of your hand. — 2

3. Place the medicine cup on a flat surface and, at eye level, pour the medication to the prescribed dose mark on the medicine cup. — 2

For Both Solid and Liquid Oral Medications

10. Recap the container and compare the label and the physician order before replacing the container in storage. — 5

11. Transport the medication to the patient. — 3

12. Greet and identify the patient by name. — 3

13. Mention the name of the drug, why it is being given, and ask the patient if she or he has any allergies to the medication. — 5

14. If necessary, help the patient into a sitting position. — 3

15. Administer tablets, capsules, or caplets with water. If the patient is receiving liquid medication, offer water after the medication has been taken, if appropriate. Make sure the patient swallows the entire dose. — 5

16. Conduct patient education on the purpose of the drug, typical side effects, and dosage and storage recommendations. Refer to the physician to clarify information if necessary. — 5

17. The patient must remain in the office for 20 to 30 minutes after drug administration as a precaution against untoward effects. — 5

18. If the patient experiences any discomfort after taking a medication, the physician should be notified immediately, and the incident should be documented completely and accurately. — 5

19. Wash hands. — 5

20. Document the administration of the drug including the date and time; the drug name, dose, strength, and route of administration; any side effects; and patient education conducted about the drug.* — 5

Documentation in the Medical Record

_____
_____
_____
_____

Comments:

Total Points Earned _____ Divided by _____ Total Possible Points = _____ % Score

Instructor's Signature _____

Procedure 10-2 Filling a Syringe from a Vial

Task: To fill a syringe with 1.5 ml of sterile water from a multidose vial by using sterile technique.

Equipment and Supplies:
• A multidose vial containing the material to be injected
• Alcohol wipes
• A sterile needle and syringe unit
• A written order, including the drug name, strength, and route

Standards: Complete the procedure and all critical steps in _____ minutes with a minimum

score of _____ % within three attempts.

Scoring: Divide points earned by total possible points. Failure to perform a critical step that is indicated with an asterisk (*), will result in an unsatisfactory overall score.

Time began _____ **Time ended** _____

Steps	Possible Points	First Attempt	Second Attempt	Third Attempt
1. Wash your hands.*	5			
2. Read the order and choose the correct vial of medication.	10			
3. Choose the correct syringe and needle size, depending on the site and the quantity of medication to be injected.	5			
4. Compare the order with both the name of the drug on the vial of medication and the amount to be withdrawn in the syringe.	10			
5. Gently agitate the medication by rolling the vial between your palms.	5			
6. Check the quality of the medication and the expiration date.*	5			
7. Cleanse the rubber stopper of the vial with the alcohol wipe, using a circular motion. Place the vial on a secure flat surface, leaving the alcohol wipe over the rubber stopper.*	5			
8. Grasp the syringe plunger and draw up an amount of air equal to the amount of medication ordered.	5			
9. Remove the needle cover and insert the needle into the center of the rubber stopper. Hold the vial firmly against a flat surface and make sure that the needle only touches the cleaned rubber area.	5			

Steps	Possible Points	First Attempt	Second Attempt	Third Attempt
10. Inject the aspirated air in the syringe into the vial.	5			
11. Pick the vial and syringe unit up and invert it. Slowly pull back on the plunger with the unit at eye level until the proper amount of medication is withdrawn.	10			
12. While the needle is still in the vial, check that there are no air bubbles in the syringe.	5			
13. If there are air bubbles, slip the fingers holding the vial down to grasp the vial and syringe as a single unit.	5			
14. With your free hand, tap the syringe until the air bubbles dislodge and float into the tip of the syringe.	5			
15. Gently expel these tiny air bubbles through the needle, then continue withdrawing the medication.	5			
16. Withdraw the needle from the vial, and replace the cover over the needle without the needle touching the sides.	5			
17. Return the medication to the shelf or the refrigerator, checking that you have the correct drug and dosage.	5			

Comments:

Total Points Earned _____ Divided by _____ Total Possible Points = _____ % Score

Instructor's Signature _____

Procedure 10-3 Filling a Syringe from an Ampule

Task: To open an ampule.

Equipment and Supplies:
• Ampule
• Two alcohol pads (It is safer to use an unopened pad while breaking the neck of the ampule.)
• Filter needle
• Syringe

Standards: Complete the procedure and all critical steps in _____ minutes with a minimum

score of _____ % within three attempts.

Scoring: Divide points earned by total possible points. Failure to perform a critical step that is indicated with an asterisk (*), will result in an unsatisfactory overall score.

Time began _____ **Time ended** _____

Steps	Possible Points	First Attempt	Second Attempt	Third Attempt
1. Wash your hands and gather appropriate syringe unit and filter needle.*	20			
2. Gently tap the top of the ampule with your fingers to settle all the medication to the bottom portion of the flask.	20			
3. Wipe the neck of the ampule clean with alcohol. It may be necessary to use a small file provided by the manufacturer to score an ampule at the breaking point to facilitate easier opening.	10			
4. Wrap the top of the ampule with a gauze square or unopened alcohol pad to protect yourself from the glass. Hold the covered ampule between your thumb and finger, in front of you and above waist level.	10			
5. Snap your wrist away from your body to break the neck of the ampule. You will hear a pop because the ampule is vacuum-sealed. The glass is designed not to shatter, and the medication will not spill out. Dispose of the glass pieces in the sharps container.	10			
6. Without touching the sides, insert the syringe unit with the filter needle into the ampule and withdraw the ordered dose. The filter needle is designed to prevent aspiration of pieces of glass into the injection unit.	20			

Steps	**Possible Points**	**First Attempt**	**Second Attempt**	**Third Attempt**
7. Change the needle for an appropriate length and gauge based on the physician order and patient characteristics.	10			

Comments:

Total Points Earned _____ Divided by _____ Total Possible Points = _____ % Score

Instructor's Signature _____

Procedure 10-4 Giving an Intradermal Injection

Task: To inject 0.1 ml of purified protein derivative (PPD) to perform a Mantoux test as ordered by the physician.

Equipment and Supplies:
- A vial of tuberculin PPD
- Alcohol wipes
- A 3/8 inch, 27-gauge sterile needle and syringe unit
- Disposable gloves
- Gauze squares
- Sharps container
- Physician order, including the patient's name, when to give the drug, the route of administration, and the name and strength of the drug.

Standards: Complete the procedure and all critical steps in _____ minutes with a minimum

score of _____ % within three attempts.

Scoring: Divide points earned by total possible points. Failure to perform a critical step that is indicated with an asterisk (*), will result in an unsatisfactory overall score.

Time began _____ **Time ended** _____

Steps	Possible Points	First Attempt	Second Attempt	Third Attempt
1. Wash your hands. Follow standard precautions. Glove yourself with nonsterile gloves.*	8			
2. Select the correct medication from the shelf or the refrigerator.	4			
3. Read the label to be sure that you have the right drug and the right strength. Perform the three label and order checks as the medication is dispensed.*	8			
4. Warm refrigerated medications by gently rolling the container between your palms.	4			
5. Prepare the syringe as described in Procedure 10-2, withdrawing the right dose.	4			
6. Transport the medication to the patient.	4			
7. Greet and identify the patient by name.	4			
8. Position the patient comfortably.	4			
9. Locate the antecubital space, then find a site several finger widths down the anterior aspect of the forearm. Avoid any scarred, discolored, or pigmented areas.	4			

Steps	Possible Points	First Attempt	Second Attempt	Third Attempt
10. Cleanse the patient's skin with an alcohol wipe, using a circular motion, moving from the center outward.	4			
11. Allow the antiseptic to dry.	4			
12. With the thumb and first two fingers of your nondominant hand, stretch the skin of the forearm apart and taut.	4			
13. Grasp the syringe between the thumb and first two fingers of your dominant hand, palm down, with the needle bevel upward. Hold the syringe close to the plunger end.	4			
14. At a 15-degree angle, carefully insert the needle through the skin just until the bevel point is under the skin surface.	4			
15. Slowly and steadily inject the medication by depressing the plunger with your little finger. A wheal should appear.	4			
16. After administering all of the medication, withdraw the needle.	4			
17. Immediately dispose of the contaminated syringe unit in a sharps container.	4			
18. Do not massage the area, but you may blot it with a cotton ball or gauze square.	4			
19. Make sure that your patient is comfortable and safe.	4			
20. Observe the patient for any adverse reaction. If you are performing allergy testing, the patient must be observed for 20 to 30 minutes.	4			
21. Dispose of the gloves in the biohazard container and wash your hands.	4			
22. Record the procedure and any reactions that occurred at the site of the injection on the patient's medical record. Include the exact site of the injection.	4			
23. Tell the patient when to return to the office for the reaction to be read or give the patient a postcard to be completed and returned.	4			

Documentation in the Medical Record

_____

_____

_____

_____

Comments:

Total Points Earned _____ Divided by _____ Total Possible Points = _____ % Score

Instructor's Signature _____

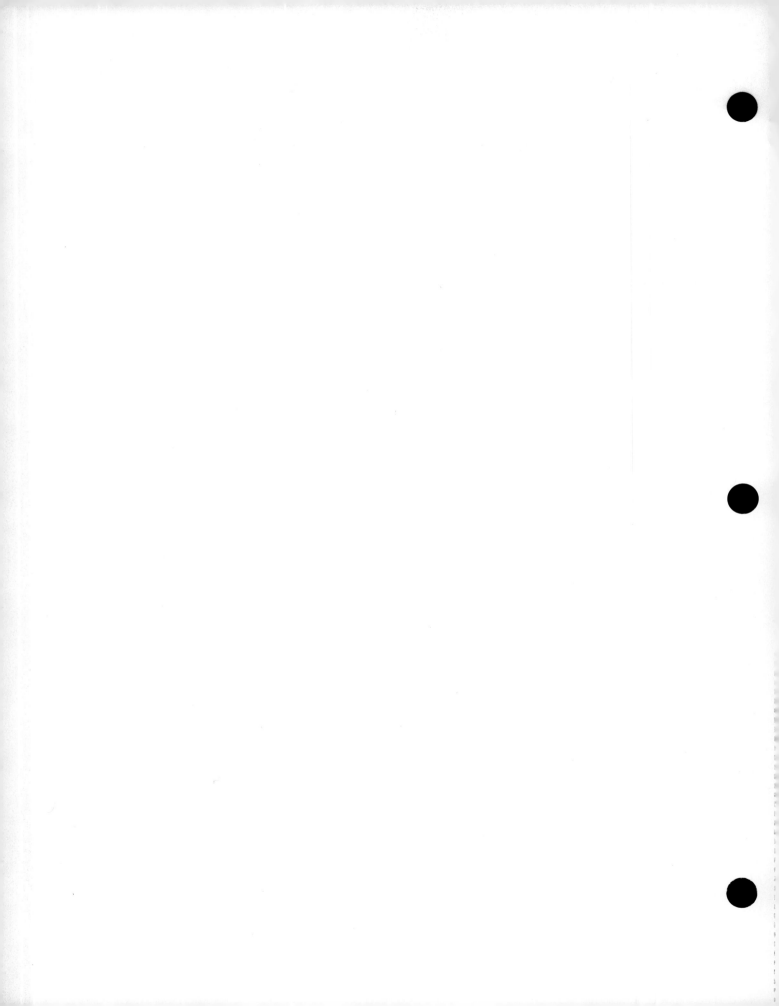

Student Name _____ Date _____ Score _____

Procedure 10-5 Administering a Tuberculin Tine Test

Task: To Administer a Tuberculin Tine Test.

Equipment and Supplies:
- Tuberculin tine test stamp
- Alcohol wipe
- Disposable gloves
- Sharps container
- Physician order

Standards: Complete the procedure and all critical steps in _____ minutes with a minimum

score of _____ % within three attempts.

Scoring: Divide points earned by total possible points. Failure to perform a critical step that is indicated with an asterisk (*), will result in an unsatisfactory overall score.

Time began _____ **Time ended** _____

Steps	Possible Points	First Attempt	Second Attempt	Third Attempt
1. Wash hands. Follow standard precautions. Glove with disposable nonsterile gloves.	10			
2. Greet the patient and verify patient name.	10			
3. Explain the procedure.	10			
4. Position the patient to reduce strain on the forearm.	5			
5. Cleanse the site with the alcohol wipe in a circular fashion from the inside outward. Allow alcohol to dry.	5			
6. Pull the site taut with the nondominant thumb and fingers.	5			
7. Press the prongs of the tine firmly against the cleansed area for 1 to 2 seconds.	10			
8. Immediately discard the stamp into the sharps container.	10			
9. Do not massage area.	5			
10. Dispose of the gloves in the biohazard container and wash hands.	10			

Steps	Possible Points	First Attempt	Second Attempt	Third Attempt
11. Observe patient for untoward reactions and document the procedure including the name of the test, time of administration, exact site of administration, and any patient complaints.	10			
12. Patient education to return to the office in 48 to 72 hours to have the results read or explain how to read results at home.	10			

Documentation in the Medical Record

_____

_____

_____

_____

Comments:

Total Points Earned _____ Divided by _____ Total Possible Points = _____ % Score

Instructor's Signature _____

Procedure 10-6 Giving a Subcutaneous Injection

Task: To inject 0.5 ml of medication into the subcutaneous tissue using a 25 gauge, 5/8 inch needle and syringe of correct size and type, as directed by the physician.

Equipment and Supplies:
• A vial or ampule containing the medication to be injected
• Alcohol wipes
• Gauze squares or cotton balls
• A sterile needle and syringe unit
• Nonsterile disposable gloves
• Sharps container
• A written order, including the patient's name, when to give the drug, the route of administration, and the name and strength of the drug

Standards: Complete the procedure and all critical steps in _____ minutes with a minimum

score of _____ % within three attempts.

Scoring: Divide points earned by total possible points. Failure to perform a critical step that is indicated with an asterisk (*), will result in an unsatisfactory overall score.

Time began _____ **Time ended** _____

Steps	Possible Points	First Attempt	Second Attempt	Third Attempt
1. Wash your hands. Follow Standard Precautions.*	5			
2. Select the correct medication from the shelf or the refrigerator.	5			
3. Read the label to be sure that you have the right drug and the right strength. Perform the 3 label and order checks while dispensing the medication and the 7 rights. Perform any necessary dose calculations.*	5			
4. Warm refrigerated medications by gently rolling the container between your palms.	5			
5. Prepare the syringe, withdrawing the right dose.	5			
6. Transport the medication to the patient.	2.5			
7. Greet and identify the patient by name.	2.5			
8. Position the patient comfortably.	5			
9. Expose the site and clean the area.	5			
10. Remove the cap from the needle.	5			

Steps	Possible Points	First Attempt	Second Attempt	Third Attempt
11. With the thumb and fingers of your nondominant hand, grasp the tissue of the posterior upper arm.	5			
12. Hold the syringe between the thumb and the first two fingers of your dominant hand, and with one swift movement, insert the entire needle up to the hub at a 45-degree angle.	5			
13. Aspirate (except when administering heparin or insulin) by withdrawing the plunger slightly to be sure that no blood enters the syringe.	5			
14. If blood appears, immediately withdraw the unit without injecting the medication, dispose of it in the sharps container. Compress the injection site with an alcohol swab or gauze bandage. Begin again with step 1.	2.5			
15. If no blood appears in the syringe, push in the plunger slowly and steadily until all medication has been administered.	2.5			
16. Place the gauze square next to the needle and withdraw it at the same angle of insertion.	5			
17. Gently massage the site with the gauze square (do not massage insulin or heparin injections).	5			
18. Discard the needle and syringe into the sharps container.	5			
19. Make sure that your patient is comfortable and safe.	5			
20. Dispose of the gloves in the biohazard waste and wash your hands.	5			
21. Observe the patient for any adverse reaction. You may need to keep the patient under observation for 20 to 30 minutes.	5			
22. Record the drug administration on the patient's medical record, and on the required DEA record if the medication is a controlled substance.	5			

Documentation in the Medical Record

_____

_____

_____

_____

Comments:

Total Points Earned _____ Divided by _____ Total Possible Points = _____ % Score

Instructor's Signature _____

Procedure 10-7 Giving an Intramuscular Injection

Task: To inject 2 ml of medication into the muscle, using a 22 gauge 1½ inch needle and 3 ml syringe, as directed by the physician.

Equipment and Supplies:
- A vial or ampule containing the medication to be injected
- Alcohol wipes
- Gauze squares or cotton balls
- A sterile needle and syringe unit
- Nonsterile disposable gloves
- Sharps container
- A written order, including the patient's name, when to give the drug, the route of administration, and the name and strength of the drug

Standards: Complete the procedure and all critical steps in _____ minutes with a minimum score of _____ % within three attempts.

Scoring: Divide points earned by total possible points. Failure to perform a critical step that is indicated with an asterisk (*), will result in an unsatisfactory overall score.

Time began _____ **Time ended** _____

Steps	Possible Points	First Attempt	Second Attempt	Third Attempt
1. Wash your hands. Follow Standard Precautions.*	5			
2. Select the correct medication from the shelf or the refrigerator.	5			
3. Read the label to be sure that you have the right drug and the right strength. Perform the 3 label and order checks while dispensing the medication and the 7 rights. Perform any necessary dose calculations.*	5			
4. Warm refrigerated medications by gently rolling the container between your palms.	5			
5. Prepare the syringe, withdrawing the right dose. Complete calculations.	5			
6. Transport the medication to the patient.	2.5			
7. Greet and identify the patient by name.	2.5			
8. Help the patient into an upright sitting position.	5			
9. Apply gloves. Expose the site.	5			
10. Clean skin. Remove the cap from the needle.	5			

Steps	Possible Points	First Attempt	Second Attempt	Third Attempt
11. With the thumb and fingers of your nondominant hand, grasp the tissue of the upper arm.	5			
12. Hold the syringe between the thumb and the first two fingers of your dominant hand, and with one swift movement, insert the entire needle up to the hub at a 90-degree* angle.	5			
13. Aspirate* by withdrawing the plunger slightly to be sure that no blood enters the syringe.	5			
14. If blood appears, immediately withdraw the unit without injecting the medication, dispose of it in the sharps container. Compress the injection site with an alcohol swab or gauze bandage. Begin again with step 1.	2.5			
15. If no blood appears in the syringe, push in the plunger slowly and steadily until all medication has been administered.	2.5			
16. Place the gauze square next to the needle and withdraw it at the same angle of insertion.	5			
17. Gently massage the site with a cotton ball.	5			
18. Discard the needle and syringe into the sharps container.	5			
19. Make sure that your patient is comfortable and safe.	5			
20. Dispose of the gloves in the biohazard waste and wash your hands.	5			
21. Observe the patient for any adverse reaction. You may need to keep the patient under observation for 20 to 30 minutes.	5			
22. Record the drug administration on the patient's medical record, and on the required DEA record if the medication is a controlled substance.	5			

Documentation in the Medical Record

_____

_____

_____

_____

Comments:

Total Points Earned _____ Divided by _____ Total Possible Points = _____ % Score

Instructor's Signature _____

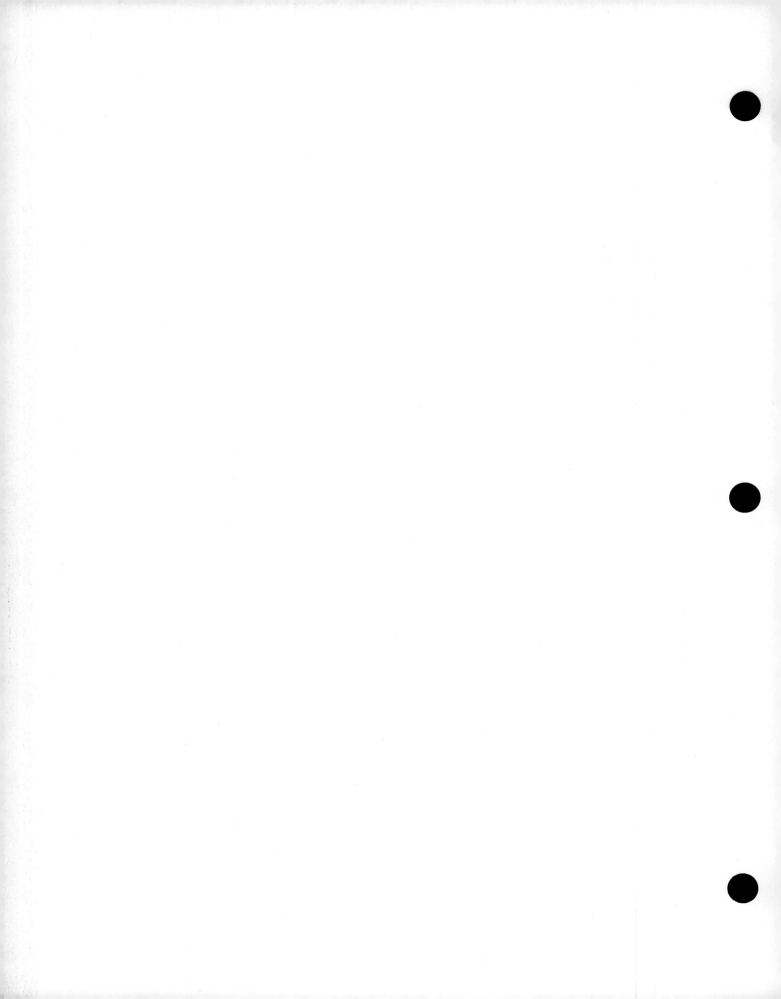

Procedure 10-8 Reconstituting a Powdered Drug for Administration

Task: To reconstitute a powdered drug for intramuscular injection as ordered by the physician.

Equipment and Supplies:
- A vial containing the ordered powdered medication
- Diluent: Sterile saline solution
- Alcohol wipes
- A cotton ball
- Two sterile needle and syringe units
- Nonsterile disposable gloves
- A sharps container
- A written order, including the patient's name, when to give the drug, the route of administration, and the name and strength of the drug.

Standards: Complete the procedure and all critical steps in _____ minutes with a minimum

score of _____ % within three attempts.

Scoring: Divide points earned by total possible points. Failure to perform a critical step that is indicated with an asterisk (*), will result in an unsatisfactory overall score.

Time began _____ **Time ended** _____

Steps	Possible Points	First Attempt	Second Attempt	Third Attempt
1. Wash your hands. Follow standard precautions.*	10			
2. Select the correct vial of powdered medication from the shelf and the recommended diluent for reconstitution. Perform the three drug label and physician order checks during preparation and apply the seven rights throughout the procedure.*	15			
3. Read the label to determine the correct amount of diluent to add to create the dose ordered by the physician. Calculate the correct dose, if necessary, and continue with the three label checks.	15			
4. Remove the top from each vial and clean each with an alcohol wipe. Leave the wipes in place on top of each vial.	5			
5. Grasp the syringe plunger and draw up an amount of air equal to the amount of diluent needed to reconstitute the drug.	5			
6. Remove the needle cover and insert the needle into the center of the rubber stopper of the vial of diluent. Hold the vial firmly against a flat surface and watch carefully that the needle only touches the cleaned rubber area.	5			
7. Inject the aspirated air in the syringe into the diluent vial.	5			

Steps	Possible Points	First Attempt	Second Attempt	Third Attempt
8. Invert the diluent vial and aspirate the calculated or recommended amount of diluent.	5			
9. Remove the needle from the diluent vial and inject the diluent into the drug vial. Remove the needle and discard it in the sharps container.	5			
10. Roll the vial with the drug and diluent mixture between the palms of your hands to mix it thoroughly. Do not shake the vial unless directed to do so on the drug label. When the medication has been completely mixed, there will be no residue or crystals on the bottom of the vial.	5			
11. Aspirate air into the second syringe unit that is equal to the calculated amount of medication to be administered.	5			
12. Inject the air into the mixed drug vial, invert the vial, and withdraw the ordered amount of medication.	15			
13. Proceed as outlined in steps 6 to 22 in Procedure 10-6.	5			

Documentation in the Medical Record

_____

_____

_____

_____

Comments:

Total Points Earned _____ Divided by _____ Total Possible Points = _____ % Score

Instructor's Signature _____

Procedure 10-9 Giving a Z-Track Intramuscular Injection

Task: To inject 1 ml of medication into the muscle by using a 23-gauge, 2½-inch needle, and 3-ml syringe and the Z-track method, as directed by the physician.

Equipment and Supplies:
- A vial or ampule containing the medication to be injected
- Alcohol wipes
- Gauze squares or cotton balls
- A sterile needle and syringe unit
- Nonsterile disposable gloves
- Sharps container
- A written order, including the patient's name, when to give the drug, the route of administration, and the name and strength of the drug
- Package insert drug reference for safety precautions

Standards: Complete the procedure and all critical steps in _____ minutes with a minimum score of _____ % within three attempts.

Scoring: Divide points earned by total possible points. Failure to perform a critical step that is indicated with an asterisk (*), will result in an unsatisfactory overall score.

Time began _____ Time ended _____

Steps	Possible Points	First Attempt	Second Attempt	Third Attempt
1. Wash your hands. Follow standard precautions.*	5			
2. Select the correct medication from the shelf or the refrigerator.	5			
3. Read the label to be sure that you have the right drug and the right strength. Perform the three label and order checks while dispensing the medication and apply the seven rights. Perform any necessary dose calculations.*	5			
4. Warm refrigerated medications by gently rolling the container between your palms.	2			
5. Prepare the syringe, withdrawing the right dose. Complete calculations.	5			
6. Replace the needle cover and give a slight turn to loosen the needle. Secure a new needle, still in its sheath, to the tip of the syringe. Discard the drug-contaminated needle.	5			
7. Transport the medication to the patient.	2			
8. Greet and identify the patient by name.	2			
9. Help the patient into a semiprone position.	5			

Steps	Possible Points	First Attempt	Second Attempt	Third Attempt
10. Apply gloves. Expose the site.	2			
11. Clean skin. Remove the cap from the needle.	5			
12. Push the skin to one side and hold it firmly in place.* If the skin is slippery, use a dry gauze sponge to hold the skin in place.	5			
13. Grasp the syringe as you would a dart, and with one swift movement, insert the entire needle up to the hub, at a 90-degree angle* into the gluteal muscle.	5			
14. Aspirate* by withdrawing the plunger slightly to be sure that no blood enters the syringe.	5			
15. If blood appears, immediately withdraw the unit without injecting the medication, and dispose of it in the sharps container. Compress the injection site with an alcohol swab or gauze bandage. Begin again with step 1.	5			
16. If no blood appears in the syringe, push in the plunger slowly and steadily until all medication has been administered.	2			
17. Wait a few seconds, then withdraw the needle at the same angle of insertion. Wait 10 seconds, then release the skin.	5			
18. If recommended by the manufacturer, gently massage the site with a cotton ball.	5			
19. Discard the needle and syringe in the sharps container.	5			
20. Make sure that your patient is comfortable and safe.	5			
21. Dispose of the gloves in the biohazard waste container and wash your hands.	5			
22. Observe the patient for any adverse reaction. You may need to keep the patient under observation for 20 to 30 minutes.	5			
23. Record the drug administration on the patient's medical record and on the required Drug Enforcement Agency (DEA) record if the medication is a controlled substance.	5			

Documentation in the Medical Record

_____

_____

_____

_____

Comments:

Total Points Earned _____ Divided by _____ Total Possible Points = _____ % Score

Instructor's Signature _____

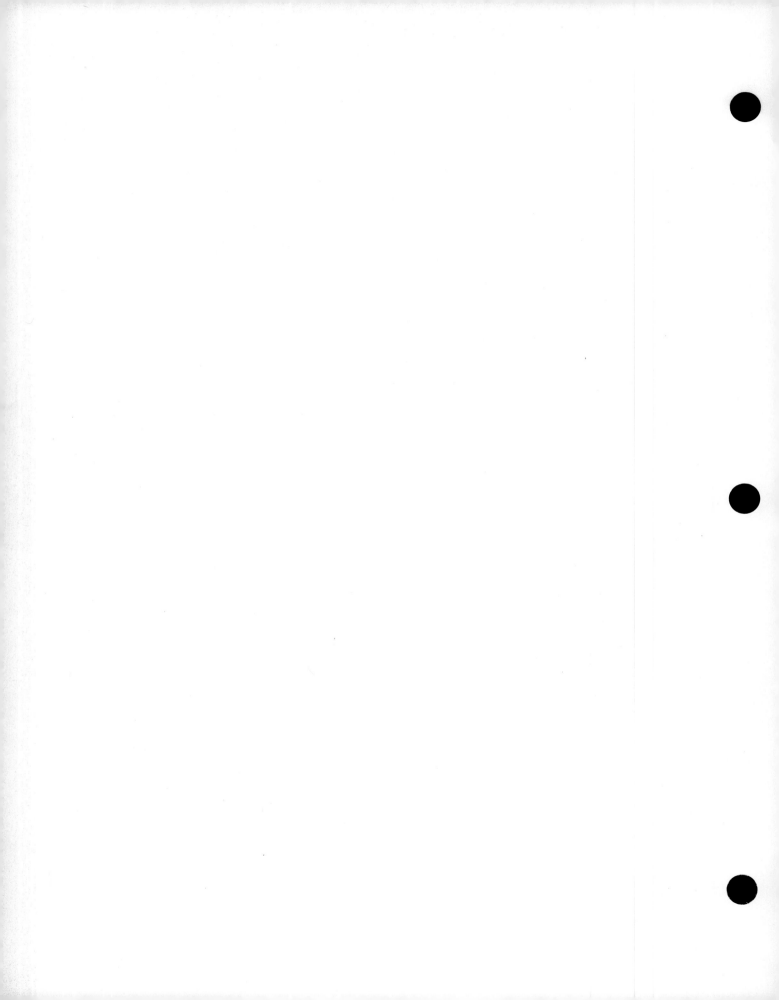

Procedure 11-1 Using an Automated External Defibrillator (AED)

Task: To defibrillate adult victims with cardiac arrest.

Equipment and Supplies:
• Practice AED
• Approved mannequin

Standards: Complete the procedure and all critical steps in _____ minutes with a minimum

score of _____ % within three attempts.

Scoring: Divide points earned by total possible points. Failure to perform a critical step that is indicated with an asterisk (*), will result in an unsatisfactory overall score.

Time began _____ **Time ended** _____

Steps	Possible Points	First Attempt	Second Attempt	Third Attempt
1. Place the AED near the victim's left ear. Turn the AED on.	20	_____	_____	_____
2. Attach electrode pads as pictured on the AED electrodes at the sternum and apex of the heart. Make sure pads have complete contact with the victim's chest and they do not overlap.	20	_____	_____	_____
3. All rescuers must clear away from the victim. Press the ANALYZE button. The AED will analyze the victim's coronary status, will announce if the victim is going to be shocked, and automatically charges the electrodes.	20	_____	_____	_____
4. All rescuers must clear away from the victim.* Press the SHOCK button if the machine is not automated. May repeat 1 to 2 more analyze-shock cycles.	20*	_____	_____	_____
5. If the machine gives the "no shock indicated" signal, assess the victim. Check the carotid pulse and breathing status and keep the AED attached until EMS arrives.	20	_____	_____	_____

Documentation in the Medical Record

_____

_____

_____

_____

Comments:

Total Points Earned _____ Divided by _____ Total Possible Points = _____ % Score

Instructor's Signature _____

Procedure 11-2 Responding to a Patient with an Obstructed Airway

Task: To remove an airway obstruction and restore ventilation.

Equipment and Supplies:
- Nonsterile gloves
- Ventilation mask (for unconscious victim)
- Approved mannequin to practice unconscious Foreign Body Airway Obstruction (FBAO).

Standards: Complete the procedure and all critical steps in _____ minutes with a minimum

score of _____ % within three attempts.

Scoring: Divide points earned by total possible points. Failure to perform a critical step that is indicated with an asterisk (*), will result in an unsatisfactory overall score.

Time began _____ **Time ended** _____

Steps	Possible Points	First Attempt	Second Attempt	Third Attempt
1. Ask, "Are you choking?" If victim indicates yes, ask "Can you speak?". If unable to speak, tell the victim you are going to help.*	10			
2. Stand behind the victim with feet slightly apart.	5			
3. Reach around the victim's abdomen and place an index finger into the victim's navel or at the level of the belt buckle. Make a fist of the opposite hand (do not tuck the thumb into the fist) and place the thumb side of the fist against the victim's abdomen above the navel. If the victim is pregnant, place the fist above the enlarged uterus. If the victim is obese, it may be necessary to place the fist higher in the abdomen. It may be necessary to perform chest thrusts on a victim who is pregnant or obese.	5			
4. Place the opposite hand over the fist and give abdominal thrusts in a quick upward movement.	5			
5. Repeat the abdominal thrusts until the object is expelled or the victim becomes unresponsive.	5			
Unresponsive Victim				
6. Activate the emergency response system.*	10			
7. Put on gloves if available and get ventilation mask. Open the victim's mouth and perform a finger sweep to determine if the foreign object is in the mouth and to remove it.	5			

Steps	Possible Points	First Attempt	Second Attempt	Third Attempt
8. Open the airway with a head-tilt, jaw-thrust maneuver and attempt to ventilate with 2 slow breaths. If breaths do not go in (chest does not rise), retilt the head and try to ventilate again.	5			
9. If ventilation is unsuccessful, move to the victim's feet and kneel across the victim's thighs. Place the heel of one hand above the navel but below the xiphoid process of the sternum. Place the other hand on top of the first, with the fingers elevated off of the abdomen. Administer 5 abdominal thrusts.	5			
10. Move back beside the head of the victim and repeat the finger sweep. If the obstruction is not found, continue cycles of 2 rescue breaths, 5 abdominal thrusts, and finger sweep until either the obstruction is removed or EMS arrives.	5			
11. If the obstruction is removed, assess the victim for breathing and circulation. If a pulse is present, but no breathing, begin rescues breathing. If there is no pulse, begin CPR.	5			
12. Once patient is either stabilized or EMS has taken over care, remove gloves and the ventilator mask valve and dispose in the biohazard container. Disinfect the ventilator mask per manufacturer recommendations. Wash hands.	5			
13. Document the procedure and patient condition.	5			

Documentation in the Medical Record

_____

_____

_____

_____

Comments:

Total Points Earned _____ Divided by _____ Total Possible Points = _____ % Score

Instructor's Signature _____

Procedure 11-3 Administering Oxygen

Task: To provide oxygen for a patient in respiratory distress.

Equipment and Supplies:
• Portable oxygen tank
• Pressure regulator
• Flow meter
• Nasal cannula with connecting tubing

Standards: Complete the procedure and all critical steps in _____ minutes with a minimum

score of _____ % within three attempts.

Scoring: Divide points earned by total possible points. Failure to perform a critical step that is indicated with an asterisk (*), will result in an unsatisfactory overall score.

Time began _____ **Time ended** _____

Steps	Possible Points	First Attempt	Second Attempt	Third Attempt
1. Gather equipment and wash hands.	10			
2. Identify the patient and explain the procedure.	10			
3. Check the pressure gauge on the tank to determine the amount of oxygen in the tank.	10			
4. If necessary, open the cylinder on the tank one full counterclockwise turn and attach the cannula tubing to the flowmeter.	20			
5. Adjust the administration of the oxygen according to the physician's order. Check to make sure the oxygen is flowing through the cannula.	10			
6. Insert the cannula tips into the nostrils and adjust the tubing around the back of the patient's ears.	10			
7. Make sure the patient is comfortable and answer any questions.	10			
8. Wash hands.	10			
9. Document the procedure including the number of liters of oxygen being administered and the patient's condition. Continue to monitor the patient throughout the procedure and document any changes in condition.	10			

Documentation in the Medical Record

_____

_____

_____

_____

Comments:

Total Points Earned _____ Divided by _____ Total Possible Points = _____ % Score

Instructor's Signature _____

Procedure 11-4 Providing Rescue Breathing and Performing One Man CPR

Task: To restore a victim's breathing and blood circulation when respiration and pulse stop.

Equipment and Supplies:
- Nonsterile gloves
- CPR ventilator mask
- Approved mannequin

Standards: Complete the procedure and all critical steps in _____ minutes with a minimum

score of _____ % within three attempts.

Scoring: Divide points earned by total possible points. Failure to perform a critical step that is indicated with an asterisk (*), will result in an unsatisfactory overall score.

Time began _____ **Time ended** _____

Steps	Possible Points	First Attempt	Second Attempt	Third Attempt
1. Establish unresponsiveness. Tap the victim and ask, Are you OK? Wait for victim to respond.	10			
2. Activate the emergency response system. Put on gloves and get ventilator mask.	5			
3. Tilt the victim's head and lift the chin. Look, listen, and feel for signs of breathing. Place your ear over the mouth and listen for breathing. Watch the rising and falling of the chest for evidence of breathing.	10			
4. If breathing is absent or inadequate, place the ventilator mask over the victim's mouth and give 2 slow breaths (2 seconds per breath), holding the ventilator mask tightly against the face while tilting the victim's chin back to open the airway. Allow time for exhalation between breaths.	10			
5. Check the carotid pulse. If a pulse is present, continue rescue breathing (1 breath every 5 seconds, about 10 to 12 breaths per minute). If no signs of circulation are present, begin cycles of 15 chest compressions (at a rate of about 100 compressions per minute) followed by 2 slow breaths.	10			
6. Kneel at the victim's side opposite the chest. Move your fingers up the ribs to the point where the sternum and the ribs join. Your middle fingers should fit into the area and your index finger should be next to it across the sternum.	10			

Steps	Possible Points	First Attempt	Second Attempt	Third Attempt
7. Place the heel of your hand on the chest midline over the sternum, just above your index finger.	5			
8. Place your other hand on top of your first hand and lift your fingers upward off of the chest.	5			
9. Bring your shoulders directly over the victim's sternum as you compress downward, and keep your arms straight.	5			
10. Depress the sternum 1½ to 2 inches for an adult victim. Relax the pressure on the sternum after each compression but do not remove your hands from the victim's sternum.	10			
11. After performing 15 compressions (at a rate of about 100 compressions per minute), open the airway and give 2 slow breaths.	5			
12. After 4 cycles of compressions and breaths (15:2 ratio, about 1 minute) recheck breathing and carotid pulse. If there is a pulse but no breathing, continue rescue breathing (1 breath every 5 seconds, about 10 to 12 breaths per minute) and reevaluate the victim's breathing and pulse every few minutes. If there are no signs of circulation, continue 15:2 cycles of compressions and ventilations, starting with chest compressions. Continue giving CPR until the EMS relieves you.	5			
13. Remove gloves and the ventilator mask valve and dispose in the biohazard container. Disinfect the ventilator mask per manufacturer recommendations. Wash hands.	5			
14. Document the procedure and patient condition.	5			

Documentation in the Medical Record

_____
_____
_____
_____

Comments:

Total Points Earned _____ Divided by _____ Total Possible Points = _____ % Score

Instructor's Signature _____

Procedure 11-5 Caring for a Patient who Fainted

Task: To provide emergency care and assessment of a patient who has fainted.

Equipment and Supplies:
- Sphygmomanometer
- Stethoscope
- Watch with second hand
- Blanket
- Foot stool or box
- Physician may order oxygen:
  - Portable oxygen tank
  - Pressure regulator
  - Flow meter
  - Nasal cannula with connecting tubing

Standards: Complete the procedure and all critical steps in _____ minutes with a minimum score of _____ % within three attempts.

Scoring: Divide points earned by total possible points. Failure to perform a critical step that is indicated with an asterisk (*), will result in an unsatisfactory overall score.

Time began _____ **Time ended** _____

Steps	Possible Points	First Attempt	Second Attempt	Third Attempt
1. If warning is given that the patient feels faint, have the patient lower the head to the knees to increase blood supply to the brain. If this does not stop the episode, either have the patient lie down on the examination table or lower the patient to the floor. If the patient collapses to the floor when fainting, treat with caution due to possible head or neck injuries.	10			
2. Immediately notify the physician of the patient's condition and assess the patient for life-threatening emergencies such as respiratory or cardiac arrest. If the patient is breathing and has a pulse, monitor the patient's vital signs.	10			
3. Loosen any tight clothing and keep the patient warm, applying a blanket if needed.	20			
4. If there is no concern about a head or neck injury, elevate the patient's legs above the level of the heart.	10			
5. Continue to monitor vital signs and apply oxygen via nasal cannula if ordered by the physician.	10			

Steps	Possible Points	First Attempt	Second Attempt	Third Attempt
6. If vital signs are unstable or the patient does not respond quickly, activate emergency medical services.	10			
7. If the patient vomits, roll the patient on his or her side to avoid aspiration of vomitus into the lungs.	10			
8. Once the patient has completely recovered, assist the patient into a sitting position. *Do not* leave the patient unattended on the examination table.	10			
9. Document the incident including a description of the episode, patient symptoms, vital signs, length of time, and any complaints. If oxygen was administered, document the number of liters and length of administration.	10			

Documentation in the Medical Record

_____

_____

_____

_____

Comments:

Total Points Earned _____ Divided by _____ Total Possible Points = _____ % Score

Instructor's Signature _____

Procedure 11-6 Controlling Bleeding

Task: To stop hemorrhaging from an open wound.

Equipment and Supplies:
- Gloves, sterile if available
- Appropriate Personal Protective Equipment according to OSHA guidelines including:
  - Impermeable gown
  - Goggles
  - Impermeable mask
- Sterile dressings
- Bandaging material
- Biohazard waste container

Standards: Complete the procedure and all critical steps in _____ minutes with a minimum

score of _____ % within three attempts.

Scoring: Divide points earned by total possible points. Failure to perform a critical step that is indicated with an asterisk (*), will result in an unsatisfactory overall score.

Time began _____ **Time ended** _____

Steps	Possible Points	First Attempt	Second Attempt	Third Attempt
1. Wash hands and apply appropriate personal protective equipment.	10			
2. Assemble equipment and supplies.	10			
3. Apply several layers of sterile dressing material directly to the wound and exert pressure.	10			
4. Wrap the wound with bandage material. Add more dressing and bandaging material if bleeding continues.	10			
5. If bleeding persists and the wound is located on an extremity, elevate the extremity above the level of the heart. Notify the physician immediately if bleeding cannot be controlled.	10			
6. If bleeding still continues, apply pressure to the appropriate artery. If bleeding is in the arm, apply pressure to the brachial artery by squeezing the inner aspect of the upper mid-arm. If bleeding is in the leg apply pressure to the femoral artery on the affected side by pushing with the heel of the hand into the femoral crease at the groin. *If bleeding cannot be controlled, it may be necessary to activate the emergency medical system.*	10			

Steps	Possible Points	First Attempt	Second Attempt	Third Attempt
7. Once the bleeding is controlled and the patient is stabilized, dispose of contaminated materials into the biohazard waste container.	10			
8. Disinfect the area, remove gloves, and dispose into biohazard waste.				
9. Wash hands.	10			
10. Document the incident including the details of the wound, when and how it occurred, patient symptoms, vital signs, physician treatment, and the patient's current condition	10			

Documentation in the Medical Record

_____

_____

_____

_____

Comments:

Total Points Earned _____ Divided by _____ Total Possible Points = _____ % Score

Instructor's Signature _____

Procedure 12-1 Measuring Distance Visual Acuity with the Snellen Chart

Task: To determine the patient's degree of visual clarity at a measured distance by using the Snellen chart.

Equipment and Supplies:
- Snellen eye chart
- Eye occluder
- Pen or pencil and paper

Standards: Complete the procedure and all critical steps in _____ minutes with a minimum

score of _____ % within three attempts.

Scoring: Divide points earned by total possible points. Failure to perform a critical step that is indicated with an asterisk (*), will result in an unsatisfactory overall score.

Time began _____ **Time ended** _____

Steps	Possible Points	First Attempt	Second Attempt	Third Attempt
1. Wash your hands.	10			
2. Prepare the examination room. Make sure that (a) the room is well lighted, (b) a distance marker is 20 feet from the chart, and (c) the chart is placed at the eye level of the patient.*	10			
3. Identify the patient and explain the procedure. Instruct the patient not to squint during the test, since this temporarily improves vision. The patient should not have an opportunity to study the chart before the test. If the patient wears corrective lenses, they should be worn during the test.	10			
4. Have the patient stand or sit at the 20-foot marker.*	10			
5. Position the Snellen chart at eye level to the patient.	5			
6. Instruct the patient to cover the left eye with the occluder and to keep both eyes open throughout the test to prevent squinting.	10			
7. Stand beside the chart and point to each row as the patient orally reads down the chart, starting with the 20/70 row.	10			
8. Proceed down the rows of the chart until the smallest row the patient can read with a maximum of two errors is reached. If one or two letters are missed, the outcome is recorded with a minus sign and the number of errors. If more than two errors are made, findings from reading the previous line should be documented.	10			

Steps	Possible Points	First Attempt	Second Attempt	Third Attempt
9. Record any patient reactions in reading the chart.	5			
10. Repeat the procedure with the left eye.	10			
11. Document the date and time, the procedure, visual acuity results, and any patient reactions on the patient's record. Also record whether corrective lenses were worn.	10			

Documentation in the Medical Record

_____

_____

_____

_____

Comments:

Total Points Earned _____ Divided by _____ Total Possible Points = _____ % Score

Instructor's Signature _____

Procedure 12-2 Assessment of Color Acuity with the Ishihara Test

Task: To correctly assess a patient's color acuity and record the results.

Equipment and Supplies:
- Appropriate room area with natural light
- Ishihara color plate book
- Pen, pencil, and paper
- Watch with a second hand

Standards: Complete the procedure and all critical steps in _____ minutes with a minimum

score of _____ % within three attempts.

Scoring: Divide points earned by total possible points. Failure to perform a critical step that is indicated with an asterisk (*), will result in an unsatisfactory overall score.

Time began _____ **Time ended** _____

Steps	Possible Points	First Attempt	Second Attempt	Third Attempt
1. Assemble the necessary equipment and prepare the room for testing. The room should be quiet and illuminated with natural light.	10			
2. Identify the patient and explain the procedure. Use a practice card during the explanation and be sure that the patient understands that he or she has 3 seconds to identify each plate.	10			
3. Hold up the first plate at a right angle to the patient's line of vision and 30 inches from the patient. Be sure both eyes are kept open during the test.	20			
4. Ask the patient to tell you what number is on the plate and record the plate number and the patient's answer.	10			
5. Continue this sequence until all 11 plates have been read. If the patient cannot identify the number on the plate, place an X in the record for that plate number. Your record should look like this: Plate 1 = pass, Plate 2 = pass, Plate 3 = x, Plate 4 = pass, and so on.	10			
6. Include any unusual symptoms such as eye rubbing, squinting, or excessive blinking in the record.	10			

Steps	Possible Points	First Attempt	Second Attempt	Third Attempt
7. Place the book back into its cardboard sleeve and return the book to its storage space. The Ishihara color plates need to be stored in a closed position away from external light to protect the colors.	10			
8. Record the procedure, including the date and time, the test results, and any patient symptoms exhibited during the test in the patient's record.	20			

Documentation in the medical record

_____

_____

_____

_____

Comments:

Total Points Earned _____ Divided by _____ Total Possible Points = _____ % Score

Instructor's Signature _____

Procedure 12-3 Irrigating a Patient's Eyes

Task: To cleanse the eye(s), as ordered by the physician.

Equipment and Supplies:
- Prescribed sterile irrigation solution
- Sterile irrigating bulb syringe and sterile basin or prepackaged solution with dispenser
- Basin for drainage
- Sterile gauze squares
- Disposable drape
- Towel
- Nonsterile gloves
- Biohazard waste container

Standards: Complete the procedure and all critical steps in _____ minutes with a minimum

score of _____ % within three attempts.

Scoring: Divide points earned by total possible points. Failure to perform a critical step that is indicated with an asterisk (*), will result in an unsatisfactory overall score.

Time began _____ **Time ended** _____

Steps	Possible Points	First Attempt	Second Attempt	Third Attempt
1. Wash your hands. Put on gloves.*	5			
2. Check the physician's orders to determine which eye (or both) requires irrigation and the type of solution to be used.*	5			
3. Assemble the materials needed.	5			
4. Check the expiration date of the solution and read the label three times.	5			
5. Identify the patient and explain the procedure.	5			
6. Assist the patient into a sitting or supine position, making certain that the head is turned toward the side of the affected eye. Place the disposable drape over the patient's neck and shoulder.	5			
7. Place or have the patient hold a drainage basin next to the affected eye to receive the solution from the eye. Place a polylined drape under the basin to avoid getting the solution on the patient.	5			
8. Moisten a gauze square with solution and cleanse the eyelid and lashes. Start at the inner canthus (near nose) and wipe toward the outer canthus (farthest from nose) and dispose of the gauze square after each wipe.	10			

Steps	Possible Points	First Attempt	Second Attempt	Third Attempt
9. If you are using a bulb syringe, pour the required volume of body-temperature irrigating solution into the basin and withdraw solution into the bulb syringe. If you are using an irrigating solution in a prepackaged dispenser, remove the lid.	10			
10. Separate and hold eyelids with the index finger and thumb of one hand. With the other hand, place the syringe or dispenser on the bridge of the nose parallel to the eye.	10			
11. Squeeze the bulb or dispenser, directing the solution toward the lower conjunctiva of the inner canthus, allowing the solution to flow steadily and slowly from the inner to outer canthus. Do not touch the eye or eyelids with the applicator.	10			
12. Refill the syringe or continue to gently squeeze the prepackaged bottle and continue the procedure until the amount of solution ordered by the physician has been administered or until the drainage is clear.	5			
13. Dry the eyelid from the inner canthus to the outer canthus with sterile gauze. Do not use cotton balls because fibers might remain in the eye.	5			
14. Clean the work area.	5			
15. Remove gloves and wash your hands.	5			
16. Document the procedure using appropriate abbreviations; include the date and time, the type and amount of solution used, which eye was irrigated, any significant patient reactions, and the results in the patient's record.	5			

Documentation in the Medical Record

_____

_____

_____

_____

Comments:

Total Points Earned _____ Divided by _____ Total Possible Points = _____ % Score

Instructor's Signature _____

Procedure 12-4 Instilling Eye Medication

Task: To apply medication to the eye(s), as ordered by the physician.

Equipment and Supplies:
- Sterile medication with sterile eye dropper or ophthalmic ointment
- Disposable drape
- Sterile gauze squares
- Nonsterile gloves

Standards: Complete the procedure and all critical steps in _____ minutes with a minimum

score of _____ % within three attempts.

Scoring: Divide points earned by total possible points. Failure to perform a critical step that is indicated with an asterisk (*), will result in an unsatisfactory overall score.

Time began _____ **Time ended** _____

Steps	Possible Points	First Attempt	Second Attempt	Third Attempt
1. Wash your hands.*	10			
2. Check the physician's order to determine which eye(s) requires medication and the name and strength of the medication you will be using.	6			
3. Assemble equipment and supplies.	6			
4. Read the medication label three times.*	10			
5. Identify the patient and explain the procedure.	6			
6. Put on nonsterile gloves and rinse your gloved hands under warm water to remove all powder from gloves.	6			
7. Assist the patient into a sitting or supine position. Ask the patient to tilt the head backward and look up.	6			
8. Pull the lower conjunctival sac downward.*	10			
9. Insert the prescribed number of drops or amount of ointment into the eye. For eye drops, place drops in the center of the lower conjunctival sac with the tip of the dropper held parallel to the eye and ½ inch above the eye sac. For eye ointment (unguent), squeeze a thin ribbon along the lower conjunctival sac from inner to outer canthus, making sure not to touch the eye with the applicator.*	10			

Steps	Possible Points	First Attempt	Second Attempt	Third Attempt
10. Instruct the patient to *gently* close the eye and rotate the eyeball.	6			
11. Dry any excess drainage from inner to outer canthus and explain that the medication may temporarily blur vision.	6			
12. Discard the unused medication and clean the procedure area.	6			
13. Remove gloves and wash hands.	6			
14. Record the procedure on the patient's chart including the date and time, the name and strength of the medication, the amount of the dose administered, which eye was treated, teaching instructions given if the treatment is to continue at home, and any observations.	6			

Documentation in the medical record

_____

_____

_____

_____

Comments:

Total Points Earned _____ Divided by _____ Total Possible Points = _____ % Score

Instructor's Signature _____

Procedure 12-5 Measuring Hearing Acuity Using an Audiometer

Task: To perform audiometric testing of hearing acuity.

Equipment and Supplies:
• Audiometer with adjustable headphones
• Quiet area

Standards: Complete the procedure and all critical steps in _____ minutes with a minimum

score of _____ % within three attempts.

Scoring: Divide points earned by total possible points. Failure to perform a critical step that is indicated
with an asterisk (*), will result in an unsatisfactory overall score.

Time began _____ **Time ended** _____

Steps	Possible Points	First Attempt	Second Attempt	Third Attempt
1. Wash hands, assemble equipment, and conduct patient into a quiet area.	10			
2. Explain the audiometer will measure if the patient can hear various sound wave frequencies through the headphones. Each ear will be tested separately. When the patient hears a frequency, he or she should raise a hand to signal the medical assistant.	10			
3. Place the headphones over the patient's ears, making sure they are adjusted for comfort.	10			
4. The audiometer tests each ear separately, starting at a low frequency. If the results are not automatically recorded by the machine, the medical assistant documents the patient response to the frequencies on a graph or audiogram. *The medical assistant requires specialized training to conduct this test.*	20			
5. Frequencies are gradually increased to test patient ability to hear. The medical assistant continues to document each response by the patient.	10			
6. The other ear is then tested and results documented.	10			
7. Patient results are given to the physician for interpretation.	10			
8. Disinfect the equipment according to manufacture guidelines.	10			
9. Wash hands.	10			

Documentation in the Medical Record

_____

_____

_____

_____

Comments:

Total Points Earned _____ Divided by _____ Total Possible Points = _____ % Score

Instructor's Signature _____

Procedure 12-6 Irrigating a Patient's Ear

Task: To irrigate a patient's ear.

Equipment and Supplies:
- Irrigating solution
- Basin for irrigating solution
- Bulb syringe or an approved otic irrigation device
- Gauze squares
- Otoscope
- Drainage basin
- Disposable drape with polylined barrier
- Cotton-tipped applicators
- Disposable gloves

Standards: Complete the procedure and all critical steps in _____ minutes with a minimum

score of _____ % within three attempts.

Scoring: Divide points earned by total possible points. Failure to perform a critical step that is indicated with an asterisk (*), will result in an unsatisfactory overall score.

Time began _____   **Time ended** _____

Steps	Possible Points	First Attempt	Second Attempt	Third Attempt
1. Wash your hands.	5			
2. Check the physician's order and assemble the materials needed.	5			
3. Check the label of the solution three times: (a) when you remove it from the shelf, (b) when you pour it, and (c) when you return it to the shelf.	5			
4. Prepare the solution as ordered. The solution temperature should be at body temperature (98.6°F to 100°F) to help loosen the cerumen.	10			
5. Identify the patient and explain the procedure.	5			
6. View the affected ear with an otoscope to locate cerumen impaction.	5			
7. Place the patient in a sitting position with the head tilted toward the affected ear. Place a water-absorbent towel over a polylined barrier on the patient's shoulder, and place the collecting basin on the towel flush against the base of the ear.	5			
8. Apply gloves and wipe any particles from the outside of the ear with gauze squares.	5			
9. Test to be certain that the solution is warm,* fill the syringe, and expel air.	5			

Steps	Possible Points	First Attempt	Second Attempt	Third Attempt
10. Straighten the external ear canal.* For adults and children over the age of 3 years, gently pull the ear up and back; for children younger than 3 years, pull the ear down and back.	10			
11. Place the tip of the syringe into the meatus of the ear.	5			
12. Gently direct the flow of the solution toward the roof of the canal.	5			
13. Refill the syringe with warm solution and continue until the material has been removed. Note the particles in the collecting basin to be evaluated when the material has been successfully removed.	5			
14. Dry the patient's external ear with gauze squares and the visible ear canal gently with cotton-tipped applicators.	5			
15. Inspect the ear with an otoscope to determine the results.	5			
16. Place a clean, absorbent towel against the freshly irrigated ear and allow the patient to rest quietly while you wait for the physician to return to check the affected ear.	5			
17. Clean the work area, and return all equipment after it has been properly disinfected. Wash your hands.	5			
18. Record the procedure including the date and time, which ear was irrigated by using the appropriate abbreviations (AU – both ears, AD – right ear, AS – left ear), the type and amount of irrigating solution used, the characteristics of the material returned from the irrigation, the isibility of the tympanic membrane after irrigation, and any patient reactions.	5			

Documentation in the Medical Record

_____
_____
_____
_____

Comments:

Total Points Earned _____ Divided by _____ Total Possible Points = _____ % Score

Instructor's Signature _____

Procedure 12-7 Instilling Medicated Ear Drops

Task: To instill the correct medication in the accurate dosage directly into the external auditory canal.

Equipment and Supplies:
- Prescribed otic drops in dispenser bottle
- Cotton balls
- Disposable gloves

Standards: Complete the procedure and all critical steps in _____ minutes with a minimum score of _____ % within three attempts.

Scoring: Divide points earned by total possible points. Failure to perform a critical step that is indicated with an asterisk (*) will result in an unsatisfactory overall score.

Time began _____ **Time ended** _____

Steps	Possible Points	First Attempt	Second Attempt	Third Attempt
1. Wash hands and gather the needed equipment and supplies.	10			
2. Check the medication label three times: (a) when you remove it from the shelf, (b) when you prepare it, and (c) when you return it to the shelf.	10			
3. Identify your patient and explain the procedure.	10			
4. Have the patient sit up and tilt the head away from the affected ear or lie down on the side with the affected ear upward.	10			
5. Check the temperature of the medication bottle. If it feels cold, gently roll the bottle back and forth between your hands to warm the drops.	10			
6. Hold the dropper firmly in your dominant hand. With the other hand, gently pull the pinna up and back if the patient is an adult or down and back if patient is younger than 3 years.*	10			
7. Place the tip of the dropper in the ear canal meatus and instill the medication drops along the side of the canal.	10			
8. Rest the patient on the opposite side of the affected ear and instruct him or her to remain in this position for about 3 minutes.	10			
9. If instructed to do so by the physician, place a moistened cotton ball into the ear canal.	10			
10. Clean the work area and wash your hands.	10			

Documentation in the Medical Record

_____

_____

_____

_____

Comments:

Total Points Earned _____ Divided by _____ Total Possible Points = _____ % Score

Instructor's Signature _____

Procedure 12-8 Collecting a Specimen for a Throat Culture

Task: To collect a specimen for throat culture with sterile technique for either immediate testing or transportation to the laboratory.

Equipment and Supplies:
- Nonsterile gloves
- Face protection barrier if the patient is coughing or if there is danger of splattering of body fluids
- Sterile swab
- Sterile tongue depressor
- Transport medium
- Biohazard waste container

Standards: Complete the procedure and all critical steps in _____ minutes with a minimum

score of _____ % within three attempts.

Scoring: Divide points earned by total possible points. Failure to perform a critical step that is indicated with an asterisk (*), will result in an unsatisfactory overall score.

Time began _____ **Time ended** _____

Steps	Possible Points	First Attempt	Second Attempt	Third Attempt
1. Wash and dry your hands.	5			
2. Gather the materials needed.	5			
3. Don gloves and face protection if needed.	10			
4. Position the patient so that the light shines into the mouth.	10			
5. Remove the sterile swab from the sterile wrap with your dominant hand, and grasp the sterile tongue depressor with your nondominant hand.	10			
6. Instruct the patient to open the mouth and say "ah." Depress the tongue with the depressor.	10			
7. Swab the back of the throat between the tonsillar pillars and especially any reddened, patchy areas of the throat, white pus pockets, purulent areas, and the tonsils.	10			
8. Place the swab into the transport medium, label it, and send it to the outside laboratory. If direct slide testing is requested, return the labeled swab to the office laboratory.	10			
9. Dispose of contaminated supplies in a biohazard waste container.	5			

Steps	Possible Points	First Attempt	Second Attempt	Third Attempt
10. Disinfect the work area.	5	_____	_____	_____
11. Remove gloves; place in biohazard waste container.	5	_____	_____	_____
12. Wash your hands.	5	_____	_____	_____
13. Record procedure in the patient's record.	10	_____	_____	_____

Documentation in the Medical Record

_____

_____

_____

_____

Comments:

Total Points Earned _____ Divided by _____ Total Possible Points = _____ % Score

Instructor's Signature _____

Procedure 13-1 Collecting a Wound Specimen for Testing and/or Culture

Task: To obtain an adequate, noncontaminated sample for culture.

Equipment and Supplies:
- Sterile culture kit containing tube, swabs, and transport media (for swabbing)
- Sterile culture kit containing syringe and transport media (for aspirating)
- Gauze flats
- Recommended wound cleansing solution
- Clean sterile dressing
- Gloves
- Biohazard container
- Face guard

Standards: Complete the procedure and all critical steps in _____ minutes with a minimum

score of _____ % within three attempts.

Scoring: Divide points earned by total possible points. Failure to perform a critical step that is indicated with an asterisk (*), will result in an unsatisfactory overall score.

Time began _____ **Time ended** _____

Steps	Possible Points	First Attempt	Second Attempt	Third Attempt
1. Wash hands, gather supplies, and don gloves and face protection.	10			
2. Remove dressing from the wound and dispose of dressing in biohazard waste container.	10			
3. Observe the wound and make note of the color, odor, and amount of exudate present.	10			
4. Swabbing. Remove the swab from the culture kit, insert the swab into the wound, and saturate it with the exudate. If necessary, use more than one swab, properly labeling each container, to obtain exudates from the entire wound. If doing an anaerobic culture, place the specimen in the culture tube as quickly as possible to avoid oxygen exposure and possible destruction of microbes.	10			
5. Aspirating. Remove the syringe from the kit, insert the tip into the wound exudate, and pull back the plunger, drawing the exudate up into the syringe.	10			
6. Place the swab into the culture tube and crush the transport media ampule, which is in the transport tube, by squeezing the walls of the transport tube slightly, or place the exudate-filled syringe directly into the transport tube.	10			

Steps	Possible Points	First Attempt	Second Attempt	Third Attempt
7. Label the culture tube accurately. Include on the laboratory slip recent antibiotic therapy, the wound site, and the suspected organism.	10			
8. Clean the wound as ordered by the physician and apply a clean sterile dressing to the area.	10			
9. Clean area and dispose of all waste materials in biohazard waste container. Remove gloves and wash hands.	10			
10. Place culture tube in the laboratory collection area. Chart the procedure and all wound data on the patient's record.	10			

Documentation in the Medical Record

_____

_____

_____

_____

Comments:

Total Points Earned _____ Divided by _____ Total Possible Points = _____ % Score

Instructor's Signature _____

Procedure 14-1 Inserting a Rectal Suppository

Task: To insert the prescribed medication accurately into the rectal mucosa.

Equipment and Supplies:
- Prescribed suppository medication
- Water-soluble lubricant
- Disposable tissues
- Biohazard waste container
- Disposable gloves

Standards: Complete the procedure and all critical steps in _____ minutes with a minimum

score of _____ % within three attempts.

Scoring: Divide points earned by total possible points. Failure to perform a critical step that is indicated with an asterisk (*), will result in an unsatisfactory overall score.

Time began _____ **Time ended** _____

Steps	Possible Points	First Attempt	Second Attempt	Third Attempt
1. Wash your hands, read the order, and obtain the necessary supplies.	5			
2. Identify the patient and explain the procedure. Purpose: Proper identification saves time and avoids possible errors.	5			
3. Ask the patient to remove clothing covering the anal area.	5			
4. Assist the patient into a Sims' position and drape the exposed area.	5			
5. Don gloves. Purpose: Infection control.	10			
6. Remove the covering from the suppository and smooth any rough edges on the suppository. Purpose: Eliminates any possible trauma to the rectal mucosa.	5			
7. Generously lubricate the suppository with a water-soluble lubricant. Purpose: Promotes ease of insertion.	10			
8. With your free hand, gently lift the uppermost buttock.	20			
9. With your index finger, guide the suppository into the anus, directing it along the rectal wall and away from any fecal masses.	10			

Steps	Possible Points	First Attempt	Second Attempt	Third Attempt
10. To prevent immediate expulsion, be sure to insert the suppository beyond the internal sphincter.	5			
11. Use tissue to gently press on the anus for a few minutes to help the patient retain the rectal medication. Then, with the same tissue, wipe any excess lubricant from the rectal area. Dispose of used tissue in a biohazard container.	5			
12. Allow the patient to rest for 20 to 30 minutes before he or she gets up and leaves the office. Purpose: Medication retention.	5			
13. Clean up the area, remove gloves, and wash your hands. Purpose: Infection Control.	5			
14. Record the procedure and any pertinent information on the patient's record. Purpose: Procedures that are not recorded are considered not done.	5			

Documentation in the medical record

_____

_____

_____

_____

Comments:

Total Points Earned _____ Divided by _____ Total Possible Points = _____ % Score

Instructor's Signature _____

Procedure 14-2 Assisting with a Colon Endoscopic Examination

Task: To assist the physician with the examination, to prepare collected specimens as requested, and to promote patient comfort and safety.

Equipment and Supplies:
- Gloves (for medical assistant and physician)
- Appropriate instrument: sigmoidoscope, anoscope, or proctoscope
- Water-soluble lubricant
- Drape and patient gown
- Long cotton-tipped swabs
- Suction source
- Sterile biopsy forceps
- Rectal speculum
- Specimen containers with appropriate preservative added
- Laboratory requisition form
- Tissue wipes
- Biohazard container

Standards: Complete the procedure and all critical steps in _____ minutes with a minimum

score of _____ % within three attempts.

Scoring: Divide points earned by total possible points. Failure to perform a critical step that is indicated with an asterisk (*), will result in an unsatisfactory overall score.

Time began _____ **Time ended** _____

Steps	Possible Points	First Attempt	Second Attempt	Third Attempt
1. Wash hands and assemble all needed equipment and supplies.	5			
2. Identify the patient and explain the procedure. Be sure patient has completed proper preparation procedures.	5			
3. Ask the patient to empty his or her bladder.	5			
4. Give the patient an examination gown and instruct him or her to remove all clothing below the waist and put on the gown with the opening to the back.	5			
5. Obtain and record the patient's vital signs.	10			
6. Assist the patient onto the table. When the physician is ready, place the patient in the appropriate position for the type of examination ordered.	5			
7. Drape the patient so that only the anus is exposed. A fenestrated drape (drape with a circular opening placed over the anus) may be used in place of the rectangular drape.	10			

Steps	Possible Points	First Attempt	Second Attempt	Third Attempt
8. Put on gloves and assist the physician as requested during the examination. This includes: • Lubricating the physician's gloved index finger for the digital examination • Lubricating the obturator tip of the instrument before insertion • Plugging in the scope's light source when the physician is ready • Handing the needed supplies to the physician • Collecting specimens by holding the container to accept the sample • Labeling specimens immediately because several specimens may be taken from different areas • Disposing of contaminated supplies as you are given them by the physician	20			
9. Throughout the examination, observe the patient for any adverse reactions. Encourage the patient to breathe slowly through pursed lips to facilitate relaxation.	10			
10. On completion of the examination, cleanse the patient's anal area with tissue wipes. Remove gloves and assist the patient into a resting position and allow the patient time to recover from the procedure.	5			
11. Assist patient off of table and instruct him or her to get dressed. Show the patient where the sink, towels, and tissues are and provide assistance if needed.	5			
12. Complete all laboratory request forms and specimen container labels, and place specimens in appropriate location for laboratory pickup.	5			
13. Clean work area and all equipment used. Endoscope is first sanitized and then sterilized according to manufacturer recommendations.	5			
14. Record procedure and any pertinent information on the patient's record.	5			

Documentation in the Medical Record

_____

_____

_____

_____

Comments:

Total Points Earned _____ Divided by _____ Total Possible Points = _____ % Score

Instructor's Signature _____

Procedure 15-1 Teaching Testicular Self-Examination

Task: To instruct the patient in the steps of testicular self-examination.

Equipment and Supplies:
- Self-examination pamphlet and shower card
- Demonstration model
- Nonsterile gloves

Standards: Complete the procedure and all critical steps in _____ minutes with a minimum

score of _____ % within three attempts.

Scoring: Divide points earned by total possible points. Failure to perform a critical step that is indicated with an asterisk (*), will result in an unsatisfactory overall score.

Time began _____ **Time ended** _____

Steps	Possible Points	First Attempt	Second Attempt	Third Attempt
1. Wash your hands and collect needed supplies.	10	_____	_____	_____
2. Explain to the patient what you are going to do.	10	_____	_____	_____
3. Begin by explaining to the patient that testicular cancer may produce no symptoms in early stages so it is important to examine the testes once a month for abnormal changes and early detection of the disease. This should begin at puberty or about 15 years of age. It is best to do the examination in the shower or in a warm bath. The total examination takes about 3 minutes.	10	_____	_____	_____
4. Examination of the testes: Start by holding the scrotum in the palms of the hands. Then feel one testicle. Apply a small amount of pressure. Slowly roll it between the fingers and try to find hard, painless lumps.	10	_____	_____	_____
5. Examination of the epididymis: This comma-shaped cord is found behind the testis. Its job is to store and transport sperm. Tender when touched, it is the location of most noncancerous problems.	10	_____	_____	_____
6. Examination of the vas deferens: Continue by examining the sperm-carrying tube that runs up the epididymis. Normally, the vas feels like a firm, movable, smooth tube.	10	_____	_____	_____
7. Now repeat the entire examination on the other side, beginning with the opposite testis.	10	_____	_____	_____

Steps	Possible Points	First Attempt	Second Attempt	Third Attempt
8. After completing the examination on the model, ask the patient to do a return-examination using the model. A male assistant can have the patient do a self–testicular examination.	10			
9. Give the pamphlet to the patient along with the shower card with instructions regarding hanging it in the shower as a monthly reminder and guide.	10			
10. Record the instructional transaction in the patient's medical record.	10			

Documentation in the Medical Record

_____

_____

_____

_____

Comments:

Total Points Earned _____ Divided by _____ Total Possible Points = _____ % Score

Instructor's Signature _____

Procedure 15-2 Catheterization of the Female Patient

Task: To successfully empty the bladder by means of sterile catheterization.

Equipment and Supplies:
- Sterile urethral catheterization kit containing a straight catheter
- Sterile drapes
- Sterile lubricant
- Sterile tray
- Sterile gloves
- Sterile cotton balls or gauze squares
- Povidone-iodine (Betadine)
- Specimen container and laboratory slip
- Waterproof pad
- Gooseneck lamp
- Extra pair of sterile gloves

Standards: Complete the procedure and all critical steps in _____ minutes with a minimum

score of _____ % within three attempts.

Scoring: Divide points earned by total possible points. Failure to perform a critical step that is indicated with an asterisk (*), will result in an unsatisfactory overall score.

Time began _____ **Time ended** _____

Steps	Possible Points	First Attempt	Second Attempt	Third Attempt
1. Wash your hands and collect necessary supplies.	4			
2. Explain the procedure to the patient and have the patient remove necessary clothing.	4			
3. Place your patient in the dorsal recumbent position.	4			
4. Drape the patient's upper body, leaving the genital area exposed.	4			
5. Position a gooseneck lamp over the genital area.	4			
6. Wash your hands and open the catheterization tray on a clean stable surface using sterile techniques. (A Mayo stand is often used.)	4			
7. Open the sterile underpad drape and hold the underpad so that the undersurface of the two corners encircles your hands. Slide it under the patient while she is lifting her hips off the table. Be careful not to touch the patient or the table with your hands. Ask patient to keep knees apart.	4			
8. Open the sterile drape and place it over the patient's exposed genital area so that the vulval area is exposed.	4			

Steps	Possible Points	First Attempt	Second Attempt	Third Attempt
9. Place the insertion kit and any other supplies on the sterile drape between the patient's legs.	4			
10. Put on sterile gloves following sterile procedure (see Chapter 54). Open the sterile povidone-iodine (Betadine) package and pour it over cotton balls or gauze squares in the tray.	8			
11. Open the sterile lubricant package and place it on the sterile field.	4			
12. Open all other items, including the catheter. Stand the specimen container on the tray.	4			
13. With the thumb and index finger of your non-dominant hand, separate the patient's labia as widely as possible. Your nondominant hand must maintain this position throughout the balance of the procedure. Take care that your dominant hand does not touch the patient during the cleansing process. With your dominant hand, pick up one of the povidone-iodine–soaked gauze squares and wipe from top to bottom on one side of the labia. Discard the used gauze.	4			
14. Pick up another gauze square and wipe from top to bottom on the other side of the labia. Discard the used gauze.	4			
15. Pick up another gauze square, and using a circular motion, wipe over the urinary meatus from the inside outward. Discard the gauze.	4			
16. With your dominant hand, pick up the catheter about 3 inches from the insertion end and dip the tip into the sterile lubricant. Position the other end of the catheter in the collection compartment of the kit tray.	4			
17. Insert the lubricated tip into the urinary meatus and continue inserting the catheter 2 to 3 inches or until urine begins flowing out the catheter into the kit tray. Never force the catheter.	4			
18. Let some of the urine flow and then place the specimen container over the end of the catheter and collect the specimen.	4			
19. When the bladder is completely emptied and the urine stops flowing, gently remove the catheter. If more than 500 ml of urine drains into the collection tray, clamp the catheter and wait 10 to 15 minutes, then reopen the catheter and allow the bladder to empty.	4			
20. Secure the lid to the urine specimen container.	4			

Steps	Possible Points	First Attempt	Second Attempt	Third Attempt
21. Remove all supplies and dispose of them according to standard precautions.	4			
22. Assist patient off table and with dressing as needed.	4			
23. Complete the laboratory requisition and record the procedure; include the number of milliliters of urine removed from the bladder.	8			

Documentation in the Medical Record

_____

_____

_____

_____

Comments:

Total Points Earned _____ Divided by _____ Total Possible Points = _____ % Score

Instructor's Signature _____

Procedure 15-3 Catheterization of a Male Patient with a Straight Catheter

Task: To successfully empty the bladder by means of sterile catheterization.

Equipment and Supplies:
- Sterile urethral catheterization kit containing a straight catheter
- Sterile drapes
- Sterile lubricant
- Sterile tray
- Sterile gloves
- Sterile cotton balls or gauze squares
- Povidone-iodine (Betadine)
- Specimen container and laboratory slip
- Waterproof pad
- Gooseneck lamp
- Extra pair of sterile gloves

Standards: Complete the procedure and all critical steps in _____ minutes with a minimum score of _____ % within three attempts.

Scoring: Divide points earned by total possible points. Failure to perform a critical step that is indicated with an asterisk (*), will result in an unsatisfactory overall score.

Time began _____ **Time ended** _____

Steps	Possible Points	First Attempt	Second Attempt	Third Attempt
1. Wash your hands and collect necessary supplies.	5			
2. Explain the procedure to the patient and have the patient remove necessary clothing.	5			
3. Place your patient in the dorsal recumbent position.	5			
4. Drape the patient's upper body, leaving the genital area exposed.	5			
5. Position a gooseneck lamp over the genital area.	5			
6. Wash your hands and open the catheterization tray on a clean stable surface using sterile techniques. (A Mayo stand is often used.)	5			
7. Put on sterile gloves following sterile procedure (see Chapter 32). Open the sterile povidone-iodine (Betadine) package and pour it over cotton balls or gauze squares in the tray.	5			
8. Open the sterile lubricant package and place it on the sterile field.	5			

Steps	Possible Points	First Attempt	Second Attempt	Third Attempt
9. Open all other items, including the catheter. Stand the specimen container on the tray.	5			
10. Open the fenestrated drape and position it so the opening exposes the penis. Be careful not to touch the patient or the table.	5			
11. Place the sterile kit on the table on top of the sterile drape and open all the supplies as in Procedure 15-2, steps 10 through 12.	5			
12. Grasp the penis below the glans with your non-dominant hand. In uncircumcised males, you must pull back the foreskin to see the meatus. You must do this and hold the penis upright with your nondominant hand only.	5			
13. Using your dominant hand and forceps, pick up a povidone-iodine (Betadine)–soaked cotton ball and clean around the meatus in circular motions from the center outward. Repeat this a total of three times using a fresh soaked cotton ball each time.	5			
14. With your dominant hand, lubricate the tip of the catheter at least 7 inches. Be sure to put the other end of the catheter into the collection compartment of the kit tray.	5			
15. Hold the shaft of the penis straight and upright with your dominant hand and apply gentle traction to straighten the urethra. Ask the patient to bear down as if to urinate. Gently insert the lubricated catheter tip into the urinary meatus 6 to 8 inches or until urine begins flowing out of the catheter. Never force the catheter; if you meet resistance, remove the catheter and notify the physician.	5			
16. Let some of the urine flow and then place the specimen container over the end of the catheter and collect the specimen.	5			
17. When the bladder is completely emptied and the urine stops flowing, gently remove the catheter. If more than 500 ml of urine drains into the collection tray, clamp the catheter and wait 10 to 15 minutes, then reopen the catheter and allow the bladder to empty.	5			
18. Secure the lid to the urine specimen container.	5			
19. Remove all supplies and dispose of them according to standard precautions.	2.5			

Steps	Possible Points	First Attempt	Second Attempt	Third Attempt
20. Assist patient off table and with dressing as needed.	2.5			
21. Complete the laboratory requisition and record the procedure; include the number of milliliters of urine removed from the bladder.	5			

Documentation in the Medical Record

_____

_____

_____

_____

Comments:

Total Points Earned _____ Divided by _____ Total Possible Points = _____ % Score

Instructor's Signature _____

Procedure 16-1 Assisting with Examination of the Female Patient and Pap Smear

Task: To assist the physician in examination of a female patient and diagnostic Pap smear.

Equipment and Supplies:
- Patient gown
- Lubricant
- 44-inch gauze squares
- Laboratory requisition slips
- Drape sheet
- Examination light
- Cervical spatula and Cytobrush
- Microscopic slides
- Vaginal speculum
- Uterine sponge forceps
- Disposable gloves
- Fixative for Papanicolaou smear
- Urine specimen container if needed
- Stool for occult blood test if needed
- Biohazard waste container

Standards: Complete the procedure and all critical steps in _____ minutes with a minimum score of _____ % within three attempts.

Scoring: Divide points earned by total possible points. Failure to perform a critical step that is indicated with an asterisk (*), will result in an unsatisfactory overall score.

Time began _____ **Time ended** _____

Steps	Possible Points	First Attempt	Second Attempt	Third Attempt
1. Assemble the materials needed and prepare the room. Prepare the equipment and supplies needed for the Pap smear.	5			
2. Wash hands. Follow standard precautions. Don gloves.	5			
3. Identify the patient and briefly explain the procedure.	5			
4. Instruct the patient to empty the bladder and collect a urine specimen if needed.	5			
5. Instruct the patient to disrobe completely and to put on a gown. Explain that gown should open in the front.	5			
6. Assist the patient into a sitting position at the end of the examination table. Drape the patient and assist the physician with the examination. Provide reassurance to the patient as needed.	5			

Steps	Possible Points	First Attempt	Second Attempt	Third Attempt
7. When the physician is ready to examine the breasts and the abdomen in the supine position, assist the patient into the supine position and drape as needed.	5			
8. When the physician is ready to begin the vaginal examination, assist the patient into the lithotomy position. Patient's knees should be relaxed and rotated outward. Remember to always position the patient underneath the drape.	5			
9. Direct the light source toward the perineal area.	5			
10. Warm the stainless steel vaginal speculum in warm water (physician may prefer disposable plastic speculum). Pass the proper instruments to the physician in proper sequence. Physician will need the Cytobrush for cervical cells and the spatula for vaginal cells.	5			
11. Assist the physician with preparation of the slides and labeling (one marked *v* for vaginal, one marked *e* for endocervical). Spray fixative immediately about 6 inches from slide. Let dry for 10 minutes.	5			
12. Apply the water-soluble lubricant to the physician's fingers.	5			
13. Physician may obtain stool for occult blood test after rectal examination has been performed. Have materials ready.	5			
14. Instruct the patient to breathe deeply through the mouth with hands crossed over the chest.	5			
15. Place the soiled instruments in a basin.	5			
16. Assist the patient off the table and with dressing if needed.	5			
17. While patient is in the dressing room, clean the room, removing used equipment.	5			
18. Sanitize and sterilize stainless steel equipment. Remove gloves and wash your hands.	5			
19. Prepare the Pap smear for transportation to the laboratory. Include patient's last menstrual period (LMP) date and indicate whether patient is receiving hormone therapy.	5			
20. Record all procedures on the patient's medical record.	5			

Documentation in the Medical Record

_____

_____

_____

_____

Comments:

Total Points Earned _____ Divided by _____ Total Possible Points = _____ % Score

Instructor's Signature _____

Procedure 16-2 Teaching the Patient Breast Self-Examination

Task: To teach the patient how to palpate her breasts for possible abnormalities.

Equipment and Supplies:
- Instruction pamphlet
- Teaching model (to use to demonstrate the technique before a return demonstration by the patient)

Standards: Complete the procedure and all critical steps in _____ minutes with a minimum

score of _____ % within three attempts.

Scoring: Divide points earned by total possible points. Failure to perform a critical step that is indicated with an asterisk (*), will result in an unsatisfactory overall score.

Time began _____ **Time ended** _____

Steps	Possible Points	First Attempt	Second Attempt	Third Attempt
1. Assemble equipment.	10			
2. Tell patient to always examine breasts while bathing or showering in warm water. The best time to perform this examination is immediately after the menstrual period is completed because at this time there is minimal breast engorgement. Nonmenstruating women should examine breasts on the first day of the month.	20			
3. Have patient raise one arm. With her fingers flat, she should press gently in small circles, starting at the outermost top edge of the breast and spiraling in toward the nipple. Instruct her to touch every part of each breast, including the axillary region, gently feeling for a lump or thickening. The right hand should be used to examine the left breast, and the left hand, to examine the right breast.	20			
4. After the bath/shower is completed, the patient should continue the examination in front of a mirror with arms at the sides. Then with arms raised above the head, she should look carefully for changes in the size, shape, and contour of each breast. She should look for puckering, dimpling, or changes in skin texture.	20			
5. The patient should gently squeeze both nipples and look for discharge.	10			

Steps	Possible Points	First Attempt	Second Attempt	Third Attempt
6. Before dressing, the patient should lie on a bed, place a towel or pillow under the right shoulder, and place the right hand behind the head. The right breast should be examined by using the left hand. Instruct the patient to press gently in small circles, starting at the outermost top edge, including the axillary region, and spiraling in toward the nipple. The procedure should be repeated with left breast.	10			
7. The patient should return the demonstration of how to do the breast examination to confirm understanding.	10			
8. Give the patient the instruction pamphlet to use at home.	10			

Documentation in the Medical Record

_____

_____

_____

_____

Comments:

Total Points Earned _____ Divided by _____ Total Possible Points = _____ % Score

Instructor's Signature _____

Procedure 16-3 Preparing the Patient for Cryosurgery

Task: To prepare the patient for cryosurgery and assist the physician in cryosurgery.

Equipment and Supplies:
- Cryosurgery machine equipped with liquid nitrogen canister
- Cryoprobe
- Cervical tenaculum
- Cervical ring forceps or disposable cervical swabs
- Vaginal speculum
- 44-inch gauze squares
- Gloves
- Gowns and face protection
- Specimen containers
- Biohazard waste container
- Cytology request forms

Standards: Complete the procedure and all critical steps in _____ minutes with a minimum score of _____ % within three attempts.

Scoring: Divide points earned by total possible points. Failure to perform a critical step that is indicated with an asterisk (*), will result in an unsatisfactory overall score.

Time began _____ **Time ended** _____

Steps	Possible Points	First Attempt	Second Attempt	Third Attempt
1. Assemble equipment.	5			
2. Wash hands and don gloves.	10			
3. Obtain the patient's temperature and blood pressure and record them on the patient's record.	10			
4. Drape and assist the patient into the lithotomy position. Don gloves.	10			
5. Assist the physician with the procedure by handing the equipment needed.	10			
6. Encourage the patient to take deep breaths to promote relaxation of the pelvic muscles during the procedure. Observe patient for any sign of distress.	10			
7. When the procedure has been completed, place the patient in a supine position and allow her to rest while you tidy the room and remove the used supplies. Retake temperature and blood pressure.	10			
8. Help patient sit up and assist her in dressing if necessary.	5			

Steps	Possible Points	First Attempt	Second Attempt	Third Attempt
9. Remove gloves and wash hands.	10			
10. Return equipment to the proper storage area.	10			
11. Record procedure and final vital sign measurements on the patient's record.	10			

Documentation in the Medical Record

_____
_____
_____
_____

Comments:

Total Points Earned _____ Divided by _____ Total Possible Points = _____ % Score

Instructor's Signature _____

Procedure 16-4 Assisting with the Prenatal Examination

Task: To promote a healthy pregnancy for the mother and fetus and screen for potential problems.

Equipment and Supplies:
- Scale with height measurement
- Sphygmomanometer
- Stethoscope
- Tape measure
- Doppler fetoscope
- Urine specimen container
- Latex gloves, vaginal speculum, and lubricant if vaginal examination conducted
- Biohazard waste container

Standards: Complete the procedure and all critical steps in _____ minutes with a minimum

score of _____ % within three attempts.

Scoring: Divide points earned by total possible points. Failure to perform a critical step that is indicated with an asterisk (*), will result in an unsatisfactory overall score.

Time began _____ **Time ended** _____

Steps	Possible Points	First Attempt	Second Attempt	Third Attempt
1. Wash hands, assemble equipment, and identify the patient.	5			
2. Measure and record the patient's weight.	10			
3. Collect a urine specimen, perform, and record urinalysis results to determine the presence of protein, glucose, or ketones in the urine.	10			
4. Measure and record the mother's blood pressure.	10			
5. Instruct the patient to disrobe form the waist down and put on a gown open to the front so the uterine fundal height can be measured.	10			
6. Assist the patient onto the examination table if needed and provide a drape for privacy.	10			
7. Assist the physician as needed throughout the examination.	10			
8. After the examination is completed, assist the patient off the examination table, making sure to observe for signs of dizziness or problems with balance.	10			
9. Answer patient questions and provide patient education materials needed.	10			

Steps	Possible Points	First Attempt	Second Attempt	Third Attempt
10. Discard supplies and disinfect the equipment according to manufacture guidelines. Wear latex gloves and follow OSHA guidelines if handling any contaminated items.	5			
11. Wash hands.	5			
12. Document pertinent information in the patient chart.	5			

Documentation in the Medical Record

_____

_____

_____

_____

Comments:

Total Points Earned _____ Divided by _____ Total Possible Points = _____ % Score

Instructor's Signature _____

Procedure 16-5 Establishing the Estimated Day of Delivery with Nagele's Rule and the Lunar Method

Task: To establish the patient's due date.

Equipment and Supplies:
- Calendar for present and following year
- Paper and pencil
- Commercial estimated day of delivery (EDD) wheel (optional)

Standards: Complete the procedure and all critical steps in _____ minutes with a minimum

score of _____ % within three attempts.

Scoring: Divide points earned by total possible points. Failure to perform a critical step that is indicated with an asterisk (*), will result in an unsatisfactory overall score.

Time began _____ **Time ended** _____

Steps	Possible Points	First Attempt	Second Attempt	Third Attempt
1. Ask patient for the date of the onset of the last menstrual period (LMP). Be sure that this is the date of the onset and not the date of the termination of the menses.	20			
2. Patient informs you that her LMP was April 12, 20XX.	20			
3. Calculate her EDD by using Nagele's method. Begin with the date of the first day of her LMP. Count back 3 months and add 1 year plus 7 days.	20			
4. Using the same LMP, calculate her EDD with the lunar rule. Example: LMP = June 7, 2002 + 9 months = March 7, 2002 + 7 days = March 14, 2003.	20			
5. Compare the results for accuracy. Did you obtain the same EDD with both methods?	20			

Documentation in the Medical Record

_____

_____

_____

_____

Comments:

Total Points Earned _____ Divided by _____ Total Possible Points = _____ % Score

Instructor's Signature _____

Procedure 17-1 Measuring the Circumference of an Infant's Head

Task: To obtain an accurate measurement of the circumference of an infant's head.

Equipment and Supplies:
- Flexible disposable tape measure
- Age-specific and gender-specific growth chart
- Patient's chart
- Pen or pencil

Standards: Complete the procedure and all critical steps in _____ minutes with a minimum

score of _____ % within three attempts.

Scoring: Divide points earned by total possible points. Failure to perform a critical step that is indicated with an asterisk (*), will result in an unsatisfactory overall score.

Time began _____ **Time ended** _____

Steps	Possible Points	First Attempt	Second Attempt	Third Attempt
1. Wash hands.	10			
2. Identify the patient and gain infant cooperation through conversation.	10			
3. Place the infant in the supine position; an older child may sit on the examination table; alternatively, the infant may be held by the parent.	10			
4. Hold the tape measure with the zero mark against the infant's forehead, slightly above the eyebrows and the top of the ears. Ask the parent for assistance if necessary.	10			
5. Bring the tape measure around the head, just above the ears, to meet at the mid forehead.	10			
6. Read to the nearest 0.01 cm or ¼ inch.	20			
7. Record the measurement on the growth chart and the patient's chart.	10			
8. Dispose of the tape measure.	10			
9. Wash hands.	10			

Documentation in the Medical Record

_____

_____

_____

_____

Comments:

Total Points Earned _____ Divided by _____ Total Possible Points = _____ % Score

Instructor's Signature _____

Procedure 17-2 Measuring Infant Length and Weight

Task: To accurately measure infant length and weight so growth patterns can be monitored and recorded.

Equipment and Supplies:
- Infant scale with paper cover
- Flexible measuring tape
- Examination table paper
- Pen
- Infant growth chart
- Biohazard waste container

Standards: Complete the procedure and all critical steps in _____ minutes with a minimum

score of _____ % within three attempts.

Scoring: Divide points earned by total possible points. Failure to perform a critical step that is indicated with an asterisk (*), will result in an unsatisfactory overall score.

Time began _____ **Time ended** _____

Steps	Possible Points	First Attempt	Second Attempt	Third Attempt
Measuring Infant Length				
1. Wash hands, assemble equipment, and explain the procedure to the infant's caregiver.	5			
2. Undress infant in preparation for measurement of length and height. May leave diaper on until length measurement is taken but it must be removed before weighing the infant.	10			
3. Ask the caregiver to place the infant on his or her back on the examination table that is covered with paper. If it is a pediatric table with a headboard, ask the caregiver to gently hold the infant's head against the board while you straighten the infant's leg and mark on the paper the location of the heel. If there is no headboard ask the caregiver to gently hold the infant's head still while you extend the leg for measurement.	10			
4. Measure and record the infant's length with the tape measure.	10			
5. Document the results in either inches or centimeters depending on office policy on the infant's growth chart, in the progress notes, and in the caregiver's record if requested. Complete the growth chart graph by connecting the dot from the last visit.	5			

Steps	Possible Points	First Attempt	Second Attempt	Third Attempt

Measuring Infant Weight

1. Wash hands, assemble equipment, and explain the procedure to the infant's caregiver. — **5** _____ _____ _____

2. Completely undress the infant including the diaper. — **10** _____ _____ _____

3. Place the infant gently onto the center of the scale, keeping your hand directly above the infant's trunk for safety. — **10** _____ _____ _____

4. Slide the weights across the scale until balance is achieved. Attempt to read the infant's weight while he or she is still. — **10** _____ _____ _____

5. Return the weights to the far left of the scale and remove the baby. Caregiver can apply a diaper while you discard the paper covering the scale. If it has become contaminated during the procedure, follow OSHA guidelines for gloves and disposal of contaminated waste. Disinfect the equipment according to manufacturer's guidelines. — **10** _____ _____ _____

6. Wash hands. — **5** _____ _____ _____

7. Document the results in either pounds or kilograms dependent on office policy on the infant's growth chart, in the progress notes, and in the caregiver's record if requested. Complete the growth chart graph by connecting the dot from the last visit. — **5** _____ _____ _____

Documentation in the Medical Record

_____

_____

_____

_____

Comments:

Total Points Earned _____ Divided by _____ Total Possible Points = _____ % Score

Instructor's Signature _____

Procedure 17-3 Obtaining Pediatric Vital Signs and Vision Screening

Task: To accurately obtain vital signs and screen vision in a pediatric patient.

Equipment and Supplies:
- Digital or tympanic thermometer
- Pediatric blood pressure cuff
- Wristwatch with sweep second-hand
- Weight scale
- Stethoscope
- Pediatric E eye chart and oculator
- Pencil and paper

Standards: Complete the procedure and all critical steps in _____ minutes with a minimum

score of _____ % within three attempts.

Scoring: Divide points earned by total possible points. Failure to perform a critical step that is indicated with an asterisk (*), will result in an unsatisfactory overall score.

Time began _____ **Time ended** _____

Steps	Possible Points	First Attempt	Second Attempt	Third Attempt
1. Gather equipment.	5			
2. Wash hands.	5			
3. Explain the procedure to the parent, and if you want the parent to help by holding the child, explain the technique you want him or her to use.	5			
4. Help child stand in the center of the scale and weigh the child. Ask child to turn around and obtain the child's height. Record your findings.	5			
5. Obtain tympanic or axillary temperature by using the procedure explained in Chapter 6.	5			
6. Record temperature. Indicate the method used: A = axillary.	5			
7. Place stethoscope on child's chest at the midpoint between the sternum and the left nipple and listen for the apical beat.	5			
8. Count the apical beat for 1 full minute.	10			
9. Record the apical pulse. Be sure to write "(A)" after the rate to indicate that this is an apical pulse reading.	5			

Steps	Possible Points	First Attempt	Second Attempt	Third Attempt
10. Place the palm of your hand flat on the child's chest and count the respirations for 1 full minute.	5			
11. Record the respiration rate.	5			
12. Check to be sure that you have the correct-size blood pressure cuff and then proceed with taking the blood pressure. Follow procedure in Chapter 28.	10			
13. Record the blood pressure.	5			
14. If vision screening is to be done, familiarize the child with the E by asking him to make an E point the same way as your E is pointing. Then position the child in front of the pediatric E Snellen chart and have him or her match the E, by using his or her hands, with the one to which you are pointing.	5			
15. Record the vision results: OD = right eye, OS = left eye, OU = both eyes.	5			
16. Compliment the child on his or her performance, and if the parent is present, share the praise with the parent.	5			
17. Wash hands.	5			
18. Return all equipment used to proper storage area.	5			

Documentation in the Medical Record

_____

_____

_____

_____

Comments:

Total Points Earned _____ Divided by _____ Total Possible Points = _____ % Score

Instructor's Signature _____

Procedure 17-4 Applying a Urinary Collection Device

Task: To properly apply a pediatric urinary collection device.

Equipment and Supplies:
Pediatric urine collection bag
Labeled laboratory urine specimen container
Laboratory test request form
Antiseptic wipes
Biohazard waste container
Disposable examination gloves

Standards: Complete the procedure and all critical steps in _____ minutes with a minimum

score of _____ % within three attempts.

Scoring: Divide points earned by total possible points. Failure to perform a critical step that is indicated with an asterisk (*), will result in an unsatisfactory overall score.

Time began _____ Time ended _____

Steps	Possible Points	First Attempt	Second Attempt	Third Attempt
1. Assemble all needed supplies.	5			
2. Wash hands and don gloves.	5			
3. Ask parent to remove the diaper from the child or lay the child in a supine position on the examination table and remove the diaper.	10			
4. Cleanse the genitalia with antiseptic wipes. Male: Cleanse the urinary meatus in a circular motion, starting directly on the meatus, and work in an outward pattern. Repeat with a clean wipe. If the child is not circumcised, retract the foreskin to expose the meatus, and when you have completed cleansing, return the foreskin to its natural position. Female: Hold the labia open with your left hand and with your right hand, cleanse the inner labia, from the clitoris to the vaginal meatus, in a superior to inferior pattern. Discard the first wipe and repeat with a clean wipe.	10			
5. Make sure the area is dry. Unfold the collection device, remove the paper from the upper portion, place this portion over the mons pubis, and press it securely into place. Continue by removing the lower portion of the paper and securing this portion against the perineum. Be sure that the device is attached smoothly and that you have not taped it to part of the infant's thigh.	10			

Steps	Possible Points	First Attempt	Second Attempt	Third Attempt
6. Re-diaper the infant, or if the parent is helping, the parent may re-diaper the infant at this time. The diaper will help hold the bag in place.	5			
7. Suggest that the parent give the child liquids if allowed and check the bag for urine at frequent intervals.	5			
8. When there is a noticeable amount of urine in the bag, remove the device, cleanse the skin area that was attached to the device, and rediaper the child.	10			
9. Pour the urine carefully into the laboratory urine container and handle the sample in a routine manner.	10			
10. Dispose of all used equipment in a biohazard waste container.	10			
11. Remove gloves, dispose of them in a biohazard container, and wash hands.	10			
12. Record the procedure in the patient's record.	10			

Documentation in the Medical Record

_____

_____

_____

_____

Comments:

Total Points Earned _____ Divided by _____ Total Possible Points = _____ % Score

Instructor's Signature _____

Student Name _____ Date _____ Score _____

Procedure 18-1 Assisting with Cold Application

Task: To instruct a patient in the correct application of cold to a body area to decrease pain, prevent further swelling, and/or decrease inflammation.

Equipment and Supplies:
- Ice bag or closeable disposable plastic kitchen food bag
- Small ice cubes or ice chips
- Towel

Standards: Complete the procedure and all critical steps in _____ minutes with a minimum score of _____ % within three attempts.

Scoring: Divide points earned by total possible points. Failure to perform a critical step that is indicated with an asterisk (*), will result in an unsatisfactory overall score.

Time began _____ **Time ended** _____

Steps	Possible Points	First Attempt	Second Attempt	Third Attempt
1. Wash your hands.	10			
2. Explain the procedure to the patient and answer any questions.	10			
3. Check the bag for possible leaks.	10			
4. Fill the bag with small cubes or chips of ice until it is about two thirds full.	10			
5. Push down on the top of the bag to expel excess air and apply the cap.	10			
6. Dry the outside and cover it with one or two layers of the towel.	10			
7. Help the patient position the ice bag on the injured area.	10			
8. Advise the patient to leave the ice bag in place for about 20 to 30 minutes or until the area feels numb, whichever is first.	10			
9. Check the skin for color, sensation, and pain.	10			
10. Record the procedure in the patient's chart.	10			

Documentation in the Medical Record

_____

_____

_____

_____

Comments:

Total Points Earned _____ Divided by _____ Total Possible Points = _____ % Score

Instructor's Signature _____

Student Name _____ Date _____ Score _____

Procedure 18-2 Assisting with Hot Moist Heat Application in the Office

Task: To instruct a patient in the correct application of moist heat to a body area to increase circulation, increase metabolism, and relax muscles.

Equipment and Supplies:
• Commercial hot moist heat packs
• Towel

Standards: Complete the procedure and all critical steps in _____ minutes with a minimum

score of _____ % within three attempts.

Scoring: Divide points earned by total possible points. Failure to perform a critical step that is indicated with an asterisk (*), will result in an unsatisfactory overall score.

Time began _____ **Time ended** _____

Steps	Possible Points	First Attempt	Second Attempt	Third Attempt
1. Wash your hands.	10			
2. Explain the procedure to the patient and answer any questions.	10			
3. Ask the patient to remove all jewelry in the area to be treated.	20			
4. Place one or two layers of towel over the area to be treated.	20			
5. Apply the commercial heated moist heat packs.	20			
6. Cover with the remaining portion of the towel.	20			

Documentation in the Medical Record

_____

_____

_____

_____

Comments:

Total Points Earned _____ Divided by _____ Total Possible Points = _____ % Score

Instructor's Signature _____

Procedure 18-3 Assisting with Therapeutic Ultrasound Application

Task: To apply ultra–high-frequency sound waves to the patient's deep tissues for therapy.

Equipment and Supplies:
• Ultrasound machine
• Ultrasound gel or lotion (the coupling agent)

Standards: Complete the procedure and all critical steps in _____ minutes with a minimum

score of _____ % within three attempts.

Scoring: Divide points earned by total possible points. Failure to perform a critical step that is indicated with an asterisk (*), will result in an unsatisfactory overall score.

Time began _____ **Time ended** _____

Steps	Possible Points	First Attempt	Second Attempt	Third Attempt
1. Prepare the equipment and wash your hands.	5			
2. Confirm the patient's identity.	5			
3. Explain the procedure and tell the patient to notify you of any discomfort immediately during the procedure.	5			
4. Question the patient about the presence of any internal or external metal objects.	5			
5. Position the patient comfortably, with the area to be treated exposed.	5			
6. Apply a warmed ultrasound gel (the coupling agent) liberally over the area to be treated and to the applicator head.	5			
7. Begin the treatment with the intensity control at the lowest setting.	5			
8. Set the timer on the machine to the ordered time.	5			
9. Slowly increase the intensity control to the ordered amount.	5			
10. Hold the applicator with the head firmly and completely against the patient's skin over the area to be treated.	5			
11. Work the applicator over the area to be treated by moving it continuously in a circular fashion at a speed of 2 inches per second or as directed by the physician.	5			

Steps	Possible Points	First Attempt	Second Attempt	Third Attempt
12. Keep the applicator head in contact with the patient's skin at all times while the machine is on and keep it moving continuously during the treatment time.	5			
13. When the timer sounds, it shuts off the machine automatically. Then you can safely lift the applicator head away from the patient.	5			
14. Return the intensity control to zero.	5			
15. Remove the ultrasound gel from the patient's skin and from the applicator head with a tissue or paper wipe.	5			
16. Assist the patient in getting dressed if necessary.	5			
17. Record the procedure in the patient's chart including the date, area treated, intensity setting, duration of treatment, and any unusual occurrences or reactions during treatment. If none occurred, indicate that also.	20			

Documentation in the Medical Record

_____

_____

_____

_____

Comments:

Total Points Earned _____ Divided by _____ Total Possible Points = _____ % Score

Instructor's Signature _____

Procedure 18-4 Assisting with Cast Application

Task: To assist the physician in applying a plaster cast.

Equipment and Supplies:
• Tubular stockinette to fit the limb to be casted
• Sheet wadding or roller padding
• Roller plaster or other appropriate casting material
• Bucket of cool or room temperature water
• Cast knife or heavy bandage scissors (used only for casting)
• Gloves

Standards: Complete the procedure and all critical steps in _____ minutes with a minimum

score of _____ % within three attempts.

Scoring: Divide points earned by total possible points. Failure to perform a critical step that is indicated with an asterisk (*), will result in an unsatisfactory overall score.

Time began _____ **Time ended** _____

Steps	Possible Points	First Attempt	Second Attempt	Third Attempt
1. Assemble equipment and supplies. Be sure that the stockinette is correct size to fit comfortably over the fractured area.	5			
2. Explain the procedure to the patient.	5			
3. Assist the physician in covering the injured limb with the stockinette leaving extra fabric above and below the proposed casting area.	5			
4. Hand the physician the sheet wadding and support the patient's limb as directed.	5			
5. Wet the roller plaster by holding it in the bucket of water until bubbles no longer appear around the ends of the roller, then gently squeeze the roller.	5			
6. Press out the extra water and hand the saturated rollers on at a time as requested.	5			
7. When the plaster cast application has been completed, hand the physician the plaster knife or heavy bandage scissors and assist as needed in trimming the rough plaster edges.	5			
8. After the edges are smooth, assist in folding the extra stockinette over the cast ends toward the center of the cast to for a cuff of stockinette at each end of the cast.	5			

Steps	Possible Points	First Attempt	Second Attempt	Third Attempt
9. Place the casted limb carefully on a pillow to begin drying. Avoid squeezing the soft cast.	10			
10. Clean the skin of all casting material.	5			
11. Instruct the patient to report odors, staining, undue warmth, changes in limb color, swelling, and numbness and to keep the limb elevated for at least the first 24 hours.	5			
12. Review case care instructions with the patient and a family member if the cast was placed on a child. Give the patient a copy of the cast care instructions and if the physician has ordered a form of isometric exercises, be certain to demonstrate the exercise technique. Be sure to reinforce any precautions the physician has informed the patient.	5			
13. Discard water down the sink drain but keep all plaster residues from the bottom of the bucket out of the drain. Discard the used plaster bandage and plaster residue in the regular trash or in a designated disposal container.	5			
14. Check the limb in 20 to 30 minutes for color, swelling, numbness, and temperature. Advise the physician and chart your finding.*	10			
15. If arm has been casted, and the physician has ordered a sling, apply the sling as ordered.	10			
16. If a foot has been casted and crutches are ordered, continue instructions with the patient in the use of crutches after fitting them appropriately.	10			

Documentation in the Medical Record

_____

_____

_____

_____

Comments:

Total Points Earned _____ Divided by _____ Total Possible Points = _____ % Score

Instructor's Signature _____

Procedure 18-5 Triangular Arm Sling Application

Task: To properly place a casted arm in a triangular sling.

Equipment and Supplies:
• Triangular-shaped arm sling

Standards: Complete the procedure and all critical steps in _____ minutes with a minimum

score of _____ % within three attempts.

Scoring: Divide points earned by total possible points. Failure to perform a critical step that is indicated with an asterisk (*), will result in an unsatisfactory overall score.

Time began _____ **Time ended** _____

Steps	Possible Points	First Attempt	Second Attempt	Third Attempt
1. Be sure that you have a physician's order for a triangular arm sling.	10			
2 Wash your hands and obtain the desired sling.	10			
3. Explain the procedure to the patient.	10			
4. Position the patient's injured arm across the chest so that it is parallel to the floor and the patient's waist with the hand slightly elevated.	10			
5. Carefully slide the triangular sling between the patient's chest and the affected arm.	10			
6. Bring the lower front corner up over the shoulder of the affected side to the neck.	10			
7. Grab the opposite corner and tie or pin the ends together at the side of the neck.	20			
8. Fold the sling edge to form a smooth edge along the wrist.	10			
9. Record the procedure in the patient's record.	10			

Documentation in the Medical Record

_____

_____

_____

_____

Comments:

Total Points Earned _____ Divided by _____ Total Possible Points = _____ % Score

Instructor's Signature _____

Procedure 18-6 Assisting with Cast Removal

Task: To remove a cast.

Equipment and Supplies:
- Cast cutter
- Cast spreader
- Large bandage scissors

Standards: Complete the procedure and all critical steps in _____ minutes with a minimum

score of _____ % within three attempts.

Scoring: Divide points earned by total possible points. Failure to perform a critical step that is indicated with an asterisk (*), will result in an unsatisfactory overall score.

Time began _____ **Time ended** _____

Steps	Possible Points	First Attempt	Second Attempt	Third Attempt
1. Explain the procedure to the patient.	10			
2. Provide adequate support for the limb throughout the entire procedure.	10			
3. Make a cut on both the medial side and the lateral side of the long axis of the cast.	10			
4. Pry the two halves apart using the cast spreader.	10			
5. Carefully remove the two parts of the cast.	10			
6. Use the large bandage scissors to cut away the stockinette and padding remaining.	10			
7. Gently wash the area that was covered by the cast with mild soap and warm water.	10			
8. Dry and apply a gentle skin lotion.	10			
9. Give the patient appropriate instructions as to exercising and using the limb.	10			
10. Record the procedure in the patient's medical record.	10			

Documentation in the Medical Record

_____

_____

_____

_____

Comments:

Total Points Earned _____ Divided by _____ Total Possible Points = _____ % Score

Instructor's Signature _____

Procedure 18-7 Assisting the Patient with Crutch Walking

Task: To properly fit crutches for your patient and teach them how to use them properly in three point walking.

Equipment and Supplies:
• Crutches

Standards: Complete the procedure and all critical steps in _____ minutes with a minimum

score of _____ % within three attempts.

Scoring: Divide points earned by total possible points. Failure to perform a critical step that is indicated with an asterisk (*), will result in an unsatisfactory overall score.

Time began _____ **Time ended** _____

Steps	Possible Points	First Attempt	Second Attempt	Third Attempt
1. Fit the crutches to the patient so the armrest is 2 inches below the armpit.	20			
2. Be sure that all wing nuts are tight.	10			
3. Make sure the foam pads at the armpits and around the handgrips are comfortable.	10			
4. Instruct the patient to keep the injured leg as relaxed as possible and slightly bent at the knee.	10			
5. The patient's elbow should be bent from 23 to 30 degrees when holding the handgrip.	10			
6. Place the crutch tips about 6 inches away from and parallel to the toes.	10			
7. Ask the patient to push down on the crutches and lift the body slightly, nearly straightening the arms.	10			
8. Swing the body forward about 12 inches.	10			
9. Standing on the good leg, move the crutches just ahead of the good foot and repeat	10			

Documentation in the Medical Record

_____

_____

_____

_____

Comments:

Total Points Earned _____ Divided by _____ Total Possible Points = _____ % Score

Instructor's Signature _____

Procedure 19-1 Assisting with the Neurological Examination

Task: To assist the physician in obtaining an accurate neurological examination of the patient.

Equipment and Supplies:
- Otoscope
- Ophthalmoscope
- Percussion hammer
- Disposable pinwheel
- Penlight
- Tuning fork
- Cotton ball
- Tongue depressor
- Small vials of warm and cold liquids prepared according to the physician's instructions
- Small vials of sweet and salty tasting liquids prepared according to the physician's instructions
- Small vials containing substances with distinct odors such as instant coffee, cinnamon, vanilla, etc. prepared according to the physician's instructions

Standards: Complete the procedure and all critical steps in _____ minutes with a minimum

score of _____ % within three attempts.

Scoring: Divide points earned by total possible points. Failure to perform a critical step that is indicated with an asterisk (*), will result in an unsatisfactory overall score.

Time began _____ **Time ended** _____

Steps	Possible Points	First Attempt	Second Attempt	Third Attempt
1. Greet the patient and help them onto the examination table. Explain the procedure to the patient.	25			
2. During the examination, be prepared to assist the patient in changing positions as necessary, have the necessary examination instruments ready for the physician at the appropriate time during the examination, and record all results from the examination as indicated by the physician.	25			
3. The neurological examination will generally follow the following order but can be modified according to physician preference. a. Mental status examination b. Proprioception and cerebellar function c. Cranial nerve assessment d. Sensory nerve function e. Reflexes	25			
4. Complete the documentation of the examination in the patient's medical record.	25			

Documentation in the Medical Record

_____

_____

_____

_____

Comments:

Total Points Earned _____ Divided by _____ Total Possible Points = _____ % Score

Instructor's Signature _____

Procedure 19-2 Preparing the Patient for an EEG

Task: To properly prepare a patient physically and psychologically to obtain an accurate and useful EEG recording.

Equipment and Supplies:
• Collodion

Standards: Complete the procedure and all critical steps in _____ minutes with a minimum

score of _____ % within three attempts.

Scoring: Divide points earned by total possible points. Failure to perform a critical step that is indicated with an asterisk (*), will result in an unsatisfactory overall score.

Time began _____ Time ended _____

Steps	Possible Points	First Attempt	Second Attempt	Third Attempt
1. Greet patient and introduce yourself. Explain to the patient you will go over what is going to happen step by step to ensure the best results.	5			
2. Explain to the patient the purpose of the EEG, how the procedure will be carried out, and what will be expected of the patient during the test.	5			
3. Tell the patient that the electrodes pick up tiny electrical signals from the body and that there is no danger of electrical shock.	10			
4. Explain that the test is painless because the electrodes are attached to the scalp with collodion.	10			
5. If this is a sleep EEG, suggest the patient stay up later than usual the night before the test so that it will be easier to fall asleep.	10			
6. Go over the physical preparation including the diet to be followed for the 48 hours before the fest. This usually includes no stimulants like coffee, chocolate or sodas and no meal skipping.	10			
7. Tell the patient that at the beginning of the test a baseline EEG will be taken and during this time the patient will be asked to avoid all movement, even eye and tongue movement.	10			
8. Explain that the brain will be stimulated by the patient viewing flickering lights. The EEG will be measuring the brain's response to this stimulation.	10			
9. Ask the patient if they have any questions. If so, answer them so the patient understands the procedure clearly.	10			

Documentation in the Medical Record

_____

_____

_____

_____

Comments:

Total Points Earned _____ Divided by _____ Total Possible Points = _____ % Score

Instructor's Signature _____

Procedure 19-3 Preparing the Patient for and Assisting with a Lumbar Puncture

Task: To properly prepare a patient physically and mentally for a lumar puncture in order to obtain a specimen of CSF for testing.

Equipment and Supplies:
- Local anesthetic
- Sterile, disposable lumbar puncture kit
- Mayo stand
- Sterile gloves
- Permanent marker to label tubes

Standards: Complete the procedure and all critical steps in _____ minutes with a minimum

score of _____ % within three attempts.

Scoring: Divide points earned by total possible points. Failure to perform a critical step that is indicated with an asterisk (*), will result in an unsatisfactory overall score.

Time began _____ **Time ended** _____

Steps	Possible Points	First Attempt	Second Attempt	Third Attempt
1. Greet patient and introduce yourself. Explain to the patient you will go over what is going to happen step by step to ensure the best results.	5			
2. Explain to the patient the purpose of the lumbar puncture, how the procedure will be carried out, and what will be expected of the patient during the test.	5			
3. Have the patient void just prior to the procedure.	5			
4. Give the patient a hospital gown and have them put it on with the opening down the back.	5			
5. Place the patient in a left, side-lying fetal position for the lumbar puncture.	5			
6. Support the patient's head with a pillow as needed and provide a pillow for between the knees if needed also.	5			
7. Do a sterile skin prep of the patient's lumbar region in the usual manner.	10			
8. Place the sterile disposable lumbar puncture kit on the mayo stand and open it establishing a sterile field. Put on sterile gloves and take the fenestrated drape from the kit and drape the lumbar region of the patient so that only the L3-L4 region of the lower spine is exposed.	10			

Steps	Possible Points	First Attempt	Second Attempt	Third Attempt
9. When the physician is ready to do the lumbar puncture, provide the local anesthetic by holding the vial for the physician or pouring it into the sterile medicine cup on the sterile field on the mayo stand.	5			
10. Reassure the patient and help them to hold still during the injection of the local anesthetic and the insertion of the spinal needle.	5			
11. Be prepared to hold the top of the manometer steady if requested by the physician.	5			
12. Using the permanent marker, label the specimens #1, #2, and #3 in the order that they were collected. This is a critically important step in this procedure.	10			
13. Complete the laboratory requisition form and prepare the CSF specimens for transport to the laboratory.	5			
14. Break down the mayo stand by disposing of the sharps, biohazard and regular waste in the normal manner.	5			
15. Monitor the patient and give liquids as directed by the physician.	5			
16. Document the procedure in the patient's chart.	10			

Documentation in the Medical Record

_____

_____

_____

_____

Comments:

Total Points Earned _____ Divided by _____ Total Possible Points = _____ % Score

Instructor's Signature _____

Procedure 21-1 Performing Spirometry Testing

Task: To perform volume capacity testing.

Equipment and Supplies:
- Balance scale with measuring device
- Volume capacity spirometer with recording paper in place
- External spirometric tubing
- Disposable mouthpiece
- Noseclip
- Biohazard waste container

Standards: Complete the procedure and all critical steps in _____ minutes with a minimum

score of _____ % within three attempts.

Scoring: Divide points earned by total possible points. Failure to perform a critical step that is indicated with an asterisk (*), will result in an unsatisfactory overall score.

Time began _____ **Time ended** _____

Steps	Possible Points	First Attempt	Second Attempt	Third Attempt
1. Introduce yourself and confirm the identity of the patient. Ascertain if any special preparation was needed by this patient and if it was followed.	5			
2. Explain the purpose of the test.	5			
3. Obtain the patient's vital signs.	5			
4. Explain the actual maneuver.	5			
5. Be certain the patient is comfortable and in proper sitting or standing position.	5			
6. Loosen any tight clothing, such as a necktie, bra, or belt. Show the patient the proper chin and neck position.	10			
7. Practice the maneuver with the patient and tell the patient, "Inhale."	10			
8. Use active, forceful coaching during testing. Begin by saying, "Blow." Then say, "Blow out hard." Then say, "Keep blowing, keep blowing." Then say, "Don't stop-blow harder."	10			
9. Give the patient feedback after the maneuver is completed.	5			

Steps	Possible Points	First Attempt	Second Attempt	Third Attempt
10. Continue testing until three acceptable maneuvers have been obtained.	10	_____	_____	_____
11. Dismiss the patient only if results are satisfactory.	5	_____	_____	_____
12. Clean and disinfect the equipment. Discard waste in a biohazard waste container.	5	_____	_____	_____
13. Wash hands.	5	_____	_____	_____
14. Record testing information on the patient's chart and place the chart with the test results on the physician's desk for interpretation.	5	_____	_____	_____

Documentation in the Medical Record

_____

_____

_____

_____

Comments:

Total Points Earned _____ Divided by _____ Total Possible Points = _____ % Score

Instructor's Signature _____

Procedure 21-2 Obtaining Sputum for Culture

Task: To collect a sputum sample while observing standard precautions.

Equipment and Supplies:
• Sterile laboratory specimen cup, accurately labeled
• Plastic laboratory specimen bag
• Biohazard waste container

Standards: Complete the procedure and all critical steps in _____ minutes with a minimum

score of _____ % within three attempts.

Scoring: Divide points earned by total possible points. Failure to perform a critical step that is indicated with an asterisk (*), will result in an unsatisfactory overall score.

Time began _____ **Time ended** _____

Steps	Possible Points	First Attempt	Second Attempt	Third Attempt
1. Assemble the equipment.	5			
2. Greet the patient and explain the procedure.	5			
3. Wash hands and put on gloves, face shield, and lab coat.	5			
4. Have the patient rinse his or her mouth with water.	10			
5. Instruct the patient to take three deep breaths and then cough deeply to bring up secretions from the lower respiratory tract.	10			
6. Tell the patient to spit directly into the specimen container and to avoid getting any sputum on the sides of the container.	10			
7. Place the lid on the container securely and then place the container into the plastic specimen bag.	10			
8. Offer the patient a glass of water or ginger ale.	10			
9. If another test is ordered for tomorrow morning, instruct the patient when to come and remind him or her to follow the same instructions for preparation.	10			
10. Clean the work area and properly dispose of all supplies.	5			

Steps	Possible Points	First Attempt	Second Attempt	Third Attempt
11. Wash your hands.	10			
12. Process the specimen immediately to ensure optimal test results.	5			
13. Record the procedure in the patient's record.	5			

Documentation in the Medical Record

_____

_____

_____

_____

Comments:

Total Points Earned _____ Divided by _____ Total Possible Points = _____ % Score

Instructor's Signature _____

Procedure 23-1 Sensorimotor Changes of Aging

Task: Role play to better understand the needs of aging persons.

Equipment and Supplies:
- Yellow glasses, ski goggles, or lab goggles
- Pink, white, yellow "pills" (various colors of tic tacs work)
- Vaseline
- Cotton balls
- Eye patches
- Tape
- Thick gloves
- Utility glove
- Tongue depressors
- Ace bandages
- Medical forms in small print
- Pennies
- Button shirts
- Walker

Standards: Complete the procedure and all critical steps in _____ minutes with a minimum

score of _____ % within three attempts.

Scoring: Divide points earned by total possible points. Failure to perform a critical step that is indicated with an asterisk (*), will result in an unsatisfactory overall score.

Time began _____ **Time ended** _____

Steps	Possible Points	First Attempt	Second Attempt	Third Attempt
1. **Role play vision and hearing loss:** • Put 2 cotton balls in each ear and eye patch over 1 eye. Follow your partner's instructions. • Partner: stand out of line of vision (to prevent lip reading) and without gestures, without change in voice volume, tell your partner to cross the room and pick up a book.	10			
2. **Role play yellowing of lens:** • Line up "pills" of different pastel colors. • Partner: pick out the different colors while wearing the yellow glasses.	10			
3. **Role-play difficulty with focusing:** • Put on goggles smeared with Vaseline and follow your partner's directions. • Partner: stand at least 3 feet in front of your partner and motion for them to come to you (your partner is deaf so talking will not help).	10			

Steps	Possible Points	First Attempt	Second Attempt	Third Attempt
4. **Loss of peripheral vision:** • Put on goggles with black paper taped to sides. • Partner: stand to the side out of the field of vision and motion for your patient to follow you.	10			
5. **Simulating aphasia and partial paralysis:** • You are unable to use your right arm or leg. Place tape over your mouth. Let your partner know you need to go to the bathroom. • Stand at least 3 feet away with your back to your partner and wait for instructions.	10			
6. **Problems with dexterity:** • Put thick gloves on your hands and try to sign your name, button a shirt, tie your shoes, and pick up pennies.	10			
7. **Problems with mobility:** • Use the walker to cross the room. • Partner: after your partner starts to use the walker, hand them a book to carry.	10			
8. **Changes in sensation:** • Put a rubber utility glove on; turn on hot water; test the difference in temperature between the gloved hand and non-gloved hand.	10			
9. **Summarize and share with the group your impressions of the affect of sensorimotor changes and aging.**	20			

Documentation in the Medical Record

_____

_____

_____

_____

Comments:

Total Points Earned _____ Divided by _____ Total Possible Points = _____ % Score

Instructor's Signature _____

Procedure 24-1 Obtaining a 12-lead ECG

Task: To obtain an accurate, artifact-free recording of the electrical activity of the heart.

Equipment and Supplies:
- ECG machine with patient lead cable
- 10 disposable, self-adhesive electrodes
- Patient gown and drape
- ECG mounting card if necessary

Standards: Complete the procedure and all critical steps in _____ minutes with a minimum

score of _____ % within three attempts.

Scoring: Divide points earned by total possible points. Failure to perform a critical step that is indicated with an asterisk (*), will result in an unsatisfactory overall score.

Time began _____ **Time ended** _____

Steps	Possible Points	First Attempt	Second Attempt	Third Attempt
1. Wash hands.	5			
2. Explain the procedure to the patient.	5			
3. Ask the patient to disrobe to the waist and remove socks, stockings, or pantyhose as necessary.	5			
4. Position the patient on the exam table and drape appropriately.	5			
5. Turn on the machine to allow the stylus to warm up.	5			
6. Label the beginning of the tracing paper with the patient's name, date, and time.	5			
7. At each site where you will place an electrode, clean the skin with an alcohol wipe.	5			
8. Apply the self-adhesive electrodes to clean, dry fleshy areas of the extremities.	10			
9. Apply the self-adhesive electrodes to clean areas on the chest	10			
10. Carefully connect the lead wires to the correct electrode with the alligator clips on the end of each lead.	10			
11. Press the AUTO button on the machine and run the ECG tracing.	5			

Steps	Possible Points	First Attempt	Second Attempt	Third Attempt
12. Watch for artifacts during the recording.	5			
13. Remove the lead wires from the electrodes, and then remove the electrodes from the patient.	5			
14. Assist the patient with getting dressed as needed. Clean and return the ECG machine to its storage area.	5			
15. Mount the ECG tape or give the unmounted ECG tape to the physician as directed.	5			
16. Wash hands.	5			
17. Record the procedure in patient's chart.	5			

Documentation in the Medical Record

_____

_____

_____

_____

Comments:

Total Points Earned _____ Divided by _____ Total Possible Points = _____ % Score

Instructor's Signature _____

Procedure 24-2 Applying a Holter Monitor

Task: To establish possible correlation between coronary disorders and daily activity.

Equipment and Supplies:
- Holter monitor and blank magnetic recording tape
- Disposable electrodes
- Razor
- Tape
- Activity diary
- Carrying case with belt or shoulder strap
- Alcohol wipes
- Cloth tape (nonallergenic)

Standards: Complete the procedure and all critical steps in _____ minutes with a minimum

score of _____ % within three attempts.

Scoring: Divide points earned by total possible points. Failure to perform a critical step that is indicated with an asterisk (*), will result in an unsatisfactory overall score.

Time began _____ **Time ended** _____

Steps	Possible Points	First Attempt	Second Attempt	Third Attempt
1. Wash your hands.	5			
2. Assemble equipment needed.	5			
3. Install new battery or fully charged rechargeable battery in the monitor.	5			
4. Greet the patient and explain the procedure.	5			
5. Ask the patient to disrobe to the waist and sit at the end of the examination table or to lie down.	5			
6. If the patient has a hairy chest, dry shave the area at each of the electrode sites.	5			
7. Clean each electrode application site with an alcohol wipe and allow the sites to air dry.	5			
8. Fold a gauze pad over your index finger and briskly rub the sites.	5			
9. Apply the electrodes to the appropriate sites, making sure to use enough pressure so that each adheres completely to the skin.	5			
10. Attach the lead wires to the electrodes and connect the end terminal to the patient cable.	5			

Steps	Possible Points	First Attempt	Second Attempt	Third Attempt
11. Place a strip of cloth tape over each electrode.	5			
12. Attach the test cable to the monitor and plug it into the electrocardiograph. Run a baseline test tracing.	5			
13. Help the patient get dressed without disturbing the connected electrodes. Be certain that the cable extends through the buttoned front or out the bottom of the shirt or blouse.	5			
14. Place the monitor in the carrying case, and attach it to the patient's belt or place it over the shoulder. Be sure the wires are not being pulled or bent in half.	5			
15. Plug the electrode cable into the monitor.	5			
16. Record the patient's name, date of birth, and starting date and time of the patient's activity diary.	5			
17. Give the patient the activity diary and advise him or her to begin by writing in the present activity.	5			
18. Give patient appointment for return in 24 hours.	5			
19. Wash hands.	5			
20. Record the procedure in patient's chart.	5			

Documentation in the Medical Record

_____

_____

_____

_____

Comments:

Total Points Earned _____ Divided by _____ Total Possible Points = _____ % Score

Instructor's Signature _____

Student Name _____ Date _____ Score _____

Procedure 25-1 General Procedure for X-Ray Examination

Task: To assist with an x-ray examination under the supervision of a physician.

Equipment and Supplies:
- Physician's order for an x-ray examination
- Patient identification card to imprint radiographs
- X-ray machine
- X-ray cassettes, loaded with film
- X-ray darkroom with automatic processor

Standards: Complete the procedure and all critical steps in _____ minutes with a minimum

score of _____ % within three attempts.

Scoring: Divide points earned by total possible points. Failure to perform a critical step that is indicated with an asterisk (*), will result in an unsatisfactory overall score.

Time began _____ Time ended _____

Steps	Possible Points	First Attempt	Second Attempt	Third Attempt
1. Check order and equipment needed. Ascertain if any special preparations were needed.	5			
2. Introduce yourself, and confirm the identity of the patient. Ascertain if any necessary preparations were implemented.	5			
3. Explain the procedure and place the x-ray cassette correctly.	5			
4. Check to make certain that the patient has removed all metal objects from the area to be examined.	5			
5. Drape the patient as necessary, and shield the pelvic area.	5			
6. Position the patient properly, and immobilize the part, if necessary.	5			
7. Align the x-ray tube to the cassette at the proper distance.	10			
8. Measure the patient's thickness through the path of the central ray and set the control panel for he correct exposure.	10			
9. Stand behind a lead shield during the exposure.	10			

471

Steps	Possible Points	First Attempt	Second Attempt	Third Attempt
10. Ask the patient to assume a comfortable position after the examination is completed, and wait until the films are processed.	10			
11. In the darkroom, remove the film from the cassette, identify the film, and process the film in the automatic processor.	10			
12. Dismiss the patient if all films are satisfactory.	10			
13. Place the dry, finished x-ray film in a properly labeled envelope and present it to the physician for interpretation. When it has been read, file it according to the policies of the office.	10			
14. Record the x-ray examination on the patient's chart, along with the final written x-ray findings.	10			

Documentation in the Medical Record

_____

_____

_____

_____

Comments:

Total Points Earned _____ Divided by _____ Total Possible Points = _____ % Score

Instructor's Signature _____

Procedure 26-1 Using the Microscope

Task: To focus the microscope properly, using a prepared slide, under low power, high power, and oil immersion

Equipment and Supplies:
• Microscope
• Lens tissue
• Lens cleaner
• Slide with stained specimen

Standards: Complete the procedure and all critical steps in _____ minutes with a minimum

score of _____ % within three attempts.

Scoring: Divide points earned by total possible points. Failure to perform a critical step that is indicated with an asterisk (*), will result in an unsatisfactory overall score.

Time began _____ **Time ended** _____

Steps	Possible Points	First Attempt	Second Attempt	Third Attempt
1. Wash your hands.	4			
2. Gather the materials needed.	4			
3. Clean the lenses with lens tissue and lens cleaner. Clean the 100x lens (oil immersion) last.	4			
4. Adjust seating to a comfortable height.	4			
5. Plug the microscope into an electric outlet, and turn on the light switch.	4			
6. Place the slide specimen on the stage and secure it.	4			
7. Turn the revolving nosepiece to low power.	4			
8. Carefully raise the stage while observing with the naked eye from the side.	4			
9. Focus the specimen, using the coarse-adjustment knob.	4			
10. Switch to fine adjustment, and focus the specimen in detail.	4			
11. Adjust the amount of light by closing the iris diaphragm and lowering the condenser.	4			
12. Turn the revolving nosepiece between the high-power objective and oil immersion.	4			

Steps	Possible Points	First Attempt	Second Attempt	Third Attempt
13. Place a small drop of oil on the slide.	4			
14. Carefully swing the oil immersion objective into place.	4			
15. Adjust the focus with the fine-adjustment knob.	4			
16. Increase the light by opening the iris diaphragm and raising the condenser.	4			
17. Identify the specimen.	4			
18. Return to low power.	4			
19. Lower the stage.	4			
20. Center the stage. Remove the slide.	4			
21. Switch off the light and unplug the microscope.	4			
22. Clean the lenses with lens tissue, and remove oil with lens cleaner.	4			
23. Wipe the microscope with a cloth.	4			
24. Cover the microscope. Clean the work area.	4			
25. Wash your hands.	4			

Documentation in the Medical Record

_____

_____

_____

_____

Comments:

Total Points Earned _____ Divided by _____ Total Possible Points = _____ % Score

Instructor's Signature _____

Student Name _____ Date _____ Score _____

Procedure 27-1 Collecting a Clean-catch Urine Specimen

Task: To collect a contaminant-free urine sample for culture or analysis using midstream clean-catch technique.

Equipment and Supplies:
• Sterile container with lid and label
• Antiseptic towelettes
• Set of written patient instructions

Standards: Complete the procedure and all critical steps in _____ minutes with a minimum

score of _____ % within three attempts.

Scoring: Divide points earned by total possible points. Failure to perform a critical step that is indicated with an asterisk (*), will result in an unsatisfactory overall score.

Time began _____ **Time ended** _____

Steps	Possible Points	First Attempt	Second Attempt	Third Attempt
1. Label the container and give the patient the supplies.	10			
2. Explain the instructions to adult patients or to the guardians of child patients.	10			
OBTAINING A CLEAN-CATCH MIDSTREAM SPECIMEN FROM A FEMALE PATIENT	40			
1. Wash hands and remove underclothing.				
2. Expose the urinary meatus by spreading apart the labia with one hand.				
3. Cleanse each side of the urinary meatus with a front-to-back motion, from the pubis to the anus. Use a fresh cotton ball on each side. (If the midstream specimen kit is used, an antiseptic wipe is provided to cleanse each side of the meatus.)				
4. Cleanse directly across the meatus, front-to-back, using a third cotton ball or antiseptic wipe				
5. Rinse with water to remove traces of the soap used to prevent its entrance into the specimen.				
6. Dry the area with a clean cotton ball using front-to-back motion. If a midstream kit has been used, the rinsing and drying procedure can be omitted.				
7. Hold the labia apart throughout this procedure.				
8. Void a small amount of urine into the toilet.				

Copyright © 2003, Elsevier Science (USA). All rights reserved. 475

Steps	**Possible Points**	**First Attempt**	**Second Attempt**	**Third Attempt**
9. Move the specimen container into position and void the next portion of urine into it. Remember this is a sterile container. Do not put your fingers on the inside of the container	_____	_____	_____	_____
10. Remove the cup and void the last amount of urine into the toilet. (This means that the first part and the last part of the urinary flow have been excluded from the specimen. Only the middle portion of the flow is included.)	_____	_____	_____	_____

Comments:

OBTAINING A CLEAN-CATCH MIDSTREAM SPECIMEN FROM A MALE PATIENT

	Possible Points	**First Attempt**	**Second Attempt**	**Third Attempt**
	__40__	_____	_____	_____
1. Wash your hands and expose the penis.	_____	_____	_____	_____
2. Retract the foreskin of the penis (if not circumcised).	_____	_____	_____	_____
3. Cleanse the area around the glans penis (meatus) and the urethral opening by washing each side of the glans with a separate cotton ball. If a midstream kit is used, antiseptic wipes are provided.	_____	_____	_____	_____
4. Cleanse directly across the urethral opening using a third cotton ball or antiseptic wipe.	_____	_____	_____	_____
5. If soap and cotton balls are used, rinse with water to remove all traces of soap.	_____	_____	_____	_____
6. Dry the area using a front-to-back motion.	_____	_____	_____	_____
7. Void a small amount of urine into the toilet or urinal.	_____	_____	_____	_____
8. Collect the next portion of the urine in the sterile container without touching the inside of the container with hands or penis.	_____	_____	_____	_____
9. Void the last amount of urine into the toilet or urinal.	_____	_____	_____	_____
10. Wipe and redress.	_____	_____	_____	_____
11. Return the specimen to the designated area provided.	_____	_____	_____	_____

Comments:

Documentation in the Medical Record

_____
_____
_____
_____

Comments:

Total Points Earned _____ Divided by _____ Total Possible Points = _____ % Score

Instructor's Signature _____

Procedure 27-2 Assessing Urine for Color and Turbidity

Task: To assess and record the color and clarity of a urine specimen.

Equipment and Supplies:
• Urine specimen
• Centrifuge tube

Standards: Complete the procedure and all critical steps in _____ minutes with a minimum score of _____ % within three attempts.

Scoring: Divide points earned by total possible points. Failure to perform a critical step that is indicated with an asterisk (*), will result in an unsatisfactory overall score.

Time began _____ **Time ended** _____

Steps	Possible Points	First Attempt	Second Attempt	Third Attempt
1. Wash and dry your hands and apply gloves.	10			
2. Mix the urine by swirling.	10			
3. Label a centrifuge tube if a complete urinalysis is being done.	10			
4. Pour the specimen into a standard-size centrifuge tube.	10			
5. Assess and record the color. • Pale straw • Yellow • Dark yellow • Amber	20			
6. Assess clarity. • Clear—no cloudiness • Slightly cloudy—can see light print through tube • Moderately cloudy—can see only dark print through tube • Very cloudy—cannot see through tube	20			
7. Clean the work area, remove gloves, and wash your hands.	10			
8. Record the results in the patient's record.	10			

Documentation in the Medical Record

_____

_____

_____

_____

Comments:

Total Points Earned _____ Divided by _____ Total Possible Points = _____ % Score

Instructor's Signature _____

Procedure 27-3 Measuring Specific Gravity Using a Urinometer

Task: To calibrate the urinometer to perform a quality control check and to obtain duplicate specific gravity readings.

Equipment and Supplies:
- Urine specimen
- Distilled water
- Urinometer and cylinder

Standards: Complete the procedure and all critical steps in _____ minutes with a minimum

score of _____ % within three attempts.

Scoring: Divide points earned by total possible points. Failure to perform a critical step that is indicated with an asterisk (*), will result in an unsatisfactory overall score.

Time began _____ **Time ended** _____

Steps	Possible Points	First Attempt	Second Attempt	Third Attempt
1. Wash and dry your hands and put on nonsterile gloves and eye protection.	5			
2. Fill the glass cylinder two-thirds full with distilled water at 20° C (room temperature).	5			
3. Read the specific gravity of the distilled water.	10			
4. Allow the specimen to come to room temperature if it was refrigerated.	10			
5. Mix the specimen well by swirling.	10			
6. Pour the specimen into the clean glass cylinder to two-thirds to three-fourths full.	10			
7. Remove any foam using filter paper.	5			
8. With the cylinder on a level surface, gently insert the urinometer in the specimen with a spinning motion.	10			
9. While the urinometer stops rotating in the specimen, read the lower curve of the meniscus, at eye level.	10			

Steps	Possible Points	First Attempt	Second Attempt	Third Attempt
10. Clean and dry the equipment, and return it to proper storage.	5			
11. Clean the work area. Wash your hands.	5			
12. Record the results on the laboratory form or in the patient's record.	15			

Documentation in the Medical Record

_____

_____

_____

_____

Comments:

Total Points Earned _____ Divided by _____ Total Possible Points = _____ % Score

Instructor's Signature _____

Procedure 27-4 Measuring Specific Gravity Using a Refractometer

Task: To measure the refractive index of urine using a refractometer. A refractometer is also known as a total solids (TS) meter.

Equipment and Supplies:
- Urinary refractometer
- Disposable pipet
- Distilled water
- Biohazard waste container

Standards: Complete the procedure and all critical steps in _____ minutes with a minimum

score of _____ % within three attempts.

Scoring: Divide points earned by total possible points. Failure to perform a critical step that is indicated with an asterisk (*), will result in an unsatisfactory overall score.

Time began _____ **Time ended** _____

Steps	Possible Points	First Attempt	Second Attempt	Third Attempt
1. Wash hands and assemble equipment while the urine specimen reaches room temperature.	10			
2. Apply gloves and mix the urine specimen in the collection container.	10			
3. Using a disposable pipet, apply a drop of water to the prism of the refractometer by lifting the plastic cover. Close the cover and point the device toward a light source such as a window or lamp. Look into the refractometer and rotate the eyepiece so the scale can be clearly read. The scale reads from 1.000 to 1.035 in increments of 0.001; distilled water should read 1.000.	30			
4. Adjust the refractometer using the small screwdriver provided by the manufacturer if the scale does not read 1.000.	10			
5. Wipe the prism with a soft, lint-free tissue and apply a drop of mixed urine. Close the cover, point the device at a light source and read the specific gravity on the scale. Discard the pipet in a biohazard waste container.	10			
6. Wipe the urine from the prism with a disposable soft, lint-free tissue between samples. When finished, clean with tissue moistened with distilled water. Discard these tissues in a biohazard waste container.	10			

Steps	Possible Points	First Attempt	Second Attempt	Third Attempt
7. Record the results and discard the urine sample.	**10**	_____	_____	_____
8. Remove and discard gloves and wash the hands.	**10**	_____	_____	_____

Documentation in the Medical Record

_____

_____

_____

_____

Comments:

Total Points Earned _____ Divided by _____ Total Possible Points = _____ % Score

Instructor's Signature _____

Student Name _____ Date _____ Score _____

Procedure 27-5 Testing Urine with Chemical Reagent Strips

Task: To test urine with chemical reagent strips

Equipment and Supplies:
- Urine specimen
- Reagent strips
- Timer

Standards: Complete the procedure and all critical steps in _____ minutes with a minimum

score of _____ % within three attempts.

Scoring: Divide points earned by total possible points. Failure to perform a critical step that is indicated with an asterisk (*), will result in an unsatisfactory overall score.

Time began _____ **Time ended** _____

Steps	Possible Points	First Attempt	Second Attempt	Third Attempt
1. Wash and dry your hands. Put on nonsterile gloves and eye protection.	5			
2. Check the time of collection, the container, and the mode of preservation.	5			
3. If the specimen has been refrigerated, allow it to warm to room temperature.	5			
4. Check the reagent strip container for the expiration date.	5			
5. Remove the reagent strip from the container. Hold it in your hand, or place it on a clean paper towel. Recap the container tightly.	5			
6. Compare nonreactive test pads with the negative color blocks on the color chart on the container.	10			
7. Thoroughly mix the specimen by swirling or inverting.	5			
8. Following manufacturer's directions, note the time, and simultaneously dip the strip into the urine and remove it.	10			
9. Quickly remove the excess urine from the strip.	10			
10. Hold the strip horizontally. After the exact amount of time specified by the manufacturer has elapsed, compare the strip with the appropriate color chart on the reagent container.	10			

Steps	Possible Points	First Attempt	Second Attempt	Third Attempt
11. Read the concentration.	10	_____	_____	_____
12. Clean the work area, remove your gloves, and wash your hands.	10	_____	_____	_____
13. Record the results in the patient's chart.	10	_____	_____	_____

Documentation in the Medical Record

_____

_____

_____

_____

Comments:

Total Points Earned _____ Divided by _____ Total Possible Points = _____ % Score

Instructor's Signature _____

Procedure 27-6 Testing Urine for Glucose with the Clinitest Method

Task: To perform confirmatory testing for glucose in the urine with the Clinitest procedure for reducing substances.

Equipment and Supplies:
- Urine specimen
- Clinitest tablet, tube, and dropper
- Distilled water
- Test tube rack
- Color chart

Standards: Complete the procedure and all critical steps in _____ minutes with a minimum

score of _____ % within three attempts.

Scoring: Divide points earned by total possible points. Failure to perform a critical step that is indicated with an asterisk (*), will result in an unsatisfactory overall score.

Time began _____ **Time ended** _____

Steps	Possible Points	First Attempt	Second Attempt	Third Attempt
1. Wash and dry your hands and put on nonsterile gloves and eye protection.	5			
2. Holding a Clinitest dropper vertically, add 10 drops of distilled water and then 5 drops of urine to a Clinitest tube.	10			
3. Place the prepared tube in the rack.	5			
4. With dry hands, remove a Clinitest tablet from the bottle by pouring the tablet into the bottle cap.	10			
5. Tap the tablet into the test tube and recap the container.	10			
6. Observe the entire reaction to detect the rapid pass-through phenomenon, which means that the glucose level in the urine is very high.	10			
7. When reaction ceases, time exactly 15 seconds; then gently shake the tube to mix the entire contents.	10			
8. Immediately compare the color of the specimen with the five-drop color chart and record your findings.	10			
9. If an orange color briefly develops during the reaction, rapid pass-through has occurred, and the test must be repeated with the use of the two-drop color chart.	10			

Steps	Possible Points	First Attempt	Second Attempt	Third Attempt
10. Clean the work area, remove gloves, and wash hands.	10	_____	_____	_____
11. Record the results in the patient's chart. Negative—Clear Trace—Slightly cloudy 1+—Can see light print through tube 2+—Can see dark print through tube 3+—Cannot see through tube 4+—Large, fluffy precipitate forms and settles on standing	10	_____	_____	_____

Documentation in the Medical Record

_____

_____

_____

_____

Comments:

Total Points Earned _____ Divided by _____ Total Possible Points = _____ % Score

Instructor's Signature _____

Procedure 27-7 Testing Urine for Protein Using the Sulfosalicylic Acid (SSA)

Task: To test urine for protein by using the sulfosalicylic acid (SSA) precipitation test.

Equipment and Supplies:
- Urine specimen
- 3% sulfosalicylic acid
- Centrifuge tube and centrifuge
- Test tube and rack
- Dropper

Standards: Complete the procedure and all critical steps in _____ minutes with a minimum

score of _____ % within three attempts.

Scoring: Divide points earned by total possible points. Failure to perform a critical step that is indicated with an asterisk (*), will result in an unsatisfactory overall score.

Time began _____ Time ended _____

Steps	Possible Points	First Attempt	Second Attempt	Third Attempt
1. Wash and dry your hands. Put on nonsterile gloves and eye protection.	10			
2. If the urine is cloudy, filter the specimen or use a centrifuged specimen.	20			
3. In a clear test tube, mix equal volumes of urine and 3% SSA.	20			
4. Observe for cloudiness and record: Negative—Clear Trace—Slightly cloudy 1+—Can see light print through tube 2+—Can see dark print through tube 3+—Cannot see through tube 4+—Large, fluffy precipitate forms and settles on standing	20			
5. Clean the work area, remove gloves and face protection, and wash hands.	10			
6. Record the results in the patient's chart.	20			

Documentation in the Medical Record

_____

_____

_____

_____

Comments:

Total Points Earned _____ Divided by _____ Total Possible Points = _____ % Score

Instructor's Signature _____

Procedure 27-8 Analyzing Urine Specimen for Microscopic Examination

Task: To perform a microscopic examination of urine to determine the presence of normal and abnormal elements.

Equipment and Supplies:
• Urine specimen
• Centrifuge tube
• Centrifuge
• Disposable pipette
• Microscope slide and coverslip
• Microscope
• Permanent marker

Standards: Complete the procedure and all critical steps in _____ minutes with a minimum score of _____ % within three attempts.

Scoring: Divide points earned by total possible points. Failure to perform a critical step that is indicated with an asterisk (*), will result in an unsatisfactory overall score.

Time began _____ **Time ended** _____

Steps	Possible Points	First Attempt	Second Attempt	Third Attempt
1. Wash and dry your hands. Put on face protection and nonsterile gloves.	5			
2. Gently mix the urine specimen.	5			
3. Pour 10 mL of urine into a labeled centrifuge tube and cap the tube.	5			
4. Place the tube in the centrifuge.	5			
5. Place another tube containing 10 mL of water in the opposite cup.	5			
6. Secure the lid, and centrifuge for 5 minutes or for the time specified for your instrument.	5			
7. Remove the tube from the centrifuge after the instrument has come to a full stop.	5			
8. Pour off the clear supernatant from the top of the specimen by inverting the centrifuge tube over the sink drain.	5			
9. Prevent the loss of sediment down the drain.	5			

Steps	Possible Points	First Attempt	Second Attempt	Third Attempt
10. Thoroughly mix the sediment by grasping the tube near the top and rapidly flicking it with the fingers of the other hand until all sediment is thoroughly resuspended.	5			
11. Transfer one drop of sediment to a clean, labeled slide.	5			
12. Place a clean coverslip over the drop, and place the slide on the microscope stage. Remove face protection.	5			
13. Focus under low power, and reduce the light.	5			
14. First, scan the entire coverslip for abnormal findings.	5			
15. Examine five low-power fields. Count and classify each type of cast seen, if any, and note mucus if present.	5			
16. Switch to high-power magnification, and adjust the light.	5			
17. In five high-power fields, count the following elements: red blood cells, white blood cells, and round, transitional, and squamous epithelial cells.	5			
18. In the same five fields, report the following as few, moderate, or many: crystals (identify and report each type seen separately), bacteria (identify as rods or cocci), sperm, yeast, and parasites.	5			
19. Average the five fields, and report the results. Do not remove the slide from the microscope until the physician has verified the results.	5			
20. Clean up the work area, remove face protection and gloves, and wash hands.	2.5			
21. Record the verified results in the patient's chart.	2.5			

Documentation in the Medical Record

_____
_____
_____
_____

Comments:

Total Points Earned _____ Divided by _____ Total Possible Points = _____ % Score

Instructor's Signature _____

Student Name _____ Date _____ Score _____

Procedure 27-9 Performing a Pregnancy Test

Task: To perform a pregnancy testing of urine with the QuickVue by Quidel pregnancy test method.

Equipment and Supplies:
• Urine specimen
• QuickVue test kit

Standards: Complete the procedure and all critical steps in _____ minutes with a minimum score of _____ % within three attempts.

Scoring: Divide points earned by total possible points. Failure to perform a critical step that is indicated with an asterisk (*), will result in an unsatisfactory overall score.

Time began _____ **Time ended** _____

Steps	Possible Points	First Attempt	Second Attempt	Third Attempt
1. Wash and dry hands. Put on face protection and nonsterile gloves.	10			
2. Prepare the testing equipment.	10			
3. Collect the needed specimen.	10			
4. Remove the test cassette from the foil pouch.	10			
5. Add 3 drops of urine using the dropper that accompanies the kit. Dispose of the dropper in a biohazard bag.	10			
6. Wait 3 minutes and read the test results.	10			
7. Interpret the results. NEGATIVE: A blue control line will be present next to the letter C. No line will be present next to the letter T. POSITIVE: A blue control line will appear next to the letter C along with a pink line next to the letter T. If a blue line does not appear in the "C" area, the test is invalid and the specimen must be retested with another kit. Check the expiration date of the kit before proceeding.	20			
8. Discard the cassette in a biohazard waste container, remove gloves, and wash hands.	10			
9. Record the results in the patient's chart as either positive or negative.	10			

Documentation in the Medical Record

_____

_____

_____

_____

Comments:

Total Points Earned _____ Divided by _____ Total Possible Points = _____ % Score

Instructor's Signature _____

Procedure 27-10 Performing a Rapid Urine Culture Test

Task: To assess the level of bacteriuria to aid in diagnosis of urinary tract infections.

Equipment and Supplies:
- Clean-catch midstream urine specimen
- Uricult test kit
- Incubator
- Biohazard waste container

Standards: Complete the procedure and all critical steps in _____ minutes with a minimum

score of _____ % within three attempts.

Scoring: Divide points earned by total possible points. Failure to perform a critical step that is indicated with an asterisk (*), will result in an unsatisfactory overall score.

Time began _____ **Time ended** _____

Steps	Possible Points	First Attempt	Second Attempt	Third Attempt
1. Wash hands and assemble equipment and specimen. Check the expiration date on the test kit. Label the vial with the patient information.	10			
2. Put on gloves. Remove the slide from the test kit. Do not touch the slide or lay it down.	10			
3. Dip the slide into the urine specimen, tipping the cup carefully if necessary. Alternatively, the urine may be poured over the slide and caught in another container.	10			
4. Allow excess urine to drain, then replace the slide in the protective vial. Screw the cap on loosely.	10			
5. Incubate the vial upright in a 35°-37° C incubator for 18 to 24 hours.	10			
6. After incubation, read the test results by removing the slide from its protective vial and assessing bacterial colony density by comparing the slide with the density chart provided. No actual colony counting is necessary.	10			
7. Interpret the results as follows NORMAL: Less than 10,000 colony-forming units (cfu)/ml of urine; no UTI is present. BORDERLINE: 10,000 to 100,000 cfu/ml of urine; a chronic or relapsing infection may be present and the test should be repeated. POSITIVE: More than 100,000 cfu/ml of urine; a UTI is likely.	10			

Steps	Possible Points	First Attempt	Second Attempt	Third Attempt
8. Return the vial to the protective case and replace the cap.	5			
9. Dispose of the test kit in a biohazard waste container.	5			
10. Remove gloves and wash hands.	5			
11. Record the results.	5			

Documentation in the Medical Record

_____

_____

_____

_____

Comments:

Total Points Earned _____ Divided by _____ Total Possible Points = _____ % Score

Instructor's Signature _____

Procedure 28-1 Collecting a Venous Blood Sample Using the Syringe Method

Task: To collect a venous blood specimen.

Equipment and Supplies:
- Needle, syringe with 21- or 22-gauge needle
- Evacuated tubes appropriate to tests ordered
- 70% isopropyl alcohol
- Sterile gauze pads
- Tourniquet
- Nonallergenic tape

Standards: Complete the procedure and all critical steps in _____ minutes with a minimum

score of _____ % within three attempts.

Scoring: Divide points earned by total possible points. Failure to perform a critical step that is indicated with an asterisk (*), will result in an unsatisfactory overall score.

Time began _____ **Time ended** _____

Steps	Possible Points	First Attempt	Second Attempt	Third Attempt
1. Check the requisition form to determine the tests ordered. Gather the correct tubes and supplies that you will need.	5			
2. Wash and dry your hands, and put on face protection and nonsterile gloves.	5			
3. Identify the patient and explain the procedure.	5			
4. Assist the patient to a seated position with the arm well supported in a slightly downward position.	2.5			
5. Assemble equipment. Choice of syringe and needle size depends on your inspection of the patient's veins. Attach the needle to the syringe. Keep the cover on the needle.	5			
6. Apply the tourniquet around the patient's arm 3 to 4 inches above the elbow. The tourniquet should never be tied so tightly that it restricts blood flow in the artery.	5			
7. Ask the patient to open and close his or her hand several times.	5			
8. Cleanse the site, starting in the center of the area and working outward in a circular pattern.	5			
9. Dry the site with a sterile gauze pad.	5			

Steps	Possible Points	First Attempt	Second Attempt	Third Attempt
10. Remove the needle sheath.	5			
11. Grasp the patient's arm with the nondominant hand while using your thumb and forefinger to draw the skin taut over the site to anchor the vein.	5			
12. Insert the needle through the skin and into the vein with the bevel of the needle up, aligned parallel to the vein, at a 15-degree angle, rapidly, and smoothly.	5			
13. Slowly pull back the plunger of the syringe with the nondominant hand. Make sure that you do not move the needle after entering the vein. Allow the syringe or tube to fill to optimum capacity.	5			
14. Release the tourniquet when venipuncture is complete. It must be released before the needle is removed from the arm.*	5			
15. Place sterile gauze over the puncture site at the time of needle withdrawal.	5			
16. Instruct the patient to apply direct pressure on the puncture site with sterile gauze. The patient may elevate the arm.	5			
17. Transfer the blood to a tube. Gently invert tubes to mix anticoagulants and blood.	5			
18. Check the puncture site for bleeding.	5			
19. Apply a hypoallergenic bandage.	2.5			
20. Dispose of the needle safely. Allow it to drop directly into the disposal unit without touching it with your fingers. Do not recap used needles.	2.5			
21. Clean the work area, remove gloves and face protection, and wash your hands.	2.5			
22. Complete the laboratory requisition form, and route the specimen to the proper place. Record the procedure in the patient's chart.	5			

Documentation in the Medical Record

_____

_____

_____

_____

Comments:

Total Points Earned _____ Divided by _____ Total Possible Points = _____ % Score

Instructor's Signature _____

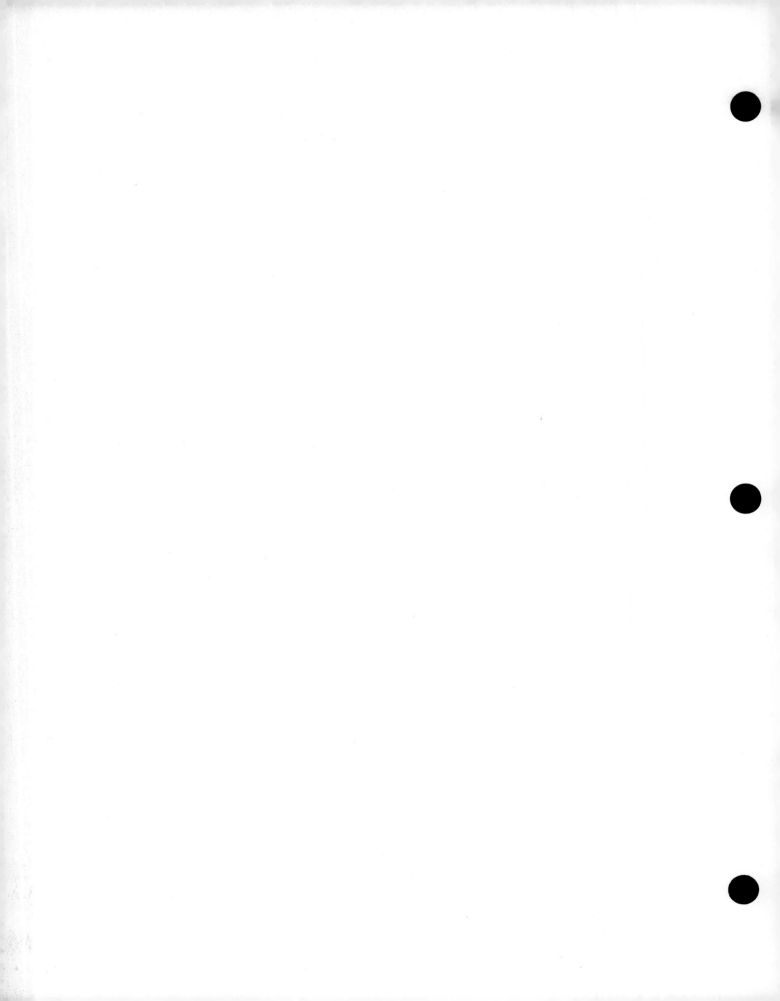

Procedure 28-2 Collecting a Venous Blood Sample Using the Evacuated Tube Method

Task: To collect a venous blood specimen.

Equipment and Supplies:
- Vacutainer needle, adapter, and proper tubes for requested tests
- 70% isopropyl alcohol
- Sterile gauze pads
- Tourniquet
- Nonallergenic tape
- Permanent marking pen

Standards: Complete the procedure and all critical steps in _____ minutes with a minimum

score of _____ % within three attempts.

Scoring: Divide points earned by total possible points. Failure to perform a critical step that is indicated with an asterisk (*), will result in an unsatisfactory overall score.

Time began _____ **Time ended** _____

Steps	Possible Points	First Attempt	Second Attempt	Third Attempt
1. Check the requisition form to determine the tests ordered. Gather the correct tubes and supplies that you will need.	4			
2. Wash and dry your hands, and put on face protection and nonsterile gloves.*	5			
3. Identify the patient and explain the procedure.	4			
4. Assist the patient to sit with the arm well supported in a slightly downward position.	4			
5 Assemble equipment.	4			
6. Apply the tourniquet around the patient's arm 3 to 4 inches above the elbow.	4			
7. Select the venipuncture site by palpating the antecubital space, and use your index finger to trace the path of the vein and to judge its depth.	4			
8. Ask the patient to open and close his or her hand several times.	4			
9. Cleanse the site, starting in the center of the area and working outward in a circular pattern.	4			

Steps	Possible Points	First Attempt	Second Attempt	Third Attempt
10. Dry the site with a sterile gauze pad.	4			
11. Remove the needle sheath.	4			
12. Anchor the vein.	4			
13. Insert the needle through the skin and into the vein with the bevel of the needle up, aligned parallel to the vein, at a 15-degree angle, rapidly, and smoothly.	5			
14. Push the tube onto the needle inside the holder.	4			
15. Allow the tube to fill to optimum capacity.	4			
16. Remove the Vacutainer tube from the adapter before removing the needle from the vein.	4			
17. Release the tourniquet when venipuncture is complete. It must be released before the needle is removed from the arm.*	5			
18. Place sterile gauze over the puncture site at the time of needle withdrawal.	4			
19. Instruct the patient to apply direct pressure on the puncture site with a sterile gauze pad.	4			
20. Gently invert tubes to mix anticoagulants and blood.	4			
21. Check the puncture site for bleeding.	4			
22. Apply a hypoallergenic bandage.	4			
23. Dispose of the needle safely.*	5			
24. Clean the work area, remove gloves and face protection, and wash your hands.	4			
25. Complete the laboratory requisition and route to the proper place. Record the procedure in the patient's record.	4			

Documentation in the Medical Record

_____

_____

_____

_____

Comments:

Total Points Earned _____ Divided by _____ Total Possible Points = _____ % Score

Instructor's Signature _____

Student Name ______________________ Date ____________ Score ________

Procedure 28-3 Collecting a Venous Blood Sample Using the Butterfly Method

Task: To accurately obtain the venous sample from a hand vein using the butterfly method.

Equipment and Supplies:
- Tourniquet
- Alcohol pads or other antiseptic preps
- Gauze pads
- Butterfly needle set
- Appropriate pediatric tubes arranged in the order of the draw or
- Luer-Lok syringe
- Sharps disposal container
- Nonallergenic bandage
- Permanent marking pen

Standards: Complete the procedure and all critical steps in ____________ minutes with a minimum score of ____________ % within three attempts.

Scoring: Divide points earned by total possible points. Failure to perform a critical step that is indicated with an asterisk (*), will result in an unsatisfactory overall score.

Time began ____________ **Time ended** ____________

Steps	Possible Points	First Attempt	Second Attempt	Third Attempt
1. Check the requisition and gather the appropriate tubes for the needed tests. Assemble the balance of your supplies.	4			
2. Wash your hands, and put on face protection and gloves.*	4			
3. Prepare your patient as for an antecubital draw.	4			
4. Remove the butterfly device from the package and stretch it slightly.	4			
5. Attach the butterfly device to the syringe or evacuated tube holder.	4			
6. Seat the first tube into the evacuated tube holder.	4			
7. Apply a tourniquet to the patient's wrist, just proximal to the wrist bone.	4			
8. Hold the hand in your nondominant hand with the fingers lower than the wrist.	4			
9. Select a vein and cleanse the site at the bifurcation.	4			

Steps	Possible Points	First Attempt	Second Attempt	Third Attempt
10. Using your thumb, pull the patient's skin taut over the knuckles.	4			
11. With the needle at a 10- to 15-degree angle, bevel up, align it with the vein.	4			
12. Insert the needle gently by threading it up the lumen of the vein.	12			
13. Push the blood collecting tube onto the end of the holder or draw blood into the syringe. Note the position of the hands while drawing the blood.	4			
14. Release the tourniquet when the blood appears in the tube.*	12			
15. Always keep the tube and the holder in a downward position so that the tube will fill from the bottom up.	4			
16. Place a gauze pad over the puncture site and gently remove the needle.	4			
17. Instruct the patient to apply direct pressure on the puncture site with a sterile gauze pad.	4			
18. Gently invert tubes to mix anticoagulants and blood.	4			
19. Check the puncture site for bleeding.	4			
20. Apply a hypoallergenic bandage.	4			
21. Dispose of the needle safely.*	12			
22. Clean the work area, remove gloves and face protection, and wash your hands.	4			

Documentation in the Medical Record

_____
_____
_____
_____

Comments:

Total Points Earned _____ Divided by _____ Total Possible Points = _____ % Score

Instructor's Signature _____

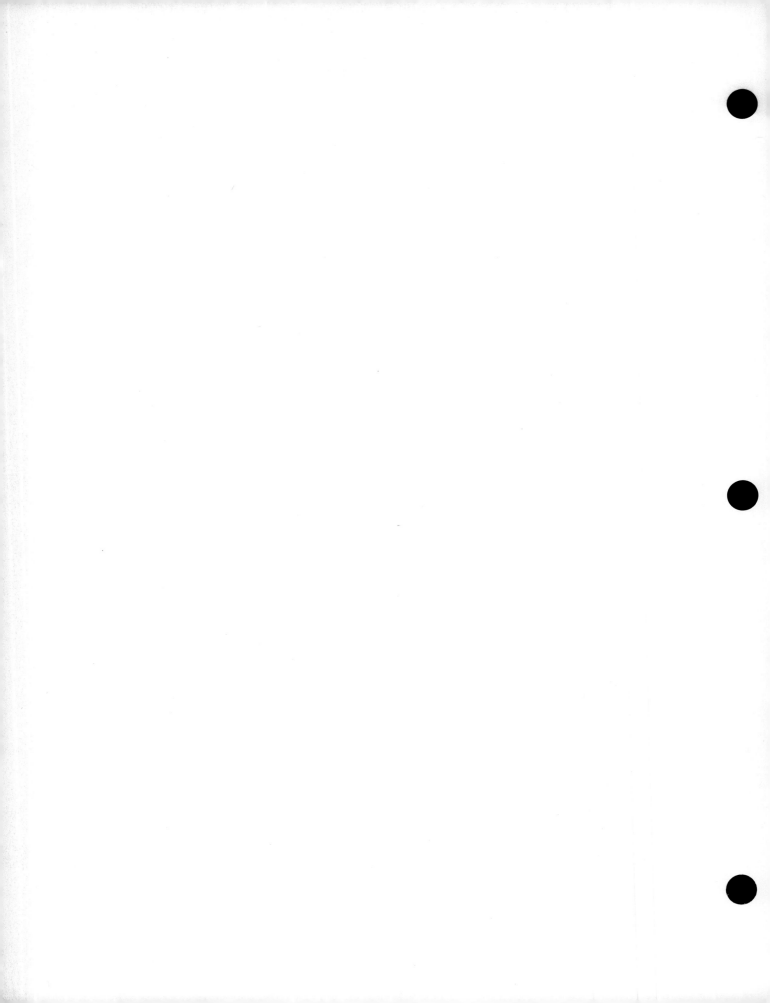

Procedure 28-4 Collecting a Capillary Blood Sample

Task: To collect a capillary blood specimen suitable for testing, using fingertip puncture technique.

Equipment and Supplies:
- Sterile disposable manual lancet or Autolet with Autolet platforms
- 70% alcohol
- Sterile gauze pads
- Nonallergenic tape
- Supplies for requested test (e.g., Unopettes or capillary tubes)
- Sealing clay or caps for capillary tubes
- Permanent marking pen

Standards: Complete the procedure and all critical steps in _____ minutes with a minimum

score of _____ % within three attempts.

Scoring: Divide points earned by total possible points. Failure to perform a critical step that is indicated with an asterisk (*), will result in an unsatisfactory overall score.

Time began _____ **Time ended** _____

Steps	Possible Points	First Attempt	Second Attempt	Third Attempt
1. Wash and dry your hands. Put on face protection and nonsterile gloves.	5			
2. Explain the procedure to your patient.	5			
3. Assemble the needed materials, based on the physician's requisition.	5			
4. Select a puncture site.	5			
5. Milk, or very gently rub, the finger along the sides.	5			
6. Milk, or very gently rub, the finger along the sides.	5			
7. Grasp the patient''s finger on the sides near the puncture site, with your nondominant forefinger and thumb.	5			
8. Hold the lancet at a right angle to the patient's finger, and make a rapid, deep puncture on the patient's fingertip.	5			
9. Wipe away the first drop of blood.	5			
10. Apply gentle pressure to cause the blood to flow freely.	5			

Steps	Possible Points	First Attempt	Second Attempt	Third Attempt
11. Collect blood samples. 　　a. Express a large drop of blood, fill capillary tubes, and seal the end of the tube in clay. 　　b. Wipe the finger with a clean sterile gauze pad, and fill a Unopette.	10			
12. Apply pressure to the site with clean sterile gauze.	5			
13. Label all samples and requisitions correctly, and forward them to the laboratory for testing.	10			
14. Check the patient for bleeding, and apply a nonallergenic bandage if indicated.	5			
15. Dispose of used materials in proper containers.	10			
16. Clean the work area. Remove face protection and gloves. Wash your hands.	5			
17. Record the procedure in the patient's record.	5			

Documentation in the Medical Record

_____

_____

_____

_____

Comments:

Total Points Earned _____ Divided by _____ Total Possible Points = _____ % Score

Instructor's Signature _____

Procedure 29-1 Performing a Microhematocrit

Task: To accurately perform a microhematocrit.

Equipment and Supplies:
• EDTA anticoagulant blood
• Capillary tubes
• Sealing clay
• Centrifuge

Standards: Complete the procedure and all critical steps in _____ minutes with a minimum

score of _____ % within three attempts.

Scoring: Divide points earned by total possible points. Failure to perform a critical step that is indicated with an asterisk (*), will result in an unsatisfactory overall score.

Time began _____ **Time ended** _____

Steps	Possible Points	First Attempt	Second Attempt	Third Attempt
1. Wash and dry your hands. Put on face protection and nonsterile gloves.	5			
2. Assemble the materials needed.	5			
3. Fill two plain (blue-tipped) capillary tubes three fourths full with well-mixed EDTA anticoagulant blood.	10			
4. Plug the dry end of each tube with a sealing clay.	10			
5. Place the tubes opposite each other in the centrifuge, with sealed ends securely against the gasket.	10			
6. Note the numbers on the centrifuge slots and record them.	10			
7. Secure the locking top, fasten the lid down, and lock.	10			
8. Set the timer, and adjust the speed as needed.	10			
9. Allow the centrifuge to come to a complete stop. Unlock the lids.	5			
10. Remove the tubes immediately.	5			

Steps	Possible Points	First Attempt	Second Attempt	Third Attempt

11. Determine the microhematocrit values, using one of the following methods:
  a. Centrifuge with built-in reader using calibrated capillary tubes.
    1) Position the tubes as directed by manufacturer's instructions.
    2) Read both tubes.
    3) The average of the two results is reported.
    4) The two values should not vary by more than 2%.
  b Centrifuge without built-in reader.
    1) Carefully remove the tubes from the centrifuge.
    2) Place a tube on the microhematocrit reader.
    3) Align the clay–red blood cell junction with the zero line on the reader. Align the plasma meniscus with the 100% line. The value is read at the junction of the red cell layer and the buffy coat.*
    4) Read both tubes.
    5) The average of the two results is reported.
    6) The two values should not vary by more than 2%.
	5			

12. Dispose of the capillary tubes in a biohazard container.	5			
13. Clean the work area and properly dispose of all biohazard materials. Remove gloves and face protection and wash your hands.	5			
14. Record the results in the patient's medical record.	5			

Documentation in the Medical Record

_____

_____

_____

_____

Comments:

Total Points Earned _____ Divided by _____ Total Possible Points = _____ % Score

Instructor's Signature _____

Student Name _____ Date _____ Score _____

Procedure 29-2 Performing a Hemoglobin Test

Task: To accurately determine the level of hemoglobin present in a blood sample with the hemoglobinometer method.

Equipment and Supplies:
- Hemoglobinometer
- Reagent applicators
- Autolet or blood lancet
- Alcohol preps
- Gauze squares

Standards: Complete the procedure and all critical steps in _____ minutes with a minimum

score of _____ % within three attempts.

Scoring: Divide points earned by total possible points. Failure to perform a critical step that is indicated with an asterisk (*), will result in an unsatisfactory overall score.

Time began _____ **Time ended** _____

Steps	Possible Points	First Attempt	Second Attempt	Third Attempt
1. Wash and dry hands.	5			
2. Collect and assemble all equipment and supplies needed.	5			
3. Explain the procedure to the patient.	5			
4. Put on gloves.*	5			
5. Prepare the clipped chamber by slightly offsetting the cover slide to expose the chamber slide surface.	5			
6. Examine the fingers and choose the site to be used to obtain the blood sample.	5			
7. Clean the site with alcohol or other recommended antiseptic preparation.	5			
8. Perform a capillary puncture and obtain the blood sample.	5			
9. Wipe away the first drop of blood.	5			
10. Place one large drop of blood on the chamber slide. Do not touch the slide with the finger.	5			
11. Agitate the blood with a reagent stick until the blood appears shiny or transparent.	5			

Copyright © 2003, Elsevier Science (USA). All rights reserved.

515

Steps	Possible Points	First Attempt	Second Attempt	Third Attempt
12. Close the chamber and insert the chamber into the hemoglobinometer.	5			
13. Hold the device horizontally at eye level and turn on the light at the base of the unit with the left hand.	5			
14. Visualize the split green field through the viewer and with the right hand move the slide adjustment until there is no visible difference between the two hemispheres in the viewer.	10			
15. Read the scale on the right side of the instrument. Your reading will be in grams of hemoglobin per 100 ml of blood.	10			
16. Dispose of the biohazard waste in correct containers, and properly clean the hemoglobinometer chamber and work area. Return equipment to proper storage location.	5			
17. Remove gloves and wash hands.	5			
18. Record the test results in the patient's medical record.	5			

Documentation in the Medical Record

_____

_____

_____

_____

Comments:

Total Points Earned _____ Divided by _____ Total Possible Points = _____ % Score

Instructor's Signature _____

Procedure 29-3 Filling a Unopette©

Task: To properly fill a Unopette pipette with blood and to transfer the sample to a Unopette reservoir.

Equipment and Supplies:
- Unopette unit: capillary pipette, pipette shield, reservoir
- EDTA anticoagulant blood
- Gauze squares
- Test tube rack

Standards: Complete the procedure and all critical steps in _____ minutes with a minimum

score of _____ % within three attempts.

Scoring: Divide points earned by total possible points. Failure to perform a critical step that is indicated with an asterisk (*), will result in an unsatisfactory overall score.

Time began _____ **Time ended** _____

Steps	Possible Points	First Attempt	Second Attempt	Third Attempt
1. Wash and dry your hands, and put on face protection and nonsterile gloves.	5			
2. Remove a Unopette reservoir from the storage container, and recap the container tightly.	5			
3. Use the pipette shield to puncture the diaphragm of the Unopette reservoir. The hole must be large enough to allow the pipette to enter freely.	5			
4. Remove the pipette shield.	5			
5. Hold the pipette nearly horizontal.	5			
6. Place the tip of the pipette into a well-mixed tube of blood, and allow the pipette to fill by capillary action until blood reaches the end of the pipette. It will stop by itself.	5			
7. Place a finger over the hole in the end of the pipette to prevent loss of any sample, and carefully wipe the outside of the pipette with gauze to remove all traces of blood.	5			
8. Squeeze the reservoir with one hand.	5			
9. While holding your index finger over the hole in the top of the pipette, insert the pipette into the reservoir and seat it firmly in place with a twisting motion.	5			

Steps	Possible Points	First Attempt	Second Attempt	Third Attempt
10. Release the pressure on the reservoir, and remove your finger from the top of the pipette. The sample will be drawn into the reservoir.	10			
11. Gently squeeze and release the reservoir several times to rinse all blood from the pipette into the reservoir. Liquid should rise to the overflow chamber but should not be forced out of the top of the pipette.	10			
12. Mix the contents of the Unopette gently by inversion or by rolling between the palms of your hands.	5			
13. Identify the Unopette.	10			
14. Allow the Unopette to sit for the specified amount of time, as stated in the directions.	5			
15. Place the shield on the top of the prepared Unopette to prevent evaporation.	5			
16. Clean the work area by properly disposing of all biohazard materials. Remove the face protection and gloves and wash your hands.	5			
17. Record the test results in the patient's medical record.	5			

Documentation in the Medical Record

_____

_____

_____

_____

Comments:

Total Points Earned _____ Divided by _____ Total Possible Points = _____ % Score

Instructor's Signature _____

Procedure 29-4 Charging (Filling) a Hemacytometer

Task: To fill the hemacytometer for a manual cell count.

Equipment and Supplies:
- Neubauer ruled hemacytometer
- Hemacytometer coverslip
- Lint-free tissue
- 70% alcohol
- Blood-diluting pipette or Unopette

Standards: Complete the procedure and all critical steps in _____ minutes with a minimum

score of _____ % within three attempts.

Scoring: Divide points earned by total possible points. Failure to perform a critical step that is indicated with an asterisk (*), will result in an unsatisfactory overall score.

Time began _____ **Time ended** _____

Steps	Possible Points	First Attempt	Second Attempt	Third Attempt
1. Wash and dry your hands. Put on face protection and nonsterile gloves.	5			
2. Clean the hemacytometer and coverslip with 70% alcohol and lint-free tissue and thoroughly dry.	10			
3. Align the coverslip on the chamber.	10			
4. Convert to dropper assembly by withdrawing the pipette from the reservoir and reseating it securely in reverse position.	10			
5. To clean the capillary bore, invert the reservoir and gently squeeze the sides, expelling two drops from the well-mixed pipette or Unopette.	10			
6. Touch the tip of the pipette to the edge of the coverslip in the loading area of the chamber.	10			
7. Controlling the flow with the finger on the pipette or by gentle squeezing of the Unopette, fill the chamber in one smooth motion.	10			
8. Stop filling when the ruled area is full, and do not overfill.	10			
9. Fill both sides of the hemacytometer.	10			

Steps	Possible Points	First Attempt	Second Attempt	Third Attempt
10. Allow the chamber to sit undisturbed for 1 or 2 minutes so that the cells settle, but do not allow the sample to dry.	5			
11. Clean the work area by properly disposing of all biohazard materials.	5			
12. Record the test results in the patient's record.	5			

Documentation in the Medical Record

_____

_____

_____

_____

Comments:

Total Points Earned _____ Divided by _____ Total Possible Points = _____ % Score

Instructor's Signature _____

Procedure 29-5 Counting Cells in the Neubauer Ruled Hemacytometer

Task: To properly focus a hemacytometer, to locate the appropriate areas to count, and to direct your field of vision through the chamber in the proper manner while counting cells.

Equipment and Supplies:
- Properly filled hemacytometer
- Microscope
- Hand tally counter

Standards: Complete the procedure and all critical steps in _____ minutes with a minimum score of _____ % within three attempts.

Scoring: Divide points earned by total possible points. Failure to perform a critical step that is indicated with an asterisk (*), will result in an unsatisfactory overall score.

Time began _____ Time ended _____

Steps	Possible Points	First Attempt	Second Attempt	Third Attempt
1. Wash and dry your hands.	5			
2. Place the hemacytometer on the lowered microscope stage under low-power magnification.	5			
3. Center the ruled area over the opening in the stage.	5			
4. Reduce the light intensity by closing the diaphragm and lowering the condenser.	5			
5. Raise the stage carefully while watching from the side to be certain that the objective lens does not hit the coverslip.	5			
6. Focus and center the correct area (top left large W square for counting white blood cells), using the coarse adjustment and mechanical stage simultaneously.	5			
7. Adjust the light until the cells are easily visible.	5			

Steps	Possible Points	First Attempt	Second Attempt	Third Attempt
8. Count white blood cells under low power, by depressing the hand tally once for each cell seen. a) Begin in the top row, on the far left. b) Count the top row, moving visually from left to right. c) Count all cells within the boundaries of the square and also cells touching the top and the left-hand lines of the square. d) Do not count cells touching the right-hand lines or the bottom lines of the square. e) When you come to the end of the top row, drop to the second row. f) Count the second row, moving visually from right to left. g) Continue counting in this zigzag pattern, ending at the bottom left small square.	25			
9. When you have finished counting a large square, record the number.	5			
10. Return the tally to zero, move to the next large square, and begin to count.	5			
11. Switch to high power and focus with the fine adjustment for counting red blood cells (top left R square).	5			
12. Locate the remaining squares to be counted and determine the number of cells in each. For white blood cells, the counts from each square should vary by no more than 10 cells. For red blood cells, the numbers should vary by no more than 20 cells. Greater variation indicates an unevenly filled hemacytometer. In such cases, the chamber should be cleaned and refilled.	5			
13. Total the cells counted in all four squares for white blood cells and in five squares for red blood cells.	5			
14. Count the second side of the chamber in the same manner.	5			
15. Average the counts from both sides.	5			
16. Calculate the results. For red blood cells: average times 10,000 For white blood cells: average times 50	5			
17. Record the results in the patient's medical record.	5			

Documentation in the Medical Record

_____
_____
_____
_____

Comments:

Total Points Earned _____ Divided by _____ Total Possible Points = _____ % Score

Instructor's Signature _____

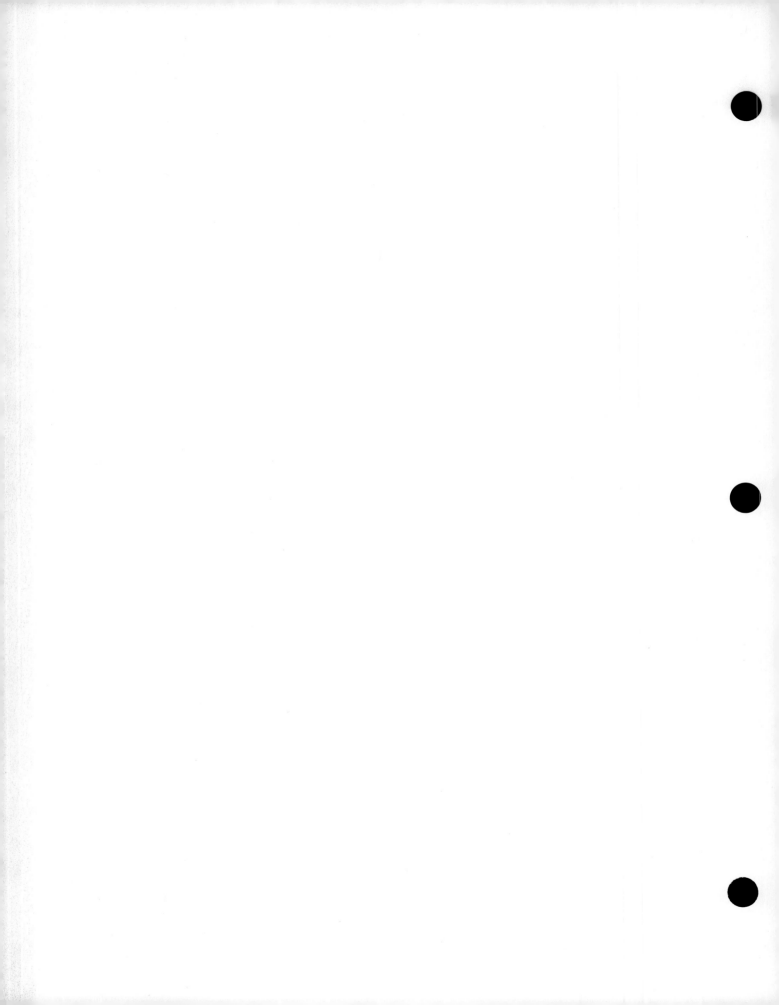

Procedure 29-6 Staining a Blood Smear with Wright's Stain

Task: To prepare and stain a slide that meets the criteria for the performance of a differential examination.

Equipment and Supplies:
- Clean glass slides
- Transfer pipette or capillary tube
- Wright's stain materials
- EDTA anticoagulant blood specimen

Standards: Complete the procedure and all critical steps in _____ minutes with a minimum score of _____ % within three attempts.

Scoring: Divide points earned by total possible points. Failure to perform a critical step that is indicated with an asterisk (*), will result in an unsatisfactory overall score.

Time began _____ Time ended _____

Steps	Possible Points	First Attempt	Second Attempt	Third Attempt
1. Wash and dry your hands. Put on face protection and nonsterile gloves.	5			
2. Assemble the materials needed.	5			
3. Mix the blood specimen.	5			
4. Use a transfer pipette or capillary tube to dispense a small drop of blood onto a slide, about ½ to ¾ inch from the right end.	5			
5. Hold one side of this slide with your nondominant hand.	5			
6. Use your dominant hand to place the spreader slide in front of the drop of blood at an angle of 30° to 35°.	5			
7. Pull back the spreader slide into the drop of blood and allow the blood to spread to the edges of the slide.	5			
8. Push the spreader slide forward with a quick smooth motion, maintaining the same angle throughout.	5			
9. Rapidly but gently wave the slide to accelerate the drying process.	5			
10. Stand the slide with the thick end down, and allow the slide to complete drying.	5			

Steps	Possible Points	First Attempt	Second Attempt	Third Attempt
11. Label the slide when it is dry. Use a pencil and write the name in the thick end of the smear.	5			
12. Stain according to method used. Two-step method: a) Place the smear on a staining rack, with the blood side up. b) Flood the smear with Wright's stain. c) Wait for 1 to 3 minutes. d) Add an equal amount of buffer, drop by drop, on top of the Wright's stain. e) Blow gently, and mix the two solutions until a green metallic sheen appears. This should appear within 2 to 4 minutes. f) Rinse thoroughly with distilled water. g) Drain water from the slide. h) Wipe the back of the smear with gauze. i) Stand the smear to dry. Quick stain: a) Place the smear into solutions according to the manufacturer's instructions b) Proceed with steps f through i just listed.	35			
13. Clean the work area. Properly dispose of all biohazard materials. Remove face protection and gloves. Wash your hands.	5			
14. Record the test results in the patient's medical record.	5			

Documentation in the Medical Record

_____

_____

_____

_____

Comments:

Total Points Earned _____ Divided by _____ Total Possible Points = _____ % Score

Instructor's Signature _____

Procedure 29-7 Performing Differential Examination of a Smear Stained with Wright's Stain

Task: To perform a differential cell count, evaluate the red blood cell morphology, and estimate the number of platelets.

Equipment and Supplies:
- Microscope
- Immersion oil
- Lens tissue
- Lens cleaner

Standards: Complete the procedure and all critical steps in _____ minutes with a minimum score of _____ % within three attempts.

Scoring: Divide points earned by total possible points. Failure to perform a critical step that is indicated with an asterisk (*), will result in an unsatisfactory overall score.

Time began _____ **Time ended** _____

Steps	Possible Points	First Attempt	Second Attempt	Third Attempt
1. Wash and dry your hands.	5			
2. Assemble the materials needed.	5			
3. Clean the microscope with lens tissue and lens cleaner.	5			
4. Place the slide on the stage, with the smear facing up.	5			
5. Locate an area of the smear where the red blood cells barely touch each other or slightly overlap, using the low-power objective.	5			
6. Focus under oil immersion with the fine-adjustment knob and increased light.	5			
7. Count 100 consecutive white blood cells in a winding pattern, identifying each cell encountered.	10			
8. Record each white cell on the differential cell counter by depressing the appropriate key for each cell.	15			

Steps	Possible Points	First Attempt	Second Attempt	Third Attempt
9. Evaluate the red blood cells observed in 10 fields. Record any variations in: Size—microcytosis, macrocytosis, anisocytosis Shape—poikilocytosis, ovalocytosis, target cells, sickle cells, etc. Content—normochromic or hypochromic	20			
10. Count the platelets in 10 fields, obtain an average, and multiply that average by 15,000 to give an estimate of the platelet count. The normal platelet count is 150,000 to 400,000/mm^3. Report the count as normal, decreased, or increased.	10			
11. Clean the microscope with lens tissue and lens cleaner.	5			
12. Clean the work area and properly dispose of all materials. Wash your hands.	5			
13. Record the testing results in the patient's record.	5			

Documentation in the Medical Record

_____

_____

_____

_____

Comments:

Total Points Earned _____ Divided by _____ Total Possible Points = _____ % Score

Instructor's Signature _____

Procedure 29-8 Determining a Sedimentation Rate by the Wintrobe Method

Task: To properly fill a Wintrobe tube and observe and record the findings of an erythrocyte sedimentation rate, using the Wintrobe method.

Equipment and Supplies:
• EDTA anticoagulant blood specimen
• Wintrobe tube
• Wintrobe rack
• Timer
• Pasteur pipette
• Bulb

Standards: Complete the procedure and all critical steps in _____ minutes with a minimum score of _____ % within three attempts.

Scoring: Divide points earned by total possible points. Failure to perform a critical step that is indicated with an asterisk (*), will result in an unsatisfactory overall score.

Time began _____ **Time ended** _____

Steps	Possible Points	First Attempt	Second Attempt	Third Attempt
1. Wash and dry your hands. Put on face protection and nonsterile gloves.	5			
2. Assemble the materials needed.	5			
3. Check the leveling bubble of the Wintrobe rack.	10			
4. Mix the blood well.	10			
5. Fill the Pasteur pipette with blood, and insert the tip of the pipette to the bottom of the Wintrobe tube.	10			
6. Fill the Wintrobe tube to the 0 mark by squeezing the bulb of the pipe.	10			
7. Slowly remove the pipette from the tube while keeping the tip of the pipette below the level of the blood.	10			
8. Place the tube in a numbered slot in the Wintrobe rack, and set the timer for 1 hour. The tube must be in a vertical position and free from all vibration.	10			
9. Measure the distance the erythrocytes have fallen after 1 hour. The ESR scale measures from 0 at the top to 100 at the bottom. Each line is 1 mm.	10			

Steps	Possible Points	First Attempt	Second Attempt	Third Attempt
10. Clean the work area and properly dispose of all biohazard materials. Remove face protection and gloves and wash your hands.	**10**			
11. Record the findings in the patient's medical record. Remember: The ESR is reported in millimeters per hour.	**10**			

Documentation in the Medical Record

_____

_____

_____

_____

Comments:

Total Points Earned _____ Divided by _____ Total Possible Points = _____ % Score

Instructor's Signature _____

Student Name _____ Date _____ Score _____

Procedure 29-9 Performing Mono-Test for Infectious Mononucleosis

Task: To perform and interpret a slide test for infectious mononucleosis.

Equipment and Supplies:
• Mono-test kit
• Blood specimen (serum or plasma)

Standards: Complete the procedure and all critical steps in _____ minutes with a minimum

score of _____ % within three attempts.

Scoring: Divide points earned by total possible points. Failure to perform a critical step that is indicated with an asterisk (*), will result in an unsatisfactory overall score.

Time began _____ **Time ended** _____

Steps	Possible Points	First Attempt	Second Attempt	Third Attempt
1. Wash and dry your hands. Glove and put on face protection.	5			
2. Remove the test kit from the refrigerator, and allow the reagents to warm to room temperature. Check the expiration date of the kit.	10			
3. Fill a disposable capillary tube to the calibration mark with serum or plasma. Using the rubber bulb included in the kit, deposit the specimen in the first circle of the clean glass slide also provided in the kit.	10			
4. Place one drop of negative control in the second circle and one drop of positive control in the third circle.	10			
5. Thoroughly mix the Mono-Test reagent by rolling the bottle gently between the palms of the hands. Squeeze the enclosed dropper to mix all the contents of the bottle.	10			
6. Hold the dropper in a vertical position, and add one drop of Mono-Test reagent to each area of the slide. Do not touch the dropper to the slide.	10			
7. Using separate stirrers, quickly and thoroughly mix each area, spreading each area out to 1 inch in diameter.	10			
8. Rock the slide gently for exactly 2 minutes; observe immediately for agglutination. A dark background is best for viewing.	10			

Steps	Possible Points	First Attempt	Second Attempt	Third Attempt
9. Interpret the test results, and record them. Agglutination is positive, and no agglutination is negative.	10			
10. Clean the work area. Remove gloves, and wash your hands.	10			
11. Record the test results in the patient's medical record.	5			

Documentation in the Medical Record

_____

_____

_____

_____

Comments:

Total Points Earned _____ Divided by _____ Total Possible Points = _____ % Score

Instructor's Signature _____

Procedure 29-10 Determining ABO Group Using a Slide Test

Task: To accurately determine a patient's ABO group using the slide test technique.

Equipment and Supplies:
- Glass slide with frosted ends
- Anti-A and anti-B serum
- Applicator sticks
- Lancet and automatic finger puncture device
- Alcohol preps
- Sterile gauze squares

Standards: Complete the procedure and all critical steps in _____ minutes with a minimum

score of _____ % within three attempts.

Scoring: Divide points earned by total possible points. Failure to perform a critical step that is indicated with an asterisk (*), will result in an unsatisfactory overall score.

Time began _____ **Time ended** _____

Steps	Possible Points	First Attempt	Second Attempt	Third Attempt
1. Reread the physician's orders and assemble all of the supplies and equipment needed to complete the testing procedure.	5			
2. Wash your hands and put on face protection and gloves.	5			
3. Explain the procedure to the patient.	5			
4. Label the slides in the frosted area with the patient's name.	5			
5. Place 1 drop of anti-A serum on slide #1, 1 drop of anti-B serum on slide #2, and 1 drop of anti-A and anti-B on slide #3.	10			
6. Select the puncture site and perform a finger puncture procedure.	10			
7. Wipe away the first drop of blood.	5			
8. Place one large drop of blood on each of the three prepared slides.	10			
9. Cover the puncture site with a sterile gauze square and instruct the patient to apply gentle pressure to the site.	10			
10. Mix the antiserum and blood thoroughly, using a clean applicator stick for each slide.	10			

Steps	Possible Points	First Attempt	Second Attempt	Third Attempt
11. Read and interpret the results of the reaction for all slides.	10			
12. Discard all biohazard testing waste in the appropriate container.	5			
13. Clean the testing area.	5			
14. Record the testing results in the patient's medical record.	5			

Documentation in the Medical Record

_____

_____

_____

_____

Comments:

Total Points Earned _____ Divided by _____ Total Possible Points = _____ % Score

Instructor's Signature _____

Procedure 29-11 Determining Rh Factor Using the Slide Method

Task: To accurately determine the presence or absence of anti-D agglutinations.

Equipment and Supplies:
- Two glass slides with frosted ends
- Anti-D serum
- Applicator sticks
- Lancet and automatic finger puncture device
- Alcohol preps
- Sterile gauze squares
- Laboratory marker or pencil

Standards: Complete the procedure and all critical steps in _____ minutes with a minimum

score of _____ % within three attempts.

Scoring: Divide points earned by total possible points. Failure to perform a critical step that is indicated with an asterisk (*), will result in an unsatisfactory overall score.

Time began _____ **Time ended** _____

Steps	Possible Points	First Attempt	Second Attempt	Third Attempt
1. Check the physician's order and assemble all of the equipment and supplies needed to complete the testing procedure.	5			
2. Wash your hands and put on face protection and gloves.	5			
3. Label one slide "D" and one slide "C."	5			
4. Place 1 drop of anti-D serum on the "D" slide.	5			
5. Place 1 drop of the appropriate control reagent on the "C" slide.	10			
6. Perform a capillary puncture to secure a blood specimen.	10			
7. To each slide, add 2 drops of the patient's blood.	10			
8. Thoroughly mix the blood with the anti-D serum, using a clean applicator stick for each slide, and spread the reaction mixture over an area measuring approximately 20 × 40 mm on each slide.	10			
9. Read the results immediately.	10			

Steps	Possible Points	First Attempt	Second Attempt	Third Attempt
10. Discard all disposable equipment in the proper biohazardous waste containers.	10			
11. Clean area. Remove gloves and wash your hands.	10			
12. Record the testing results in the patient's medical record.	10			

Documentation in the Medical Record

_____

_____

_____

_____

Comments:

Total Points Earned _____ Divided by _____ Total Possible Points = _____ % Score

Instructor's Signature _____

Procedure 29-12 Performing a Blood Glucose Accu-Check Test

Task: To accurately perform a blood test for possible diabetes mellitus.

Equipment and Supplies:
- Accu-Check glucose monitor or similar glucose monitoring device
- Accu-Check glucose testing strip
- Lancet and autoloading finger-puncturing device
- Alcohol preps
- Gauze squares

Standards: Complete the procedure and all critical steps in _____ minutes with a minimum

score of _____ % within three attempts.

Scoring: Divide points earned by total possible points. Failure to perform a critical step that is indicated with an asterisk (*), will result in an unsatisfactory overall score.

Time began _____ **Time ended** _____

Steps	Possible Points	First Attempt	Second Attempt	Third Attempt
1. Reread the physician's order and collect the necessary equipment and supplies needed to complete the testing procedure.	5			
2. Wash your hands and put on gloves.	5			
3. Ask the patient to wash his or her hands in warm soapy water, then to rinse them in warm water, and dry them completely.	5			
4. Check the patient's index and ring fingers and select the site for puncture.	5			
5. Turn on the Accu-Check monitor by pressing the ON button.	5			
6. Make sure the code number on the LED display matches the code number on the container of testing strips.	5			
7. Remove a testing strip from the vial and immediately replace the vial cover.	5			
8. Check the strip for discoloration by comparing the color of the round window on the back of the testing strip with the designated "unused" color chart provided on the test strip vial label.	5			

Steps	Possible Points	First Attempt	Second Attempt	Third Attempt
9. When the test strip symbol begins flashing in the lower right-hand corner of the display screen, insert the test strip into the designated testing slot until it locks into place. When the test strip is inserted correctly, the arrows on the test strip will be facing up and pointing toward the monitor.	5			
10. Cleanse the selected site on the patient's finger-tip with the alcohol wipe and allow the finger to air dry.	5			
11. Perform the finger puncture and wipe away the first drop of blood.	5			
12. Apply a large hanging drop of blood to the center of the yellow testing pad. a. Do not touch the pad with the patient's finger. b. Do not apply a second drop of blood. c. Do not smear the blood with your finger. d. Be certain the yellow test pad is saturated with blood.	30			
13. Give the patient a gauze square to hold securely over the puncture site.	5			
14. The monitor will automatically begin the measurement process as soon as it senses the drop of blood.	5			
15. Read the test result when it is displayed in the display window in milligrams per deciliter. Turn off the monitor by pressing the "O" button.	5			

Documentation in the Medical Record

_____

_____

_____

_____

Comments:

Total Points Earned _____ Divided by _____ Total Possible Points = _____ % Score

Instructor's Signature _____

Procedure 29-13 Determining Cholesterol Level Using a ProAct Testing Device

Task: To accurately perform and report a ProAct test for cholesterol level.

Equipment and Supplies:
• ProAct testing device
• Lithium heparin capillary tube and capillary pipettor
• Lancets and lancet device
• Sterile gauze
• Alcohol preps
• Biohazard waste container
• Biohazard sharps container

Standards: Complete the procedure and all critical steps in _____ minutes with a minimum

score of _____ % within three attempts.

Scoring: Divide points earned by total possible points. Failure to perform a critical step that is indicated with an asterisk (*), will result in an unsatisfactory overall score.

Time began _____ **Time ended** _____

Steps	Possible Points	First Attempt	Second Attempt	Third Attempt
1. Reread the physician's order and assemble all the supplies and equipment needed to complete the test.	5			
2. Wash your hands and put on gloves.	5			
3. Explain the procedure to the patient.	5			
4. Load the lancet device with a sterile lancet.	5			
5. Examine the patient's index and ring fingers and pick a puncture site.	5			
6. Cleanse the chosen puncture site with alcohol and allow the site to air dry.	5			
7. Puncture the site and wipe away the first drop of blood with a sterile gauze square.	5			
8. Give the patient a clean gauze square and ask the patient to apply pressure to the puncture site.	5			
9. Remove a cholesterol testing strip from the container and close the container immediately	5			

Steps	Possible Points	First Attempt	Second Attempt	Third Attempt
10. Remove the foil protecting the test area of the strip and place the strip on a dry, hard, flat surface.	5			
11. Attach the capillary tube filled with blood to the pipettor.	5			
12. Squeeze the plunger of the pipettor completely to allow a drop of blood to form at the end of the capillary tube.	5			
13. Allow the drop of blood to fall onto the center of the red mesh application zone. Make sure that the tip of the capillary tube does not touch the test strip and that all blood is dispensed.	5			
14. Allow the sample to soak into the red mesh for 3 to 15 seconds.	5			
15. Insert the cholesterol strip into the test port. The ProAct device will count down approximately 160 seconds.	5			
16. Remove the capillary tube from the pipettor and discard it in a biohazard container.	5			
17. When the measurement time is completed, REMOVE STRIP will appear in the LED display window. Remove the used test strip and the test result will appear on the display.	5			
18. Examine the test area of the used testing strip for uneven color development before discarding it into the biohazard waste container.	5			
19. Discard all biohazard testing waste in appropriate containers, clean the testing area, remove gloves, and wash your hands.	5			
20. Record the test results in the patient's medical record.	5			

Documentation in the Medical Record

_____

_____

_____

_____

Comments:

Total Points Earned _____ Divided by _____ Total Possible Points = _____ % Score

Instructor's Signature _____

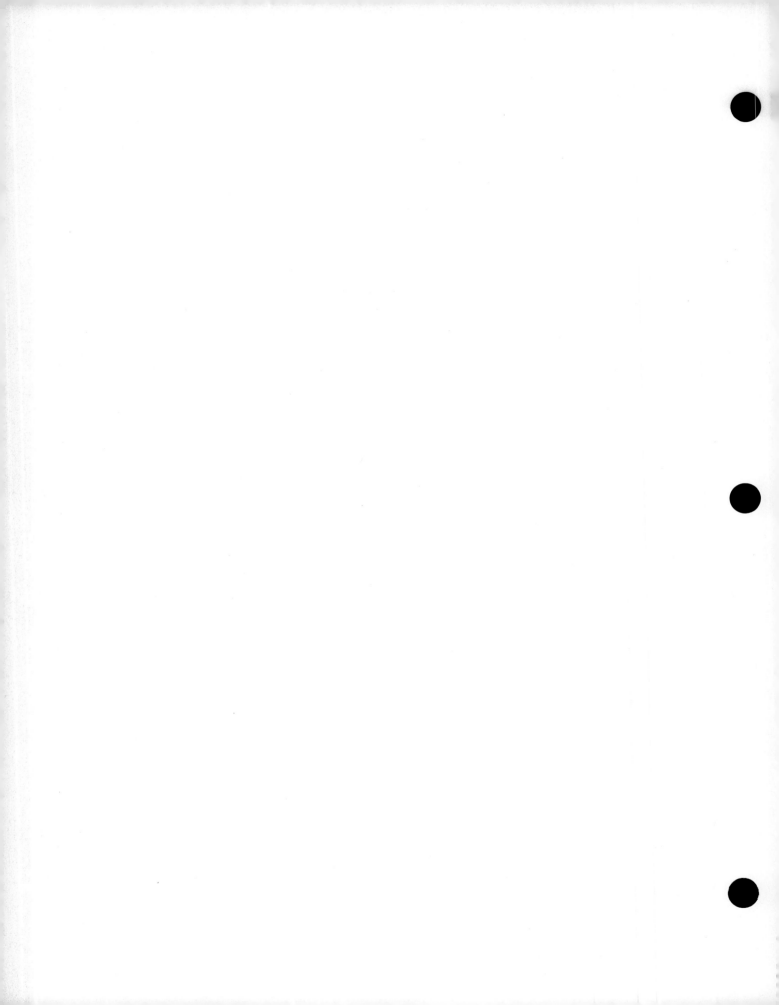

Procedure 30-1 Preparing a Direct Smear or Culture Smear for Staining

Task: To prepare a smear for staining from a clinical specimen or from a culture medium.

Equipment and Supplies:
- Clean glass slides
- Permanent marker
- Incinerator
- Normal saline solution
- Specimen collected on a smear
- 24 hour culture on agar

Standards: Complete the procedure and all critical steps in _____ minutes with a minimum

score of _____ % within three attempts.

Scoring: Divide points earned by total possible points. Failure to perform a critical step that is indicated with an asterisk (*), will result in an unsatisfactory overall score.

Time began _____ Time ended _____

Steps	Possible Points	First Attempt	Second Attempt	Third Attempt
1. Wash and dry your hands. Glove and put on face protection.	5			
2. Label the slide with a permanent marking pen.	5			
Direct Smear				
3. Prepare a thin smear by rolling the swab on the slide. Make certain that all areas of the swab touch the slide.	10			
4. Allow the smear to air dry. Do not wave it or heat-dry it.	10			
5. Hold the slide with the smear up. Heat-fix the slide using an incinerator. Check the heating process by touching the slide to the back of the hand. The slide should feel warm, not hot. Check it often by touching the back of the slide to the back of the hand. Cool the slide.	10			
Culture Smear				
6. Identify the colonies to be stained by circling them on the back of the plate and numbering them with a permanent marker. Label the slide accordingly.	10			

Steps	Possible Points	First Attempt	Second Attempt	Third Attempt
7. Apply a small drop of saline solution to the slide, using a loop.	10			
8. Touch, with a sterile loop, only the top of the colony chosen. Transfer the material picked up to the appropriate area of the slide, and spread it in a circular motion to the size of a dime. Repeat for each colony chosen using a separate slide.	10			
9. Allow the smear to air dry.	10			
10. Heat-fix the smear.	10			

Both Methods

Steps	Possible Points	First Attempt	Second Attempt	Third Attempt
11. Properly dispose of all biohazard materials and clean the work area.	5			
12. Remove gloves and wash your hands.	5			

Documentation in the Medical Record

_____

_____

_____

_____

Comments:

Total Points Earned _____ Divided by _____ Total Possible Points = _____ % Score

Instructor's Signature _____

Procedure 30-2 Staining a Smear with Gram Stain

Task: To stain a slide, using the Gram stain, so that the organisms present are colored appropriately.

Equipment and Supplies:
- Gram stain reagents
- Staining rack
- Forceps
- Wash bottle of water
- Prepared smear for staining
- Absorbent paper

Standards: Complete the procedure and all critical steps in _____ minutes with a minimum

score of _____ % within three attempts.

Scoring: Divide points earned by total possible points. Failure to perform a critical step that is indicated with an asterisk (*), will result in an unsatisfactory overall score.

Time began _____ **Time ended** _____

Steps	Possible Points	First Attempt	Second Attempt	Third Attempt
1. Wash and dry your hands.	5			
2. Place the slide face up on a level staining rack.	5			
3. Flood the slide with crystal violet. Time for 30 seconds.	10			
4. Flood the stain off with a sharp stream of water from the wash bottle. With forceps, tip the slide to remove the water.	10			
5. Flood the slide with Gram's iodine (mordant). Time for 30 seconds.	10			
6. Flood the iodine off with water. Grasp the slide with forceps, and hold it nearly vertical.	10			
7. Decolorize by running the decolorizer (alcohol) down the slide until the smear stops, giving off purple stain in all but the thickest portions (about 10 seconds).	10			
8. Rinse the slide with water, and return it to the staining rack.	5			
9. Flood the slide with safranin, and time for 30 seconds.				

Steps	Possible Points	First Attempt	Second Attempt	Third Attempt
10. Rinse the slide well with water.	5			
11. Wipe off the back of the slide with an alcohol tissue.	5			
12. Blot the slide dry between sheets of absorbent paper.	5			
13. Clean the work area. Remove gloves and wash your hands.	5			
14. Record the procedure in the patient's record.	5			

Documentation in the Medical Record

_____

_____

_____

_____

Comments:

Total Points Earned _____ Divided by _____ Total Possible Points = _____ % Score

Instructor's Signature _____

Procedure 30-3 Inoculating a Blood Agar Plate for Culture of *Streptococcus pyogens*

Task: To inoculate a blood agar plate for the detection of the etiologic agent of strep throat.

Equipment and Supplies:
- Blood agar plate
- Bacitracin disk or
- Blood agar plate
- Bacitracin disk or strep A disk
- Incinerator
- Inoculating loop
- Permanent marker
- Swab from patient's throat

Standards: Complete the procedure and all critical steps in _____ minutes with a minimum

score of _____ % within three attempts.

Scoring: Divide points earned by total possible points. Failure to perform a critical step that is indicated with an asterisk (*), will result in an unsatisfactory overall score.

Time began _____ **Time ended** _____

Steps	Possible Points	First Attempt	Second Attempt	Third Attempt
1. Wash and dry your hands. Glove and apply face protection.	5			
2. Remove the swab from the container. Grasp the plate by the bottom (media side), and lift the cover, or lift the cover while the plate is on the table.	10			
3. Roll the swab down the middle of the top half of the plate, then use the swab to streak the same half of the plate. Dispose of the swab properly.	10			
4. Sterilize the loop in the Bacti-cinerator, and allow it to cool.	10			
5. Streak for isolation of colonies in the third and fourth quadrants, using the loop. Use the loop to make three slices in the agar in the area of heavy inoculum. Sterilize the loop.	10			
6. Sterilize the forceps and remove one disk from the vial. Place the disk on the agar in the first quadrant. Sterilize the forceps.	10			

Steps	Possible Points	First Attempt	Second Attempt	Third Attempt
7. Label with permanent marker the agar side of the plate with the patient's name and identification number and the date.	10			
8. Place the plate in the incubator, with the agar side of the plate on the top.	10			
9. Record all information in the patient's medical record.	10			
10. Incubate for 24 hours and then examine. Incubate negative cultures for an additional 24 hours.	10			
11. Clean the work area and properly dispose of all biohazard waste. Remove your gloves and wash your hands.	5			

Documentation in the Medical Record

_____

_____

_____

_____

Comments:

Total Points Earned _____ Divided by _____ Total Possible Points = _____ % Score

Instructor's Signature _____

Procedure 30-4 Performing a Rapid Strep Test

Task: To perform a rapid strep test to assist in the diagnosis of strep throat.

Equipment and Supplies:
- Directigen Strep A test kit
- Timer or wristwatch with sweep second hand
- Throat swab specimen

Standards: Complete the procedure and all critical steps in _____ minutes with a minimum

score of _____ % within three attempts.

Scoring: Divide points earned by total possible points. Failure to perform a critical step that is indicated with an asterisk (*), will result in an unsatisfactory overall score.

Time began _____ **Time ended** _____

Steps	Possible Points	First Attempt	Second Attempt	Third Attempt
1. Collect all supplies and equipment needed to perform the test. Bring all reagents and reaction disks to room temperature (minimum of 30 minutes).	5			
2. Wash and dry your hands. Put on gloves and face protection.	5			
3. Position all bottles vertically, and dispense reagents slowly as free-falling drops. Avoid reagent contact with your eyes because the reagent is an irritant.	5			
4. Add 3 drops of reagent 1 to an extraction tube. This solution is pink.	10			
5. Add 3 drops of reagent 2 to the same tube. The solution should turn yellow.	10			
6. Place the specimen swab in the tube, twirling the swab in the mix.	5			
7. Let stand for exactly 1 minute.	5			
8. Add 3 drops of reagent 3 to the same tube, again twirling the swab in the tube to mix. This solution should be pink.	10			
9. Express the liquid from the swab by squeezing the tube with the thumb and forefinger and rotating the swab as it is withdrawn. The liquid must be thoroughly removed from the swab. Best results are achieved when the liquid reaches or exceeds the line on the tube.	10			

Steps	Possible Points	First Attempt	Second Attempt	Third Attempt
10. Discard the swab in a biohazard waste container.	5			
11. Remove the reaction disk from the pouch and place it on a dry, flat surface.	5			
12. Pour the entire contents of the tube into the reaction disk.	5			
13. Read the test results when the entire end of assay window turns red (5 to 10 minutes).	5			
14. Properly dispose of all contaminated waste.	5			
15. Clean work area, remove gloves, and wash your hands.	5			
16. Record the test results in the patient's medical record.	5			

Documentation in the Medical Record

_____

_____

_____

_____

Comments:

Total Points Earned _____ Divided by _____ Total Possible Points = _____ % Score

Instructor's Signature _____

Procedure 30-5 The Urine Culture

Task: To include three plates with one microliter of urine in order to quantitate the number of bacteria and aid in the diagnosis of a urinary tract infection.

Equipment and Supplies:
- Urine specimen, collected CCMS in a sterile container
- Bacti-cinerator
- Microliter calibrated inoculating loop
- Blood agar plate, MacConkey agar plate, and Columbia nutrient agar plate

Standards: Complete the procedure and all critical steps in _____ minutes with a minimum score of _____ % within three attempts.

Scoring: Divide points earned by total possible points. Failure to perform a critical step that is indicated with an asterisk (*), will result in an unsatisfactory overall score.

Time began _____ **Time ended** _____

Steps	Possible Points	First Attempt	Second Attempt	Third Attempt
1. Wash and dry your hands. Glove and apply face protection.	5			
2. With the screw cap lid in place, mix the urine specimen thoroughly by swirling.	5			
3. Sterilize the calibrated loop, cool, and dip the tip into the specimen.	10			
4. Deposit the specimen on the plate.	10			
5. Inoculate the second and third plates in the same manner.	10			
6. Label the bottom of the plates with the patient's name and identification number and the date.	10			
7. Record all information in the patient's medical record.	10			
8. Place the plates in the incubator, with the agar sides of the plates facing up.	10			
9. Incubate for 24 hours, then count the colonies on the all-purpose medium.	10			

Steps	Possible Points	First Attempt	Second Attempt	Third Attempt
10. Interpret the count • >100 colonies = >100,000 colony forming units (cfu)/ ml of urine indicates a urinary tract infection • 10–100 colonies = 10,000 to 100,000 cfu/ml of urine indicates suspicion. The urine may have been allowed to stand at room temperature which facilitated overgrowth of bacteria or the patient may have a subclinical infection. Recollection of the specimen is recommended. • (10 colonies = 10,000 cfu/ml of urine and indicates normal urethral microbiota)	10			
11. Clean the work area, dispose of all biohazard waste, remove gloves, and wash your hands.	5			
12. Record procedure in patient's medical record.	5			

Documentation in the Medical Record

_____

_____

_____

_____

Comments:

Total Points Earned _____ Divided by _____ Total Possible Points = _____ % Score

Instructor's Signature _____

Procedure 30-6 Performing a Cellulose Tape Collection for Pinworms

Task: To obtain a rectal sample using cellulose tape for the purpose of testing for pinworm eggs.

Equipment and Supplies:
- Glass slide
- Clear cellulose tape
- Wooden tongue depressor
- Toluene
- Microscope
- Gauze or cotton balls

Standards: Complete the procedure and all critical steps in _____ minutes with a minimum score of _____ % within three attempts.

Scoring: Divide points earned by total possible points. Failure to perform a critical step that is indicated with an asterisk (*), will result in an unsatisfactory overall score.

Time began _____ **Time ended** _____

Steps	Possible Points	First Attempt	Second Attempt	Third Attempt
1. Gather and prepare supplies and equipment needed for obtaining the specimen.	5			
2. Place a strip of cellulose tape on a glass slide, starting 1/2 inch from one end and running toward the same end. Continuing around this end lengthwise. Tear off the strip so that it is even with the other end. Note: Do not use Magic transparent tape; use regular clear cellulose tape.	10			
3. Place a strip of paper measuring 1/2 × 1 inch between the slide and the tape at the end where the tape is torn flush. This will be the specimen labeling area.	10			
4. Wash hands, glove, and apply face protection.	10			
5. Remove the clothing and diaper from the child and lay the child in a prone position, over the parent's lap, with the buttocks in a superior plane.	10			
6. To obtain the perianal sample, first peel back the tape on the slide by gripping the label. With the tape looped (adhesive side outward) over a wooden tongue depressor that is held against the slide and extended about 1 inch beyond it, press the tape firmly against the right and left anal folds.	10			

Steps	Possible Points	First Attempt	Second Attempt	Third Attempt
7. Spread the tape back on the slide, adhesive side down.	5			
8. Smooth the tape using a cotton ball or gauze square.	5			
9. Write the patient's name and date on the slide label.	5			
10. Advise the parent that the child can be dressed or assist with dressing the child if needed.	5			

Testing the Sample

11. Lift one side of the tape and apply 1 drop of toluene before pressing the tape back down on the glass slide.	10			
12. Place the prepared slide under the microscope's low-power objective and examine it under low illumination.	5			
13. Report and record your findings in the patient's record as a positive result if pinworm eggs were visualized and a negative result if no eggs were seen.	5			
14. Dispose of all biohazard waste, clean the work area, remove gloves, and wash your hands.	5			

Documentation in the Medical Record

_____

_____

_____

_____

Comments:

Total Points Earned _____ Divided by _____ Total Possible Points = _____ % Score

Instructor's Signature _____

Procedure 31-1 Identifying Surgical Instruments

Task: To identify, correctly spell, and determine the use(s) of standard office instruments or those selected by your instructor.

Equipment and Supplies:
• Curved hemostat
• Straight hemostat
• Dressing (thumb) forceps
• Paper and pencil
• Scalpel and blade
• Dissecting scissors
• Towel clamp
• Vaginal speculum
• Bandage scissors
• Allis tissue forceps

Standards: Complete the procedure and all critical steps in _____ minutes with a minimum score of _____ % within three attempts.

Scoring: Divide points earned by total possible points. Failure to perform a critical step that is indicated with an asterisk (*), will result in an unsatisfactory overall score.

Time began _____ **Time ended** _____

Steps	Possible Points	First Attempt	Second Attempt	Third Attempt
1. Look for the following parts that determine usage: box-lock, serrations, finger rings, cutting edge, noncutting edge, thumb type, teeth ratchets, and electric attachments.	10			
2. Consider the general classification of the instrument: cutting and dissection, grasping and clamping, retracting, or probing and dilating.	10			
3. Carefully examine the teeth and serrations.	10			
4. Look at the length of the instrument to determine the area of the body for which it is used.	10			
5. Try to remember whether the instrument was named for a famous physician, university, or clinic.	10			
6. If the instrument is a pair of scissors, look at the points and determine whether the tips are sharp-sharp, sharp-blunt, or blunt-blunt.	10			
7. Carefully compare the instrument with similar instruments that you know, to determine whether it is in the same category or has the same name.	10			
8. Write, with correct spelling, the complete name of each instrument, including its category and usage.	30			

Documentation in the Medical Record

_____

_____

_____

_____

Comments:

Total Points Earned _____ Divided by _____ Total Possible Points = _____ % Score

Instructor's Signature _____

Procedure 32-1 Wrapping Instruments and Supplies for Steam Sterilization in an Autoclave

Task: To place dry, checked, sanitized supplies and instruments inside appropriate wrapping materials for sterilization and storage without contamination.

Equipment and Supplies:
- Dry, checked, sanitized items
- Assorted wrapping materials
- Autoclave tape
- Indicator tape
- A waterproof felt-tipped pen

Standards: Complete the procedure and all critical steps in _____ minutes with a minimum

score of _____ % within three attempts.

Scoring: Divide points earned by total possible points. Failure to perform a critical step that is indicated with an asterisk (*), will result in an unsatisfactory overall score.

Time began _____ **Time ended** _____

Steps	Possible Points	First Attempt	Second Attempt	Third Attempt
1. Collect and assemble items to be wrapped.	5			
2. Place the wrapper to be used on a clean flat surface.	5			
3. Place the item(s) diagonally at the approximate center of the wrapping material. Make sure the size of the square is large enough for the items.	10			
4. With the squares that are cloth fabric, use two pieces if the cloth is single-layered, or follow the manufacturer's recommendation when using commercial autoclave wrapping paper.	10			
5. Open slightly any hinged instruments. If the instrument is sharp, its teeth or tip should be shielded with cotton or gauze.	10			
6. If the package is to contain several items, place a commercial sterilization indicator inside the package at the approximate center.	10			
7. Bring up the bottom corner of the wrap and fold back a portion of it.	10			
8. Fold over the right corner and turn back a portion of it. Fold over the left corner and turn back a portion of it.	10			

Steps	Possible Points	First Attempt	Second Attempt	Third Attempt
9. Fold the last flap over.	10			
10. Secure with autoclave tape.	10			
11. Secure with autoclave tape and label package with the date including year, contents, and your initials.	10			

Documentation in the Medical Record

_____

_____

_____

_____

Comments:

Total Points Earned _____ Divided by _____ Total Possible Points = _____ % Score

Instructor's Signature _____

Procedure 32-2 Operating the Autoclave

Task: To sterilize properly prepared supplies and instruments by using the autoclave.

Equipment and Supplies:
• An autoclave
• Wrapped items ready to be sterilized

Standards: Complete the procedure and all critical steps in _____ minutes with a minimum

score of _____ % within three attempts.

Scoring: Divide points earned by total possible points. Failure to perform a critical step that is indicated with an asterisk (*), will result in an unsatisfactory overall score.

Time began _____ **Time ended** _____

Steps	Possible Points	First Attempt	Second Attempt	Third Attempt
1. Check the water level in the reservoir and add distilled water as necessary.	5			
2. Turn the control to "fill" to allow water to flow into the chamber. The water will flow until you turn the control to its next position. Do not let the water overflow.	5			
3. Load the chamber with wrapped items, then space them for maximum circulation and penetration.	5			
4. Close and seal the door.	5			
5. Turn the control setting to "on" or "autoclave" to start the cycle.	5			
6. Watch the gauges until the temperature gauge reaches at least 250°F (121°C) and the pressure gauge reaches 15 pounds of pressure.	10			
7. Set the timer for the desired time.	10			
8. At the end of the timed cycle, turn the control setting to "vent."	10			
9. Wait for the pressure gauge to reach zero.	10			
10. Open the chamber door a fourth of an inch.	10			
11. Leave the autoclave control at "vent" to continue producing heat.	10			
12. Allow complete drying of all items.	5			

Steps	Possible Points	First Attempt	Second Attempt	Third Attempt
13. Using heat-resistant gloves or pads, remove the items from the chamber and place the sterilized packages on dry, covered shelves, or open door and allow items to cool.	5			
14. Turn the control knob to "off" and keep the door slightly ajar.	5			

Documentation in the Medical Record

_____

_____

_____

_____

Comments:

Total Points Earned _____ Divided by _____ Total Possible Points = _____ % Score

Instructor's Signature _____

Procedure 32-3 Performing Surgical Hand Scrub

Task: To scrub your hands with surgical soap, using friction, running water, and a sterile brush to sanitize your skin before assisting with any procedure that requires surgical asepsis

Equipment and Supplies:
- Sink with foot or arm control for running water
- Surgical soap in a dispenser
- Towels
- Nail file or orange stick
- Sterile brush

Standards: Complete the procedure and all critical steps in _____ minutes with a minimum

score of _____ % within three attempts.

Scoring: Divide points earned by total possible points. Failure to perform a critical step that is indicated with an asterisk (*), will result in an unsatisfactory overall score.

Time began _____ **Time ended** _____

Steps	Possible Points	First Attempt	Second Attempt	Third Attempt
1. Remove all jewelry.	5			
2. Inspect your fingernails for length and your hands for skin breaks.	5			
3. Turn on the faucet and regulate the water to a comfortable temperature.	5			
4. Keep your hands upright and held at or above waist level.	5			
5. Clean your fingernails with a file, discard it, and rinse your hands under the faucet without touching the faucet or the insides of the sink basin.	5			
6. Allow water to run over your hands, apply acceptable solution, lather while holding your fingertips upward, and remember to rub between the fingers.	5			
7. Wash wrists and forearms while holding your hands above waist level. Rinse arms and forearms without touching the faucet or the insides of the sink basin.	10			
8. Apply more solution and repeat the scrub on the other side, remembering to wash and use friction between each finger with a firm, circular motion.	10			

Steps	Possible Points	First Attempt	Second Attempt	Third Attempt
9. Scrub all surfaces with a brush, being careful not to abrade your skin. The second washing process should take at least 3 minutes.	10			
10. Rinse thoroughly, keeping your hands up and above waist level. Discard scrub brush.	10			
11. Turn off the faucet with the foot or forearm lever, if available.	10			
12. Dry one hand with a sterile towel; use the opposite end of the towel for the other hand.	10			
13. Using a patting motion, continue to dry the forearms. Discard the towel and keep your hands up and above waist level.	10			

Comments:

Total Points Earned _____ Divided by _____ Total Possible Points = _____ % Score

Instructor's Signature _____

Procedure 32-4 Putting on Sterile Gloves

Task: To apply your own sterile gloves before performing sterile procedures.

Equipment and Supplies:
• A pair of packaged sterile gloves in your size

Standards: Complete the procedure and all critical steps in _____ minutes with a minimum

score of _____ % within three attempts.

Scoring: Divide points earned by total possible points. Failure to perform a critical step that is indicated with an asterisk (*), will result in an unsatisfactory overall score.

Time began _____ **Time ended** _____

Steps	Possible Points	First Attempt	Second Attempt	Third Attempt
1. Open your glove pack. Remember, a 1-inch area around the perimeter of the glove wrapper is considered not sterile.	5			
2. Perform the surgical hand scrub.	5			
3. Dry your hands well.	5			
4. Glove your dominant hand first.	5			
5. With your nondominant hand, pick up the glove for your dominant hand with your thumb and forefinger, grabbing the top of the folded cuff, which is the inside of the glove.	10			
6. Lift the glove up and away from the sterile package.	10			
7. Hold your hands away from you and slide your dominant hand into the glove.	10			
8. Leave the cuff folded.	5			
9. With your gloved dominant hand, pick up the second glove by slipping your gloved fingers under the cuff so that your gloved hand only touches the outside of the second glove.	10			
10. Slide your nondominant hand into the glove, without touching the exterior of the glove or any part of your hand.	10			

Steps	Possible Points	First Attempt	Second Attempt	Third Attempt
11. Still holding your hands away from you, unroll the cuff by slipping the fingers up and out. Stay away from your bare arm.	10			
12. Now, slip your gloved fingers up under the first cuff and unroll it, using the same technique.	5			

Comments:

Total Points Earned _____ Divided by _____ Total Possible Points = _____ % Score

Instructor's Signature _____

Procedure 32-5 Donning a Sterile Gown

Task: To don a sterile gown before assisting with a surgical procedure.

Equipment and Supplies:
• terile gown and gloves (opened on a counter or Mayo stand, in an open area to dress)

Note: A mask and goggles and hair cover are also worn.

Standards: Complete the procedure and all critical steps in _____ minutes with a minimum

score of _____ % within three attempts.

Scoring: Divide points earned by total possible points. Failure to perform a critical step that is indicated with an asterisk (*), will result in an unsatisfactory overall score.

Time began _____ **Time ended** _____

Steps	Possible Points	First Attempt	Second Attempt	Third Attempt
1. Scrub, using aseptic technique. Remember to keep hands up and above waist level.	10			
2. Grasp the sterile gown by the collar and gently lift it from the sterile gown wrapper.	20			
3. Hold the gown away from your body. Allow it to gently unfold, grasping only the inside of the gown.	20			
4. Slip your hands into the sleeve openings. Remember to touch only the inside of the gown.	20			
5. The hands and forearms are advanced only to the edge of the gown cuff.	10			
6. The circulating assistant touches only the inside of the gown, pulling the gown over the scrub assistant's shoulders.	10			
7. The waistline and neck ties are tied.	10			

Comments:

Total Points Earned _____ Divided by _____ Total Possible Points = _____ % Score

Instructor's Signature _____

Procedure 32-6 Gloving with a Sterile Gown On

Task: To apply sterile gloves while dressed in a sterile gown before assisting with a surgical procedure.

Equipment and Supplies:
• Sterile gloves, opened on a sterile field

Note: A mask, goggles, hair cover, and a sterile gown are worn. The gloves are applied with the hands covered by the sterile gown to avoid contamination.

Standards: Complete the procedure and all critical steps in _____ minutes with a minimum

score of _____ % within three attempts.

Scoring: Divide points earned by total possible points. Failure to perform a critical step that is indicated with an asterisk (*), will result in an unsatisfactory overall score.

Time began _____ **Time ended** _____

Steps	Possible Points	First Attempt	Second Attempt	Third Attempt
1. Glove your nondominant hand first.	5	_____	_____	_____
2. Lift the glove with your dominant hand and use your thumb and forefinger to grasp the top of the folded cuff. Remember, your hands are covered with the sterile gown sleeves.	10	_____	_____	_____
3. Place the glove in the palm of your nondominant hand, with glove fingers pointing to elbows.	10	_____	_____	_____
4. Grasp the inside of the cuff with your fingers and gently stretch the glove cuff.	10	_____	_____	_____
5. Pull the glove over your hand as you push your arm through the gown cuff.	10	_____	_____	_____
6. Gently slide your fingers in the glove.	10	_____	_____	_____
7. With your nondominant gloved hand, slip your fingers under the cuff of the second glove.	10	_____	_____	_____
8. Follow steps 3, 4, 5, and 6 for the second glove.	10	_____	_____	_____
9. The cuffs may now be adjusted.	10	_____	_____	_____

Steps	Possible Points	First Attempt	Second Attempt	Third Attempt
10. The outside sterile gown ties may now be tied with the circulator's assistance.	10			
11. The circulator grasps the red part of the tag by the corner.	5			

Comments:

Total Points Earned _____ Divided by _____ Total Possible Points = _____ % Score

Instructor's Signature _____

Procedure 32-7 Removal of Contaminated Gloves

Task: To properly remove and dispose of contaminated gloves after a procedure has been completed.

Equipment and Supplies:
- Contaminated gloved (sterile or nonsterile) hands
- (Note: The following procedure is written for someone who is right-handed. If you are left-handed, simply reverse each one of the hand designations for this procedure.)

Standards: Complete the procedure and all critical steps in _____ minutes with a minimum

score of _____ % within three attempts.

Scoring: Divide points earned by total possible points. Failure to perform a critical step that is indicated with an asterisk (*), will result in an unsatisfactory overall score.

Time began _____ **Time ended** _____

Steps	Possible Points	First Attempt	Second Attempt	Third Attempt
1. Using your right hand, grasp the outside of the cuff of the glove on the left hand. Be careful not to touch the left arm during this step.	20			
2. Take the glove completely off of the left hand by pulling it away from the fingers and pulling it inside out.	20			
3. Now the contaminated left glove is inside out in the right hand. Using only the right hand, ball this dirty glove in the palm of the hand.	20			
4. Now use your left hand to carefully grasp the cuff of the right glove and pull it off over the hand (and the other glove), turning it inside out as this is done.	20			
5. Dispose of the gloves in the proper disposal receptacle or a biohazard bag if they are contaminated with blood or body fluids.	10			
6. Wash your hands.	10			

Comments:

Total Points Earned _____ Divided by _____ Total Possible Points = _____ % Score

Instructor's Signature _____

Procedure 32-8 Skin Preparation for Surgery

Task: To prepare the patient's skin for a surgical procedure to reduce the risk of wound contamination.

Equipment and Supplies:
- Gauze sponges
- Cotton-tipped applicators
- Antiseptic soap
- Sterile gloves
- Two small stainless-steel bowls
- Antiseptic
- Optional: cotton balls, nail pick, scrub brush
- A waste receptacle

Standards: Complete the procedure and all critical steps in _____ minutes with a minimum

score of _____ % within three attempts.

Scoring: Divide points earned by total possible points. Failure to perform a critical step that is indicated with an asterisk (*), will result in an unsatisfactory overall score.

Time began _____ **Time ended** _____

Steps	Possible Points	First Attempt	Second Attempt	Third Attempt
1. Wash your hands and dry them carefully. Follow standard precautions.	5			
2. Open your skin preparation pack.	5			
3. Arrange the items with sterile gloved hands.	5			
4. Add the surgical soap and antiseptic solutions to the two bowls.	5			
5. Explain the scrub procedure to the patient.	5			
6. Expose the site. Use a light if necessary.	5			
7. Don gloves using aseptic technique.	5			
8. Place two sterile towels at the edges of the area to be scrubbed.	5			
9. Start at the incision site, and begin washing with the antiseptic soap on a gauze sponge in a circular motion, moving from the center to the edges of the area to be scrubbed.	10			
10. After one complete wipe, discard the sponge, and begin again with a new sponge soaked in the antiseptic solution.	10			

Steps	Possible Points	First Attempt	Second Attempt	Third Attempt
11. Repeat the process using sufficient friction for 5 minutes (or follow office policy for the length of time required for a particular preparation).	10			
12. Dry the area using the same circular technique with dry sponges. The area may be dried by blotting with a third sterile towel.	10			
13. Check that no solutions are pooling under the patient.	10			
14. Paint on the antiseptic with the cotton-tipped applicators or gauze sponges, using the same circular technique, and never returning to an area that has already been painted.	10			

Comments:

Total Points Earned _____ Divided by _____ Total Possible Points = _____ % Score

Instructor's Signature _____

Procedure 32-9 Opening a Sterile Pack and Creating a Sterile Field

Task: To open a sterile pack that contains a table drape with correct aseptic technique.

Equipment and Supplies:
- A sterile pack (autoclaved linen or disposable) that will serve as a sterile table drape or field
- A Mayo stand or countertop
- Disinfectant and gauze sponges

Standards: Complete the procedure and all critical steps in _____ minutes with a minimum

score of _____ % within three attempts.

Scoring: Divide points earned by total possible points. Failure to perform a critical step that is indicated with an asterisk (*), will result in an unsatisfactory overall score.

Time began _____ **Time ended** _____

Steps	Possible Points	First Attempt	Second Attempt	Third Attempt
1. Check that the Mayo stand or countertop is dust-free and clean. If it is not, clean with 70% alcohol or another disinfectant and towel.	10			
2. Wash your hands and dry them carefully.	10			
3. Place the sterile pack on the Mayo stand or countertop and read the label.	10			
4. Check the expiration date. If using an autoclaved pack, check the indicator tape for color change.	10			
5. Position the package so that the outer envelope flap is face up and at the top as you look at the package.	10			
6. Open the first flap away from yourself.				
7. Pull away the two side flaps, one at a time. Be careful to lift each flap by reaching under the small folded-back tab without touching the inner surface of the pack or its contents.	20			
8. Pull the last flap toward you by its tab, exposing the towel.	10			
9. You now have a sterile drape to be used as a sterile work field and for the distribution of additional sterile supplies and instruments.	10			

Comments:

Total Points Earned _____ Divided by _____ Total Possible Points = _____ % Score

Instructor's Signature _____

Procedure 32-10 Using Transfer Forceps

Task: To move sterile items on a sterile field or transfer sterile items to a gloved team member.

Equipment and Supplies:
- A sterile item to move or transfer
- A pair of packaged sterile gloves
- A pair of sterile wrapped transfer forceps
- A Mayo stand set-up with a sterile field and sterile instruments

Standards: Complete the procedure and all critical steps in _____ minutes with a minimum

score of _____ % within three attempts.

Scoring: Divide points earned by total possible points. Failure to perform a critical step that is indicated with an asterisk (*), will result in an unsatisfactory overall score.

Time began _____ **Time ended** _____

Steps	Possible Points	First Attempt	Second Attempt	Third Attempt
1. Wash your hands and dry them carefully.	10			
2. Put on sterile gloves or open a package containing a pair of sterile transfer forceps.	10			
3. Using aseptic technique, handle sterile forceps by ring handle only. Always point forceps' tips down.	20			
4. Grasp an item on the sterile field with your sterile gloved hand or the sterile forceps, points down, and move it to its proper position for the procedure.	20			
5. Or transfer an instrument from the autoclave to the sterile field.	20			
6. Remove the transfer forceps after one-time use.	20			

Comments:

Total Points Earned _____ Divided by _____ Total Possible Points = _____ % Score

Instructor's Signature _____

Procedure 32-11 Pouring Solutions onto a Sterile Field(s)

Task: As a circulating assistant, pour a sterile solution into a stainless-steel bowl or medicine glass that is sitting at the edge of a sterile field.

Equipment and Supplies:
- A bottle of sterile solution
- A stainless-steel bowl or medicine glass
- A sterile field
- A sink or waste receptable

Note: A medicine glass or bowl on the sterile field should be near one edge of the field and the perimeter of the 1-inch barrier.

Standards: Complete the procedure and all critical steps in _____ minutes with a minimum score of _____ % within three attempts.

Scoring: Divide points earned by total possible points. Failure to perform a critical step that is indicated with an asterisk (*), will result in an unsatisfactory overall score.

Time began _____ **Time ended** _____

Steps	Possible Points	First Attempt	Second Attempt	Third Attempt
1. Wash your hands and dry them carefully.	10			
2. Read the label.	10			
3. Place your hand over the label and lift the bottle. Note: If the container has a double cap, set the outer cap on the counter inside up, then proceed.	10			
4. Lift the lid of the bottle straight up, and then slightly to one side, and hold the lid in your nondominant hand facing downward.	10			
5. Pour away from the label.	10			
6. If the container does not have a double cap, pour off a small amount of the solution into a waste receptacle.	10			
7. Pour away from the label, into the bowl, without allowing any part of the bottle to touch the bowl.	10			
8. Tilt the bottle up to stop the pouring while it is still over the bowl.	10			
9. Remove the bottle from over the sterile field.	10			
10. Replace the cap(s) off to the side, away from the sterile field.	10			

Comments:

Total Points Earned _____ Divided by _____ Total Possible Points = _____ % Score

Instructor's Signature _____

Procedure 32-12 Assisting with Minor Surgery

Task: To maintain the sterile field and to pass instruments in a prescribed sequence during a surgical procedure that involves the creation of a surgical incision and the removal of a growth.

Equipment and Supplies:
- An open patient drape pack on the side counter
- A Mayo stand covered with a sterile drape
- Packaged sterile gloves (two pairs)
- A needle and syringe for anesthesia medication
- A vial of local anesthetic medication
- One medicine glass or small bowl
- A scalpel handle and a No. 15 blade
- A pair of Allis tissue forceps
- One skin retractor
- Three hemostats
- A supply of gauze sponges
- A waste receptacle

Standards: Complete the procedure and all critical steps in _____ minutes with a minimum

score of _____ % within three attempts.

Scoring: Divide points earned by total possible points. Failure to perform a critical step that is indicated with an asterisk (*), will result in an unsatisfactory overall score.

Time began _____ **Time ended** _____

Steps	Possible Points	First Attempt	Second Attempt	Third Attempt
1. Wash your hands. Dry thoroughly.	2.5			
2. Don gloves using aseptic technique. Set up the sterile field, with instruments and supplies arranged in the sequence to be used.	2.5			
3. Remove your gloves. Read the label of the local anesthetic medication and pour the medication into a medicine glass.	5			
4. Don gloves using aseptic technique, and prepare the patient's skin with surgical soap and antiseptic solution. Explain the prep procedure to the patient.	5			
5. Scrub, using the surgical hand wash procedure. Follow standard precautions.	5			
6. Dry your hands thoroughly.	2.5			
7. Don gloves using aseptic technique.	5			

Steps	Possible Points	First Attempt	Second Attempt	Third Attempt
8. Position the Mayo stand near the patient and the operative site.	5			
9. Lift the patient drape from the open pack without touching the drape to any of the pack edges.	5			
10. Grasp the patient drape by holding one edge or corner in each hand.	5			
11. Drape the surgical site without touching any part of the patient or the operating area with your gloved hands.	5			
12. The surgeon injects the local anesthetic, after looking at the empty vial on the counter and confirming the type, strength, and expiration date. Note: The surgeon may drape the patient while you don gloves.	5			
13. Position yourself across from the surgeon. Arrange the sterile field. Check instrument placement condition.	5			
14. Place two sponges on the patient, next to the site where the incision will be made.	5			
15. Grasp the scalpel blade with a hemostat and mount the scalpel blade onto the scalpel handle. Keep all sharp equipment conspicuously placed on the sterile field.	5			
16. Pass the scalpel, blade down, to the surgeon or allow the surgeon to reach for it himself or herself. The surgeon will take the scalpel with the thumb and forefinger in the position ready for use.	5			
17. Grasp a pair of Allis tissue forceps by the tips, and pass it to the surgeon to grasp a piece of the tissue to be excised.	5			
18. Pass the forceps' handles into the surgeon's open palm with a firm and purposeful motion. A gentle "snap" is heard as the instrument makes contact with the surgeon's gloved hand.	5			
19. Dispose of soiled sponges, using the waste receptacle.	5			
20. Hold clean sponges in your hand to be passed to the surgeon, or to sponge the wound, as necessary.	5			
21. Safely position the specimen (if any) where it will not be disturbed on the sterile field.	5			

Steps	Possible Points	First Attempt	Second Attempt	Third Attempt
22. If there is a bleeding vessel or if a hemostat is requested, pass the hemostat in the manner described in steps 17 and 18.	5			
23. Receive instruments and place them on the sterile field.	5			
24. Continue to sponge blood from the wound site.	5			
25. Retract the wound edge, as needed, with a skin retractor.	5			
26. Continue to monitor the sterile field and assist the surgeon as necessary.	2.5			
27. Pass the suture to the surgeon for closure of the wound.	5			

Comments:

Total Points Earned _____ Divided by _____ Total Possible Points = _____ % Score

Instructor's Signature _____

Procedure 32-13 Assisting with Suturing

Task: To assist the surgeon in wound closure, using sterile technique.

Equipment and Supplies:
- A sterile field on a Mayo stand
- Surgical scissors
- Suture material
- Sterile gloves
- Needle holder
- Gauze sponges

Note: This procedure may be a continuation of Procedure 32-12. If this procedure is done independently, you must perform the surgical scrub and glove before beginning step 1.

Standards: Complete the procedure and all critical steps in _____ minutes with a minimum

score of _____ % within three attempts.

Scoring: Divide points earned by total possible points. Failure to perform a critical step that is indicated with an asterisk (*), will result in an unsatisfactory overall score.

Time began _____ **Time ended** _____

Steps	Possible Points	First Attempt	Second Attempt	Third Attempt
1. Hold the curved needle point in your nondominant hand, 4 to 5 inches over the sterile field.	10			
2. Always work over a sterile field.	10			
3. With your dominant hand, hold the needle holder halfway down its shaft, at the box-lock, with the suture needle point up.	10			
4. With your nondominant hand, hold the suture strand, and pass the needle holder into the surgeon's hand.	10			
5. Pick up the surgical scissors with your dominant hand and a gauze sponge with your nondominant hand.	20			
6. After the surgeon has placed a closure suture and knotted it, he or she will hold the two strands taut. Cut both suture strands in one motion. Cut between the knot and the surgeon, at the length requested, about 1/8 inch.	20			
7. Gently blot the closure once with the gauze sponge in your nondominant hand.	10			
8. If additional strands of suture are needed, repeat the process.	10			

Comments:

Total Points Earned _____ Divided by _____ Total Possible Points = _____ % Score

Instructor's Signature _____

Procedure 32-14 Suture Removal

Task: To remove sutures from a healed incision with sterile technique and without injury to the closed wound.

Equipment and Supplies:
- ture removal scissors
- Gauze sponges
- Thumb forceps
- Steri-Strips or Band-Aids
- Skin antiseptic

Standards: Complete the procedure and all critical steps in _____ minutes with a minimum

score of _____ % within three attempts.

Scoring: Divide points earned by total possible points. Failure to perform a critical step that is indicated with an asterisk (*), will result in an unsatisfactory overall score.

Time began _____ **Time ended** _____

Steps	Possible Points	First Attempt	Second Attempt	Third Attempt
1. Assemble necessary supplies.	5			
2. Wash and dry your hands. Follow standard precautions.	5			
3. Open the suture removal pack.	5			
4. Explain the procedure to the patient and instruct patient to lie or sit still during procedure.	5			
5. Place dry towels under the area from which sutures will be removed.	5			
6. Position patient comfortably and support the area.	5			
7. Place a gauze sponge next to the wound site.	5			
8. Grasp the knot of the suture with the dressing forceps, without pulling.	15			
9. Cut the suture at skin level.	15			
10. Lift—do not pull—the suture toward the incision and out with the dressing forceps.	5			
11. Place the suture on the gauze sponge, and check that the entire suture strand has been removed.	5			

Steps	Possible Points	First Attempt	Second Attempt	Third Attempt
12. If there is any bleeding, blot the area with a new gauze sponge before continuing.	5			
13. Continue in the same manner until all the other sutures have been removed.	5			
14. Remove the gauze sponge with the sutures on it.	5			
15. The surgeon may apply a Steri-Strip or Band-Aid for added support, strength, and protection.	5			
16. The patient is instructed to keep the wound edges clean and dry and not place excessive strain on the area.	5			

Documentation in the Medical Record

_____

_____

_____

_____

Comments:

Total Points Earned _____ Divided by _____ Total Possible Points = _____ % Score

Instructor's Signature _____

Procedure 32-15 Applying/Changing a Dressing

Task: To properly apply a dressing at the completion of a surgical procedure.

Equipment and Supplies:
• Sterile dressing material or Telfa

Standards: Complete the procedure and all critical steps in _____ minutes with a minimum

score of _____ % within three attempts.

Scoring: Divide points earned by total possible points. Failure to perform a critical step that is indicated with an asterisk (*), will result in an unsatisfactory overall score.

Time began _____ **Time ended** _____

Steps	Possible Points	First Attempt	Second Attempt	Third Attempt
1. Before the sterile drape is removed from the patient, pick up the dressing from the sterile field, place it on the wound, and hold it there.	25			
2. Remove the drape while switching hands to hold the dressing in place.	25			
3. Secure the dressing with paper tape and/or an appropriate bandage.	25			
4. Document the procedure in the patient's medical record.	25			

Documentation in the Medical Record

_____

_____

_____

_____

Comments:

Total Points Earned _____ Divided by _____ Total Possible Points = _____ % Score

Instructor's Signature _____

Procedure 32-16 Bandaging with Gauze and Elastic Dressings

Task: To apply an elastic bandage to the forearm.

Equipment and Supplies:
• One 3- or 4-inch elastic bandage

Standards: Complete the procedure and all critical steps in _____ minutes with a minimum

score of _____ % within three attempts.

Scoring: Divide points earned by total possible points. Failure to perform a critical step that is indicated with an asterisk (*), will result in an unsatisfactory overall score.

Time began _____ **Time ended** _____

Steps	Possible Points	First Attempt	Second Attempt	Third Attempt
1. Choose the proper size bandage for the size of the arm you are bandaging.	10			
2. Start at the distal point and hold the roll so the bandage can be rolled away from you.	10			
3. Keep the roll close to the patient and keep it facing upward.	10			
4. Maintain even tension and spacing as you continue to apply the bandage up the forearm.	10			
5. When crossing a joint, slightly flex the joint.	10			
6. Fasten the end of the bandage with clips or tape.	10			
7. Check the patient's nail beds for cyanosis.	10			
8. Check the radial pulse.	10			
9. Have the patient move his or her fingers.	10			
10. Document the procedure in the patient's medical record.	10			

Documentation in the Medical Record

_____

_____

_____

_____

Comments:

Total Points Earned _____ Divided by _____ Total Possible Points = _____ % Score

Instructor's Signature _____

Procedure 33-1 Preparing a Resumé

Task: To write an effective resume for use as a tool in gaining employment.

Equipment and Supplies:
- Scratch paper
- Pen or pencil
- Former job descriptions, if available
- List of addresses of former employers, schools, and names of supervisors
- Computer or word processor
- Quality stationary and envelopes

Standards: Complete the procedure and all critical steps in _____ minutes with a minimum

score of _____ % within three attempts.

Scoring: Divide points earned by total possible points. Failure to perform a critical step that is indicated with an asterisk (*), will result in an unsatisfactory overall score.

Time began _____ **Time ended** _____

Steps	Possible Points	First Attempt	Second Attempt	Third Attempt
1. Perform a self-evaluation by making notes about your strengths as a medical assistant. Consider job skills, self-management skills, and transferable skills.	10			
2. Explore formatting and decide on a professional resume appearance that best highlights your skills and experience. Use the templates available in word processing software or design your own.	10			
3. Place your name, address, and two telephone numbers where you can be contacted at the top of the resume.	10			
4. Write a job objective that specifies your employment goals.	10			
5. Provide details about your educational experience. List degrees and/or certifications obtained.	10			
6. Provide details about your work experience. Include all contact information and names of supervisors. Do not include salary expectations or reasons for leaving former jobs.	10			
7. Prepare a cover letter and a list of references. Send the references with the resume only when requested.	10			

Steps	Possible Points	First Attempt	Second Attempt	Third Attempt
8. Type the resume carefully and make certain that there are no errors on the document.	10			
9. Proofread the resume. Allow another person to read it as well and look for missed errors.*	5			
10. Print the resume on quality paper. Review the resume again for errors and to assure that it looks attractive on the printed page.	5			
11. Target each resume to a specific person or position. Do not send generic resumes to each prospective employer.	5			
12. Follow up on all resumes that are distributed with a phone call to arrange an interview.	5			

Documentation in the Medical Record

_____

_____

_____

_____

Comments:

Total Points Earned _____ Divided by _____ Total Possible Points = _____ % Score

Instructor's Signature _____

English-Spanish Terms for the Medical Assistant

abscess Localized collection of pus that causes tissue destruction and may be either under the skin or deep within the body.
absceso Cantidad de pus localizada en un lugar que puede estar bajo la piel o a más profundidad en el interior del cuerpo y causa la destrucción de los tejidos.

accommodation Adjustment of the eye for seeing various sizes of objects at different distances.
acomodación Ajuste del ojo para ver distintos tamaños de objetos a distancias diferentes.

acute Having a rapid onset and severe symptoms.
agudo Que tiene un comienzo rápido y síntomas serios.

adhesions Bands of scar tissue that bind together two anatomic surfaces that are normally separate.
adhesiones Bandas de tejido de una cicatriz que unen dos superficies anatómicas que están normalmente separadas.

adrenocorticotropic hormone (ACTH) A hormone, released by the anterior pituitary gland, that stimulates the production and secretion of glucocorticoids.
hormona adrenocorticotropina (ACTH) Hormona, liberada por la glándula pituitaria anterior, que estimula la producción y secreción de glucocorticoides.

advent A coming into being or use.
advenimiento Próximo a ser o a usarse.

albuminuria Abnormal presence of albumin in the urine.
albuminuria Presencia anómala de albúmina en la orina.

aliquot A portion of a well-mixed sample removed for testing.
alícuota Porción de una muestra bien mezclada, separada para ser analizada.

allopathy A method of treating a disease by introducing a condition that is intended to cause a pathologic reaction, which will be antagonistic to the condition being treated.
alopatía Método de tratar una enfermedad provocando una afección con el fin de causar una reacción patológica, la cual será opuesta a la enfermedad que se está tratando.

alopecia Partial or complete lack of hair.
alopecia Pérdida de cabello, parcial o total.

amblyopia Reduction or dimness of vision with no apparent organic cause; often referred to as lazy eye syndrome.
ambliopía Reducción o disminución de la visión sin causa orgánica aparente; con frecuencia se conoce como síndrome del ojo vago.

ambulatory Able to walk about and not be bedridden.
ambulatorio Capaz de caminar y no tiene que estar postrado en la cama.

amino acids Organic compounds that form the chief constituents of protein and are used by the body to build and repair tissues.
aminoácidos Compuestos orgánicos que son los constituyentes principales de la proteína y son usados por el cuerpo para formar y reparar tejidos.

amorphous Lacking a defined shape.
amorfo Que carece de forma definida.

analyte The substance or chemical being analyzed or detected in a specimen.
analito La sustancia o producto químico que se analiza o que se detecta en una muestra.

anaphylaxis Exaggerated hypersensitivity reaction that, in severe cases, leads to vascular collapse, bronchospasm, and shock.
anafilaxia Reacción de hipersensibilidad exagerada, la cual, en casos graves, conduce a colapso vascular, broncospasmo y choque.

anastomosis The surgical joining together of two normally distinct organs.
anastomosis Unión quirúrgica de dos órganos normalmente diferentes.

anemia A condition marked by deficiency of red blood cells.
anemia Enfermedad caracterizada por una deficiencia de glóbulos rojos en la sangre.

angiocardiography Radiography of the heart and great vessels using an iodine contrast medium.
angiocardiografía Radiografía del corazón y los vasos sanguíneos mayores usando un medio de contraste yodado.

angiography Radiography of blood vessels using an iodine contrast medium.
angiografía Radiografía de los vasos sanguíneos usando un medio de contraste yodado.

angioplasty Interventional technique using a catheter to open or widen a blood vessel to improve circulation
angioplastia Técnica quirúrgica que usa un catéter para abrir o hacer más ancho un vaso sanguíneo a fin de mejorar la circulación.

anomalies Faulty development of the fetus resulting in deformities or deviations from normal.
anomalías Desarrollo defectuoso del feto que tiene como resultado deformidades o desviaciones de lo normal.

anorexia Lack or loss of appetite for food.
anorexia Falta o pérdida del apetito.

anoxia Absence of oxygen in the tissues.
anoxia Ausencia de oxígeno en los tejidos.

anteroposterior (AP) Frontal projection in which the patient is supine or facing the x-ray tube.
anteroposterior (AP) Proyección frontal en la cual el paciente está en posición supina o frente al tubo de rayos X.

antibody Immunoglobulin produced by the immune system in response to bacteria, viruses, or other antigenic substances.
anticuerpo Inmunoglobulina producida por el sistema inmunológico en respuesta a bacterias, virus u otras substancias antigénicas.

anticoagulant A chemical added to the blood after collection to prevent clotting.
anticoagulante Producto químico que se añade a la sangre después de extraerla para que no forme coágulos.

antidiuretic hormone (ADH) A hormone secreted at the posterior pituitary gland; causes water retention in the kidneys; and an elevation of blood pressure also known as vasopressin.
hormona antidiurética (ADH) Hormona secretada por la glándula pituitaria posterior y que provoca retención de agua en los riñones y aumento de la presión sanguínea. Es conocida también como vasopresina.

antigen Foreign substance that causes the production of a specific antibody.
antígeno Substancia extraña que provoca la producción de un anticuerpo específico.

antimicrobial agent A drug that is used to treat infection.
agente antimicrobiano Substancia que se usa para tratar infecciones.

antiseptic Pertaining to substances that inhibit the growth of microorganisms such as alcohol and betadine.
antiséptico Perteneciente o relativo a las substancias que inhiben el crecimiento de microorganismos como el alcohol y la betadina.

antiseptic substance that kills **microorganisms.**
antiséptico Substancia que mata **microorganismos.**

antiseptic An agent that inhibits bacterial growth and that can be used on human tissue.
antiséptico Agente que inhibe el crecimiento bacteriano y que puede usarse en los tejidos humanos.

aortagram Radiography of the aorta using an iodine contrast medium.
aortograma Radiografía de la aorta usando un medio de contraste yodado.

apnea Absence or cessation of breathing.
apnea Ausencia o cese de la respiración.

appraisal To give an expert judgment of the value or merit of; judging as to quality.
evaluación Acción de emitir un juicio experto sobre el valor o mérito de algo; juzgar la calidad de algo; evaluar el rendimiento en el trabajo.

arrhythmia Abnormality or irregularity in the heart rhythm.
arritmia Anomalía o irregularidad en el ritmo cardiaco.

arteriography Radiography of arteries using an iodine contrast medium.
arteriografía Radiografía de las arterias usando un medio de contraste yodado.

arthritis Inflammation of a joint.
artritis Inflamación de una articulación.

arthrogram Fluoroscopic examination of the soft tissue components of joints with direct injection of a contrast medium into the joint capsule.
artrografía Examen fluoroscópico de los componentes de los tejidos blandos de las articulaciones con una inyección directa de un medio de contraste en la cápsula de la articulación.

articular Pertaining to a joint.
articulatorio Perteneciente o relativo a una articulación.

asepsis Being free from infection or infectious materials.
asepsia Que está libre del infecciones.

asystole The absence of a heartbeat.
asistolia Ausencia de latidos del corazón.

ataxia Failure or irregularity of muscle actions and coordination.
ataxia Fallo o irregularidad del movimiento y coordinación musculare.

atherosclerosis A form of arteriosclerosis distinguished by fatty deposits within the inner layers of larger arterial walls.
aterosclerosis Forma de arteriosclerosis que se distingue por la presencia de depósitos de grasa en las capas internas de las paredes de las arterias mayores.

atria The two upper chambers of the heart.
aurículas Las dos cavidades superiores del corazón.

atrioventricular (AV) node Part of the cardiac conduction system located between the atria and the ventricles
nódulo aurioventricular (AV) Parte del sistema cardiaco que se encuentra entre las aurículas y los ventrílculos.

atrophy Decrease in the size of a normally developed organ.
atrofia Disminución del tamaño de un órgano desarrollado de forma normal.

atrophy Wasting away, decreasing size.
atrofia Desgastado, disminuido en tamaño.

attenuated Weakened, or change in virulence of, a pathogenic microorganism.
atenuado Cambio o debilitación en la virulencia de un microorganismo.

audiologist An allied health care professional specializing in evaluation of hearing function, detection of hearing impairment, and determination of the anatomic site of impairment.
audiólogo Profesional del cuidado de la salud que se especializa en evaluar la función auditiva, detectar las dificultades auditivas y determinar el lugar físico en el que se produce el problema auditivo.

augment To make greater, more numerous, larger, or more intense.
aumentar Hacer mayor, más numeroso, más grande o más intenso.

aura Peculiar sensation preceding the appearance of more definite disturbance.
aura Sensación peculiar que precede a la aparición de un trastorno definido.

autoimmune Disturbance in the immune system in which the body reacts against its own tissue. Examples of autoimmune disorders include Multiple Sclerosis, Rheumatoid Arthritis, and Systemic Lupus Erythematosus.
autoinmune Trastorno del sistema inmunológico en el cual el cuerpo reacciona contra sus propios tejidos. Algunos ejemplos de trastornos autoinmunes incluyen la esclerosis múltiple, la artritis reumatoide y el lupus eritematoso sistémico.

autoimmune Development of an immune response to one's own tissues; act against own cells to cause localized and systemic reactions.
autoinmune Desarrollo de una respuesta inmunológica a los propios tejidos; actuar contra sus propias células para originar reacciones sistémicas localizadas.

axial projection Radiograph taken with a longitudinal angulation of the x-ray beam; sometimes referred to as a semi-axial projection.
proyección axial Radiografía que se toma con un ángulo longitudinal del haz de rayos X; a veces se llama proyección semi-axial.

azotemia Retention in the blood of excessive amounts of nitrogenous wastes.
azotemia Retención en la sangre de cantidades de desperdicios nitrogenados.

benign Not cancerous and not recurring.
benigno No canceroso y no recurrente.

bevel Angled tip of a needle.
bisel Punta de aguja en ángulo.

bifurcate Divide from one into two branches.
bifurcar Dividir una unidad en dos ramas.

bifurcation The point of forking or separating into two branches
bifurcación Lugar en el que se separan dos ramas.

bilirubin Orange-colored pigment in bile, which, when it accumulates, leads to jaundice
bilirrubina Pigmento de color naranja que se encuentra en la bilis; cuando se acumula produce ictericia.

bilirubinuria Presence of bilirubin in the urine.
bilirrubinuria Presencia de bilirrubina en la orina.

biophysical Pertaining to the science dealing with the application of physical methods and theories to biologic problems.
biofísico Perteneciente o relativo a la ciencia que trata de la aplicación de métodos y teorías físicas a los problemas biológicos.

bounding pulse Pulse that feels full because of increased power of cardiac contractions or due to increased blood volume.
pulso saltón Pulso que se siente lleno debido a un aumento de potencia en las contracciones cardiacas o debido a un aumento del volumen de la sangre.

bradycardia A slow heartbeat; a pulse below 60 beats per minute.
bradicardia Latido lento; pulso por debajo de 60 pulsaciones por minuto.

bradypnea Respirations that are regular in rhythm but slower than normal in rate.
bradipnea Respiración que tiene un ritmo regular pero es más lenta de lo normal.

broad-spectrum antimicrobial agent A drug used to treat a broad range of infections.
agente antimicrobiano de amplio espectro Sustancia que se usa para tratar una amplia gama de infecciones.

bronchiectasis Dilation of the bronchi and bronchioles associated with secondary infection or ciliary.
broncoectasia Dilatación de los bronquios y bronquiolos asociada con una infección secundaria o ciliar.

bronchoconstriction Narrowing of the bronchiole tubes.
broncoconstricción Estrechamiento de los bronquiolos.

bruit Abnormal sound or murmur heard on auscultation of an organ, vessel, or gland.
ruido Sonido o murmullo anómalo que se oye al auscultar un órgano, vaso sanguíneo o glándula.

bucky Moving grid device that prevents scatter radiation from fogging the film.
bucky Dispositivo de rejilla móvil que evita que la difusión de la radiación empañe la película.

bundle of His Fibers that conduct electrical impulses from AV node to ventricular myocardium.
haz de His Fibras que conducen impulsos eléctricos del nódulo aurioventricular al miocardio ventricular.

bursa A fluid-filled sac-like membrane that provides for cushioning and frictionless motion between two tissues.
bursa Membrana con forma de saco llena de fluido que proporciona amortiguación y movimiento sin fricción entre dos tejidos.

C&S–culture and sensitivity A procedure performed in the microbiology laboratory through which a specimen is cultured on artifical media to detect bacterial or fungal growth, followed by appropriate screening for antibiotic sensitivity.
C&S–cultivo y sensibilidad Procedimiento llevado a cabo en el laboratorio de microbiología en el cual se cultiva un espécimen en un medio artificial para detectar el crecimiento de bacterias u hongos y después investigar su sensibilidad los antibióticos.

candidiasis Infection caused by a yeast-like fungus which typically effects the vaginal mucosa and skin.
candidiasis Infección causada por una levadura (una especie de hongo) que típicamente afecta la mucosa y la piel vaginal.

cannula Rigid tube that surrounds a blunt trocar or a sharp, pointed trocar inserted into the body; when it is withdrawn, fluid may escape from the body through the cannula, depending on where it is inserted.
cánula Tubo rígido que envuelve un trocar romo o un trocar de punta afilada que se inserta en el cuerpo; cuando se saca, puede salir fluido corporal a través de la cánula, según en donde haya sido insertada.

carbohydrates Chemical substances, including sugars, glycogen, starches, dextrins, and celluloses, that contain only carbon, oxygen, and hydrogen.
carbohidratos Sustancias químicas, en las que se incluyen azúcares, glucógenos, almidones, dextrinas y celulosas, y están formadas sólo por carbono, oxígeno e hidrógeno.

carcinogenic A substance that is known to cause cancer.
cancerígeno Sustancia que se sabe que produce cáncer.

carcinogens Substances or agents that cause the development of or increase the incidence of cancer.
carcinógeno Sustancia o agente que origina el desarrollo de cáncer o aumenta su incidencia.

cardiac arrest Cardiac contractions completely stop.
paro cardiaco Detención completa de las contracciones cardiacas.

cardiac arrhythmias Irregular heartbeat resulting from a malfunction of the electrical system of the heart.
arritmias cardiacas Pulso irregular que es resultado de un mal funcionamiento del sistema eléctrico del corazón.

cardioversion Utilizing an electroshock to convert an abnormal cardiac rhythm to a normal one.
cardioversión Utilización de un electrochoque para normalizar un ritmo cardiaco anómalo.

cartilage Rubbery, smooth, somewhat elastic connective tissue covering the ends of bones.
cartílago Tejido de unión similar a la goma, suave y un tanto elástico, que cubre los extremos de los huesos.

casts Fibrous or protein material molded to the shape of the part in which it has accumulated and thrown off into the urine in kidney disease.
cálculos Materiales fibrosos o proteínicos que han tomado la forma de la parte del cuerpo en la que han sido acumulados y que se expulsan a través de la orina en los casos de enfermedades renales.

caustic A remark or phrase dripping with sarcasm.
cáustico Comentario o frase dicha con sarcasmo.

caustic A substance that burns or destroys tissue by chemical action.
cáustico Sustancia que quema o destruye tejidos por acción química.

centrifuge An apparatus consisting essentially of a compartment spun about a central axis to separate contained materials of different specific gravities, or to separate colloidal particles suspended in a liquid.
centrifugadora Aparato que consiste básicamente de un compartimiento que gira alrededor de un eje central para separar materiales con diferentes pesos específicos, o para separar partículas coloidales suspendidas en un líquido.

cerebrospinal fluid Fluid within the subarachnoid space, the central canal of the spinal cord, and the four ventricles of the brain.
fluido cerebroespinal Fluido del interior del espacio subaracnoideo, el canal central de la médula espinal y los cuatro ventrículos del cerebro.

cerumen A waxy secretion in the ear canal, commonly called *ear wax.*
cerumen Secreción cerosa del canal del oído, comúnmente se conoce como *cera de los oídos.*

cervical Neck region containing seven cervical vertebrae.
cervical Región del cuello en la que hay siete vértebras cervicales.

chief complaint Reason for patient seeking medical care.
problema principal Razón por la cual un paciente solicita atención médica.

chiropractic A medical discipline in which a chiropractic physician focuses on the nervous system and manually and painlessly adjusts the vertebral column in order to affect the nervous system, resulting in healthier patients.
quiropráctica Disciplina médica en la que los médicos quiroprácticos se centran en el sistema nervioso y ajustan la columna vertebral manualmente y sin dolor, para lograr un efecto sobre el sistema nervioso, dando como resultado pacientes más sanos.

cholesterol Substance produced by the liver, found in plant and animal fats, that can produce fatty deposits or atherosclerotic plaques in the blood vessels.
colesterol Sustancia que produce el hígado y que se halla en las grasas animales y vegetales, y que puede producir depósitos grasos o placas **ateroscleróticas** en los vasos sanguíneos.

chronic Persisting for a prolonged period of time.
crónico Que persiste por largo tiempo.

chronic bronchitis Recurrent inflammation of the membranes lining the bronchial tubes.
bronquitis crónica Inflamación recurrente de las membranas que recubren los tubos bronquiales.

clinical trials A research study that tests how well new medical treatments or other interventions work in the subjects, usually human beings.
ensayos clínicos Estudio de investigación que prueba cómo actúan los nuevos tratamientos médicos u otras intervenciones en los sujetos, normalmente en los seres humanos.

clitoris Small, elongated erectile body situated above the urinary meatus at the superior point of the labia minora.
clítoris Órgano eréctil pequeño y alargado situado sobre el meato urinario a la altura de los labios menores.

clubbing Abnormal enlargement of the distal phalanges (fingers and toes), associated with cyanotic heart disease or advanced chronic pulmonary disease.
hipocratismo digital (dedos en palillo de tambor) Engrosamiento anómalo de las falanges distales (en los dedos de las manos y de los pies), relacionado con una enfermedad cardiaca cianótica o una enfermedad pulmonar crónica avanzada.

coagulate Capable of being formed into clots.
coagular Formar coágulos.

cognitive Pertaining to the operation of the mind process by which we become aware of perceiving, thinking, and remembering.
cognitivo Perteneciente o relativo a la operación del proceso mental por el cual nos damos cuenta de cómo, percibimos, pensamos y recordamos.

coitus Sexual union between male and female; also known as intercourse.
coito Unión sexual entre un macho y una hembra.

collagen Protein that forms the inelastic fibers of tendons, ligaments, and fascia.
colágeno Proteína que forma las fibras no elásticas de los tendones, los ligamentos y la fascia.

collodion Preparation of cellulose nitrate that, when applied to the skin, dries to a strong, thin, protective, transparent film.
colodión Preparación de nitrato de celulosa que, cuando se aplica a la piel, se seca formando una película fina resistente, protectora y transparente.

colloidal Pertaining to a gluelike substance.
coloidal Perteneciente o relativo a una substancia parecida a la cola.

colostrum Thin, yellow, milky fluid secreted by the mammary glands a few days before and after delivery.
calostro Fluido lácteo poco espeso y amarillo que segregan las glándulas mamarias unos días antes y después del parto.

coma An unconscious state from which the patient cannot be aroused.
coma Estado inconsciente del cual el paciente no puede ser despertado.

comorbidities Preexisting conditions that will, because of their presence with a specific principal diagnosis, cause an increase in length of stay by at least 1 day in approximately 75 percent of cases.
patologías coexistentes Enfermedades preexistentes que, debido a su presencia junto al diagnóstico principal, causan un aumento en la duración de la estadía de al menos un día en aproximadamente 75 por ciento de los casos.

compression The state of being pressed together.
compresión Condición de estar apretado.

computed tomography (CT) Computerized x-ray imaging modality providing axial and three-dimensional scans.
tomografía asistida por computadora (TAC) Modalidad de formación computarizada de imágenes de rayos X que proporciona imágenes de escáner axiales y tridimensionales.

cones Structures found in the retina that make the perception of color posible.
conos Estructuras que se encuentran en la retina y que hacen posible la percepción del color.

congruence The verbal expression of the message matches the sender's nonverbal body language.
congruencia Expresión verbal del mensaje que corresponde al lenguaje corporal no verbal del emisor.

congruent Being in agreement, harmony, or correspondence; conforming to the circumstances or requirements of a situation.
congruente Que está en acuerdo, armonía o correspondencia; conforme a las circunstancias o requisitos de una situación.

contaminated Soiled with pathogens or infectious material; nonsterile.
contaminado Manchado con materiales patógenos o infecciosos; no estéril.

contamination Becoming unsterile by contact with any nonsterile material.
contaminación Pasar al estado de no estéril por contacto con cualquier material no estéril.

contamination To make impure or unclean; to make unfit for use by the introduction of unwholesome or undesirable elements.
contaminación Volver impuro o sucio; hacer que algo sea inadecuado para el uso por la introducción de elementos insalubres o indeseables.

contralateral Pertaining to the opposite side of the body.
colateral Perteneciente o relativo a la parte opuesta del cuerpo.

contrast media Substances used to enhance visualization of soft tissues in imaging studies.
medios de contraste Substancias usadas para mejorar la visualización de los tejidos blandos en estudios de formación de imágenes.

COPD chronic obstructive pulmonary disease A progressive and irreversible lung condition that results in diminished lung capacity.
COPD enfermedad pulmonar obstructiva crónica Enfermedad pulmonar progresiva e irreversible que conlleva una reducción de la capacidad pulmonar.

copulation Sexual intercourse.
copulación Cópula sexual.

coronal plane Plane that divides the body into anterior and posterior parts.
plano coronal Plano que divide el cuerpo en una anterior y una posterior.

corticosteroids Anti-inflammatory hormones, natural or synthetic.
corticosteroides Hormonas antiinflamatorias, naturales o sintéticas.

costal Pertaining to the ribs.
costal Perteneciente o relativo a las costillas.

coulombs per kilogram (C/kg) International unit of radiation exposure.
culombios por kilogramo (C/kg) Unidad internacional de exposición a la radiación.

creatinine Nitrogenous waste from muscle metabolism excreted in urine.
creatinina Residuo nitrogenado del metabolismo muscular que se excreta en la orina.

crenate Forming notches or leaflike scalloped edges on an object.
crenar Formar muescas o bordes en forma de concha o de hoja en un objeto.

crepitation Dry, crackling sound or sensation.
crepitación Sonido o sensación seca y crujiente.

critical thinking The constant practice of considering all aspects of a situation when deciding what to believe or what to do.
razonamiento crítico Práctica constante de considerar todos los aspectos de una situación al decidir qué creer o qué hacer.

cryosurgery Technique of exposing tissue to extreme cold to produce a well-defined area of cell destruction.
criocirugía Técnica que consiste en exponer los tejidos a un frío extremo para producir una destrucción de células en un área bien definida.

cryptogenic Hidden origin.
criptogénico De origen oculto.

curettage Act of scraping a body cavity with a surgical instrument such as a curette.
curetaje Acción de raspar una cavidad corporal con un instrumento quirúrgico, como una cureta o cucharilla cortante.

cyanosis Blue color of the mucous membranes and body extremities caused by lack of oxygen.
cianosis Color azul de las membranas mucosas y las extremidades provocado por una falta de oxígeno.

cyst A small capsule-like sac that encloses certain organisms in their dormant or larval stage.
quiste Pequeño saco en forma de cápsula que encierra ciertos organismos en estado letárgico o larval.

debridement Removal of foreign material and dead, damaged tissue from a wound.
desbridamiento Eliminación de materiales extraños y tejidos muertos y deteriorados de una herida.

decubitus ulcer A sore or ulcer over a bony prominence that is due to ischemia from prolonged pressure; a bed sore.
úlcera por decúbito Llaga o úlcera sobre una prominencia ósea debida a una isquemia por presión prolongada; escara.

deferment A postponement, especially of a student loan.
aplazamiento Postergación de un pago, especialmente en un préstamo de estudiante.

defibrillator Machine used to deliver electroshock to the heart through electrodes placed on the chest wall.
desfibrilador Máquina usada para dar un electrochoque al corazón por medio de electrodos colocados en la pared torácica.

deficiencies Conditions caused by a below-normal intake of a particular substance.
deficiencias Estados causados por un consumo menor del normal de una sustancia específica.

diabetes mellitus type 2 Inability to utilize glucose for energy due to either a lack of insulin production in the pancreas or resistance to insulin on the cellular level.
diabetes mellitus tipo 2 Incapacidad de utilizar la glucosa para producir energía, debido a una falta de producción de insulina en el páncreas o a una resistencia a la insulina en el nivel celular.

diagnosis Concise technical description of the cause, nature, or manifestations of a condition or problem. *Initial:* Physician's temporary impression, sometimes called a *working diagnosis. Differentiated diagnosis:* comparison of two or more diseases with similar signs and symptoms. *Final:* Conclusion physician reaches after evaluating all findings, including laboratory and other test results.
diagnóstico Descripción técnica y concisa de la causa, naturaleza o manifestaciones de una enfermedad o problema. *Inicial:* Impresión momentánea del médico, a veces se llama *diagnóstico de trabajo. Diagnóstico diferenciado:* comparación de dos o más enfermedades con signos y síntomas similares. *Final:* Conclusión médica a la que se llega tras evaluar todos los datos, incluyendo los resultados de análisis de laboratorio y otras pruebas.

"diagnosis" The determination of the nature of a disease, injury, or congenital defect.
"diagnóstico" Determinación del origen de una enfermedad, lesión o defecto congénito.

diaphoresis The profuse excretion of sweat.
diaforesis Excreción profusa de sudor.

diaphysis Middle portion of a long bone containing the medullary cavity.
diafisis Parte intermedia de un hueso largo en la que está la cavidad medular.

digestion Process of converting food into chemical substances that can be used by the body.
digestión Proceso de transformar alimentos en sustancias químicas que pueden ser usadas por el cuerpo.

dilatation Opening or widening the circumference of a body orifice with a dilating instrument.
dilatación Proceso de abrir o ensanchar un orificio corporal con un instrumento dilatador.

dilation The opening of the cervix through the process of labor; measured as 0 to 10 centimeters dilated.
dilatación Ensanchamiento del cuello del útero durante el proceso del parto; se mide en centímetros, de 0 a 10.

dilation & curettage The widening of the cervix and scraping of the endometrial wall of the uterus.
dilatación y curetaje Proceso de hacer más ancho el cuello del útero y raspar su pared endometrial.

diluent A liquid used to dilute a specimen or reagent.
diluyente Líquido usado para diluir un espécimen o un reactivo.

diplopia Double vision.
diplopía Visión doble.

disease Pathologic process having a descriptive set of signs and symptoms.
enfermedad Proceso patológico que tiene una serie descriptiva de signos y síntomas.

disinfection Destruction of **pathogens** by physical or chemical means.
desinfección Destrucción de **agentes patógenos** con medios físicos o químicos.

disorder A disruption of normal system functions.
trastorno Interrupción de las funciones normales de un sistema.

dissect To cut or separate tissue with a cutting instrument or scissors.
diseccionar Cortar o separar tejidos con tijeras u otro instrumento cortante.

dissection To separate into pieces and expose parts for scientific examination.
disección Separar en piezas y dejar las partes a la vista para realizar un estudio científico.

diurnal rhythm Patterns of activity or behavior that follow day-night cycles.
ritmo diurno Patrones de actividad o comportamiento que siguen a los ciclos nocturnos.

dosimeter Badge for monitoring exposure to radiation of personnel.
dosímetro Placa para controlar la exposición a la radiación del personal.

dyspnea Difficult or painful breathing.
disnea Respiración difícil o dolorosa.

ecchymosis A hemorrhagic skin discoloration, commonly called bruising.
equimosis Descoloramient o hemorrágico de la piel comúnmente conocido como magulladura.

edema Abnormal accumulation of fluid in the interstitial spaces of tissue; swelling between layers of tissue.
edema Acumulación anómala de fluido en los espacios intersticiales de los tejidos; inflamación entre capas de tejidos.

effacement The thinning of the cervix during labor, measured in percentages from 0 to 100 percent effaced.
borramiento Adelgazamiento del cuello del útero durante el parto. Se mide en porcentaje, borrado de 0 a 100 por ciento.

elastic pulse Pulse with regular alterations of weak and strong beats, without changes in cycle.
pulso elástico Pulso con alteraciones regulares de latidos fuertes y débiles sin cambios en el ciclo.

elastin Essential part of elastic connective tissue that, when moist, is flexible and elastic.
elastina Parte esencial del tejido conectivo elástico que cuando está húmedo es flexible y elástico.

electrodesiccation Destructive drying of cells and tissue by means of short, high-frequency electrical sparks.
electrodesecación Secado destructivo de células y tejidos por medio de cortas descargas eléctricas de alta frecuencia.

electrolytes Small molecules that conduct an electrical charge. Electrolytes are necessary for proper functioning of muscle and nerve cells.
electrolitos Pequeñas moléculas que conducen una carga eléctrica. Los electrolitos son necesarios para un funcionamiento correcto de los músculos y las células nerviosas.

embolization Interventional technique using a catheter to block off a blood vessel to prevent hemorrhage.
embolización Técnica de intervención usando un catéter para bloquear un vaso sanguíneo y evitar una hemorragia.

embolus Foreign material blocking a blood vessel, frequently a blood clot that has broken away from some other part of the body.
émbolo Material extraño que bloquea un vaso sanguíneo, con frecuencia un coágulo de sangre procedente de otra parte del cuerpo.

emetic A substance that causes vomiting.
emético Sustancia que causa vómito.

empathy Sensitivity to the individual needs and reactions of patients.
empatía Sensibilidad ante las necesidades y reacciones individuales de los pacientes.

emphysema Pathologic accumulation of air in the tissues or organs; in the lungs, the bronchioles become plugged with mucus and lose elasticity.
enfisema Acumulación patológica de aire en los tejidos u órganos; en los pulmones, los bronquiolos se obstruyen con mucosidade y pierden elasticidad.

emulsification Dispersement of ingested fats into small globules by bile.
emulsionamiento Dispersión (llevada a cabo por la bilis) en pequeños glóbulos de las grasas ingeridas.

endemic Disease or microorganism that is specific to a particular geographic area.
endémico Enfermedad o microorganismo que es específico de una zona geográfica en particular.

endocervical curettage The scraping of cells from the wall of the uterus.
curetaje endocervical Raspado de células de la pared uterina.

enteric-coated An oral medication with a coating that resists the effects of stomach juices; designed so medicine is absorbed in the small intestine; drug formulation in which tablets are coated with a special compound that does not dissolve until the tablet is exposed to the fluids of the small intestine
cubierta entérica Capa exterior que se añade a un medicamento que se toma por vía oral, la cual es resistente a los efectos de los jugos gástricos; recubrimiento diseñado para que la medicina sea absorbida en el intestino delgado; formulación usada en medicinas en la cual las tabletas se recubren con un componente especial que no se disuelve hasta que la tableta es expuesta a los fluidos del intestino delgado.

enzymatic reaction Chemical reaction controlled by an enzyme.
reacción enzimática Reacción química controlada por una enzima.

enzyme Any of several complex proteins produced by cells that act as catalysts in specific biochemical reactions.
enzima Cualquiera de las varias proteínas complejas que producen las células y que actúan como catalíticos en reacciones bioquímicas específicas.

epiphysis End of a long bone.
epífisis Extremo de un hueso largo.

erythropoietin Substance released from the kidney and liver that promotes red blood cell formation.
eritropoyetina Sustancia liberada por los riñones y el hígado y que promueve la formación de glóbulos rojos.

essential hypertension Elevated blood pressure of unknown cause that develops for no apparent reason; sometimes called *primary hypertension*.
hipertensión esencial Presión sanguínea alta de causa desconocida que surge sin razón aparente; a veces se llama *hipertensión primaria*.

eukaryote A single-celled or multicellular organism whose cells contain a distinct membrane-bound nucleus.
eucariote Organismo unicelular o multicelular cuyas células tienen un núcleo diferenciado **rodeado** por una membrana.

exacerbation An increase in the seriousness of a disease marked by greater intensity in the signs and symptoms. Worsening of disease symptoms.
exacerbación Aumento en la gravedad de una enfermedad, caracterizado por una mayor intensidad de los signos y síntomas. Empeoramiento de los síntomas de una enfermedad.

exudates Fluids with high concentration of protein and cellular debris that has escaped from the blood vessels and has been deposited in tissues or on tissue surfaces.
exudados Fluidos con una alta concentración de proteínas y restos celulares extravasados de los vasos sanguíneos y depositados en los tejidos o en sus superficies.

familial Occurring in or affecting members of a family more than would be expected by chance.
familiar Que sucede o afecta a miembros de una familia más de lo que podría esperarse por azar.

fascia Sheet or band of fibrous tissue located deep in the skin that covers muscles and body organs.
fascia Lámina o banda de tejido fibroso localizada bajo la piel y que cubre los músculos y los órganos.

fastidious Requiring specialized media or growth factors to grow.
exigente Que requiere un medio o factores especiales para crecer.

fat Stored as adipose tissue in the body and serving as a concentrated energy reserve.
grasa Sustancia que se almacena como tejido adiposo en el cuerpo y sirve como reserva de energía concentrada.

febrile Pertaining to an elevated body temperature.
febril Perteneciente o relativo a una temperatura corporal elevada.

fecalith A hard, impacted mass of feces in the colon.
fecaloma Masa de heces endurecidas e impactadas en el colon.

fermentation An enzymatically controlled transformation of an organic compound.
fermentación Transformación de un compuesto orgánico controlada por enzimas.

fibrillation Rapid, random, ineffective contractions of the Herat.
fibrilación Contracciones cardiacas rápidas, aleatorias e inefectivas.

filtrate Fluid that remains after a liquid is passed through a membranous filter.
filtrado Fluido que queda después de pasar un líquido a través de un filtro membranoso.

fissures Narrow slits or clefts in the abdominal wall.
fisuras Grietas o hendiduras estrechas en la pared abdominal.

fistulas Abnormal, tubelike passages within the body tissue, usually between two internal organs, or from an internal organ to the body surface.
fístulas Pasajes anómalos en forma de tubos entre los tejidos corporales, por lo general entre dos órganos internos, o de un órgano interno a la superficie del cuerpo.

flatus Gas expelled through the anus.
flato Gas expulsado a través del ano.

fluoroscopy Direct observation of the x-ray image in motion.
fluoroscopía Observación directa de una imagen de rayos x en movimiento.

follicle-stimulating hormone (FSH) A hormone secreted by the anterior pituitary; stimulates oogenesis and spermatogenesis.
hormona foliculoestimulante (FSH) Hormona que segrega la pituitaria anterior y que estimula los procesos de formación y desarrollo de óvulos y de espermatozoides.

fovea centralis A small pit in the center of the retina that is considered the center of clearest vision.
fóvea central Pequeña concavidad en el centro de la retina que se cree que es el centro de visión más claro.

frontal projection Radiographic view in which the coronal plane of the body or body part is parallel to the film plane; AP or PA.
proyección frontal Vista radiográfica en la cual el plano coronal del cuerpo o de la parte del cuerpo está paralelo al plano de la película; AP o PA.

gait Manner or style of walking.
andares Forma o estilo de caminar.

gamete A mature male or female germ cell, usually possessing a haploid chromosome set and capable of initiating formation of a new diploid individual.
gameto Célula germinal madura, tanto masculina como femenina, que por lo general tiene un conjunto cromosómico haploide y es capaz de iniciar la formación de un nuevo individuo diploide.

gangrene Death of body tissue due to loss of nutritive supply and followed by bacteria invasion and putrefaction.
gangrena Muerte de tejido corporal debido a la pérdida de suministro de nutrientes por invasión bacteriana y putrefacción.

gantry Doughnut-shaped portion of a scanner than surrounds the patient and that functions, at least in part, to gather imaging data.
gantry Parte de un escáner con forma de rosquilla que rodea al paciente y funciona, al menos en parte, reuniendo datos de formación de imágenes.

generic Drugs that are not protected by trademark.
genéricas Medicinas que no están protegidas por una marca registrada.

genome The genetic material of an organism.
genoma El material genético de un organismo.

germicides Agents that destroy **pathogenic** organisms.
germicidas Agentes químicos que destruyen o matan organismos **patógenos**.

girth A measure around a body or item.
contorno Medida alrededor de un cuerpo o artículo.

glucagon A hormone produced by the alpha cells of the pancreatic islets; stimulates the liver to convert glycogen into glucose.
glucagón Hormona producida por las células alfa de los islotes pancreáticos; estimula al hígado para que convierta el glucógeno en glucosa.

glucosuria The abnormal presence of glucose in the urine.
glucosuria Presencia anómala de glucosa en la orina.

glycogen The sugar (starch) formed from glucose and stored mainly in the liver.
glucógeno Azúcar (almidón) formado a partir de la glucosa y almacenado principalmente en el hígado.

glycohemoglobin or hemoglobin A1c A type of hemoglobin that is made slowly during the 120-day life span of the red blood cell (RBC). Glycohemoglobin makes up 3 to 6 percent of hemoglobin in a normal RBC, in diabetes mellitus it makes up to 12 percent.
glucohemoglobina o hemoglobina A1c Tipo de hemoglobina que se produce lentamente durante el periodo de los 120 días de vida de los glóbulos rojos (RBC). La glucohemoglobina constituye de un 3 a un 6 por ciento de la hemoglobina en un RBC normal; en los casos de diabetes mellitus constituye hasta un 12 por ciento.

glycosuria Presence of glucose in the urine.
glucosuria Presencia de glucosa en la orina.

goniometer Instrument for measuring the degrees of motion in a joint.
goniómetro Instrumento para medir los grados de movimiento de una articulación.

gray (Gy) International unit of radiation dose.
gray (Gy) Unidad internacional de dosis de radiación.

growth hormone (GH) Also called somatotropic hormone, stimulates tissue growth and restricts tissue glucose dependence when nutrients are not available.
hormona del crecimiento (GH) También llamada hormona somatotrópica, estimula el crecimiento de los tejidos y restringe la dependencia de la glucosa de los tejidos cuando no hay nutrientes disponibles.

hematemesis Vomiting of bright red blood, indicating rapid upper gastrointestinal bleeding, associated with esophageal varices or peptic ulcer.
hematemesis Vómito de sangre roja brillante que indica hemorragia rápida del sistema gastrointestinal superior, relacionado con varices esofágicas o úlcera péptica.

hematocrit The percentage by volume of packed red blood cells in a given sample of blood after centrifugation. Volume percentage of erythrocytes in whole blood.
hematocrito Porcentaje por volumen de glóbulos rojos en una muestra de sangre dada después de ser centrifugada. Porcentaje del volumen de eritrocitos en la sangre completa.

hematoma A sac filled with blood that may be the result of trauma.
hematoma Saco lleno de sangre que puede ser el resultado de una lesión.

hematuria Blood in the urine.
hematuria Sangre en la orina.

hemoconcentration A situation in which the concentration of blood cells is increased in proportion to the plasma.
hemoconcentración Situación en la cual la concentración de glóbulos rojos ha aumentado en proporción al plasma.

hemoglobin Protein found in erythrocytes that transports molecular oxygen in the blood.
hemoglobina Proteína que se encuentra en los eritrocitos que transportan el oxígeno en la sangre.

hemolysis The destruction or dissolution of red blood cells, with subsequent release of hemoglobin.
hemolisis Destrucción o disolución de los glóbulos rojos, con la subsiguiente liberación de hemoglobina.

hemolyzed A term used to describe a blood sample in which the red blood cells have ruptured.
hemolizado Término usado para describir una muestra de sangre en la cual los glóbulos rojos se han roto.

hepatomegaly Abnormal enlargement of the liver.
hepatomegalia Agrandamiento anómalo del hígado.

hereditary Pertaining to a characteristic, condition, or disease transmitted from parent to offspring on the DNA chain.
hereditario Perteneciente o relativo a una característica, estado o enfermedad transmitida de padres a hijos en la cadena de ADN.

hermetically sealed Sealed so no air is allowed to enter or escape.
herméticamente sellado Sellado de forma que el aire no pueda entrar o escapar.

holistic Related to or concerned with all of the systems of the body, rather than breaking it down into parts.
holístico Relacionado con todos los sistemas corporales y no dividido en partes.

homeostasis Maintenance of constant internal ambient conditions compatible with life.
homeostasis Mantenimiento de unas condiciones ambientales internas constantes compatibles con la vida.

homeostatic Maintaining a constant internal environment.
homeostático Que mantiene un ambiente interno constante.

hormone A substance, usually a peptide or steroid, produced by one tissue and conveyed by the bloodstream to another to effect physiological activity such as growth or metabolism; a chemical transmitter produced by the body and transported to target tissue or organs by the bloodstream.
hormona Sustancia química transmisora, por lo general un péptido o un esteroide, que es producida por un tejido y transportada por la corriente sanguínea hasta el tejido u órgano objetivo para provocar un efecto en la actividad fisiológica, como el crecimiento o el metabolismo.

hydrocephaly Enlargement of the cranium caused by abnormal accumulation of cerebrospinal fluid within the cerebral system.
hidrocefalia Agrandamiento del cráneo causado por una acumulación anómala de fluido cerebroespinal en el interior del sistema cerebral.

hydrogenated Combined with, treated with, or exposed to hydrogen.
hidrogenado Combinado con hidrógeno, tratado con él o expuesto a él.

hyperlipidemia Excess of fats or lipids in the blood plasma.
hiperlipemia Exceso de grasas o lípidos en el plasma sanguíneo.

hyperplasia An increase in the number of cells.
hiperplasia Aumento del número de células.

hyperpnea Increase in the depth of breathing.
hiperpnea Aumento en la profundidad de la respiración.

hypertension High blood pressure (systolic pressure consistently above 140 mm Hg and diastolic pressure above 90 mm Hg).
hipertensión Presión sanguínea alta (presión sistólica continuamente por encima de 140 mm Hg y presión diastólica por encima de 90 mm Hg).

hyperventilation Abnormally prolonged and deep breathing, usually associated with acute anxiety or emotional tension.
hiperventilación Respiración profunda anómalamente prolongada, que suele estar asociada con una ansiedad aguda o con tensión emocional.

hypotension Blood pressure that is below normal (systolic pressure below 90 mm Hg and diastolic pressure below 50 mm Hg).
hipotensión Presión sanguínea que está por debajo de lo normal (presión sistólica por debajo de 90 mm Hg y presión diastólica por debajo de 50 mm Hg).

idiopathic Unknown cause
idiopático Causa desconocida.

ileocecal valve Valve guarding the opening between the ileum and cecum; also called the ileocolic valve.
válvula ileocecal Válvula que controla la abertura entre el íleo y el intestino ciego; también se llama válvula ileocólica.

ileostomy Surgical formation of an opening of the ileum onto the surface of the abdomen through which fecal material is emptied.
ileostomía Formación quirúrgica de una abertura del íleo en la superficie del abdomen, a través de la cual se vacían los materiales fecales.

immunotherapy Administering repeated injections of diluted extracts of the substance that causes an allergy; also called desensitization.
inmunoterapia Administración de repetidas inyecciones de extractos diluidos de la substancia que provoca una alergia; también se conoce como desensibilización.

impenetrable Incapable of being penetrated or pierced; not capable of being damaged or harmed.
impenetrable Que no puede ser penetrado o traspasado; que no puede ser dañado o perjudicado.

in vitro Refers to conditions outside of a living body.
in vitro Expresión que se refiere a condiciones exteriores de un ser vivo.

incontinence Inability to control excretory functions.
incontinencia Incapacidad de controlar las funciones excretoras.

induration An abnormally hard, inflamed area.
induración Área anómalamente dura, inflamada.

infarction Area of tissue that has died due to lack of blood supply.
infarto Área de tejido que ha muerto debido a una falta de suministro de sangre.

infection Invasion of body tissues by **microorganisms**, which then proliferate and damage tissues.
infección Invasión de los tejidos corporales por **microorganismos**, los cuales entonces proliferan y dañan los tejidos.

infertile Not fertile or productive; not capable of reproducing.
estéril Que no es fértil o productivo; que no tiene la capacidad de reproducirse.

inflammation Tissue reaction to trauma or disease that includes redness, heat, swelling, and pain.
inflamación Reacción de los tejidos ante una lesión o enfermedad que incluye enrojecimiento, calentamiento, hinchazón y dolor.

innate Existing in, belonging to, or determined by factors present in an individual since birth.
innato Que existe en un individuo, que le pertenece o que está determinado por factores existentes en ese individuo desde el momento de su nacimiento.

insulin Hormone secreted by the beta cells of the pancreatic islets in response to increased levels of glucose in the blood.
insulina Hormona que segregan las células beta de los islotes pancreáticos en respuesta a la presencia de altos niveles de glucosa en la sangre.

intermittent claudications Recurring cramping in the calves caused by poor circulation of blood to the muscles of the lower leg.
cojeras intermitentes Calambres recurrentes en las pantorrillas causados por una mala circulación de la sangre de los músculos de la parte inferior de la pierna.

intermittent Coming and going at intervals; not continuous
intermitente Que va y viene a intervalos; de forma no continua.

intermittent pulse Pulse in which beats are occasionally skipped.
pulso intermitente Pulso en el cual de vez en cuando se salta algún latido.

intolerable Not tolerable or bearable.
intolerable Que no se puede tolerar o soportar.

intravenous urogram (IVU) Radiographic examination of the urinary tract using intravenous injection of an iodine contrast medium.
urograma intravenoso (IVU) Examen radiográfico del tracto urinario usando una inyección intravenosa de un medio de contraste yodado.

invasive Involving entry into the living body, as by incision or insertion of an instrument.
invasivo Que entra en un organismo vivo, como por incisión o inserción de un instrumento.

ipsilateral Pertaining to the same side of the body.
isolateral Perteneciente a la misma parte del cuerpo.

irregular pulse Pulse that varies in force and frequency.
pulso irregular Pulso que varía en fuerza y frecuencia.

ischemia Decreased blood flow to a body part or organ, caused by constriction or plugging of the supplying artery; temporary interruption in blood supply to a tissue or organ.
isquemia Disminución del flujo sanguíneo a una parte del cuerpo u órgano provocada por la constricción o atasco de la arteria suministradora; interrupción temporal del suministro de sangre a un tejido u órgano.

islets (of Langerhans) Cells of the pancreas that produce insulin (beta cells) and glucagon (alpha cells); also called pancreatic islets.
islotes (de Langerhans) Células del páncreas que producen insulina (células beta) y glucagón (células alfa); también llamados islotes pancreáticos

jaundice Yellowness of the skin and mucous membranes caused by deposition of bile pigment. It is not a disease, but a symptom of a number of diseases, especially liver disorders.
ictericia Coloración amarilla en la piel y las membranas mucosas causada por deposición del pigmento biliar. No es una enfermedad pero es un síntoma de muchas enfermedades, sobre todo de trastornos hepáticos.

keratin Very hard, tough protein found in hair, nails, and epidermal tissue.
queratina Proteína muy dura que se encuentra en el pelo, uñas y tejidos epidérmicos.

keratinocytes Any one of the skin cells that synthesize keratin.
queratinocitos Cualquiera de las células de la piel que sintetizan queratina.

ketosis Abnormal production of ketone bodies in the blood and tissues resulting from fat catabolism in cells. Ketones accumulate in large quantities when fat, instead of sugar, is used as fuel for energy in cells.
quetosis Producción anormal de cuerpos de quetosis en la sangre y tejidos como resultado de un catabolismo graso en las células. Los quetones se acumulan en grandes cantidades cuando se usa grasa, en lugar de azúcar, como combustible para las células.

kyphosis Abnormal convex curvature of the thoracic spine region.
cifosis Curvatura convexa anómala de la región espinal torácica.

lacrimation The secretion or discharge of tears.
lagrimeo Secreción o descarga de lágrimas.

laryngoscopy Visual examination of the voice box area through an endoscope equipped with a light and mirrors for illumination.
laringoscopia Examen visual de la laringe por medio de un endoscopio equipado con una luz y espejos.

latent image Invisible changes in exposed film that will become a visible image when the film is processed.
imagen latente Cambios invisibles en la película que se convertirán en una imagen visible cuando se procese la película.

leukoderma White patches on the skin.
leucodermia Manchas blancas en la piel.

ligament A tough connective tissue band that holds joints together by attaching to the bones on either side of the joint.
ligamento Banda de tejido conectivo resistente que sostiene las articulaciones uniendo los huesos de cada lado de la articulación.

ligation The process of tying off something to close it—for example, a blood vessel during surgery—with a tie called a ligature.
ligado Proceso de atar algo, por ejemplo, un vaso sanguíneo durante una cirugía, con una atadura llamada ligadura.

limited radiography A limited-scope radiography practice, usually in an outpatient setting, that does not require the same credentials needed for professional radiologic technology; also called practical radiography.
radiografía limitada Práctica radiográfica de alcance limitado que se suele usar con pacientes externos y que no requiere las mismas credenciales que se necesitan para la tecnología radiográfica profesional. También se llama radiografía práctica.

lithotripsy A procedure for eliminating a stone (as in the bladder) by crushing or dissolving it in situ through the use of high-intensity sound waves.
litotripsia Procedimiento para eliminar una piedra rompiéndola o disolviéndola in situ por medio del uso de ondas sonoras de alta intensidad.

loading dose A double dose of medication administered as the first dose. It is usually done with antibiotic therapy to reach therapeutic blood levels quickly.
dosis de ataque Dosis doble de una medicación ladministrada como primera dosis. Suele hacerse con terapia antibiótica para alcanzar rápidamente los niveles terapéuticos en sangre.

lordosis Abnormal concave curvature of the cervical and lumbar spine regions.
lordosis Curvatura cóncava anómala de la espina cervical y lumbar.

lower GI series Fluoroscopic examination of the colon, usually employing rectal administration of barium sulfate (also called barium enema) as a contrast medium.
serie GI inferior Examen fluoroscópico del colon, por lo general usando una administración rectal de sulfato de bario (también llamado enema de bario) como medio de contraste.

lumbar The lower back region, containing five lumbar vertebrae.
lumbar Región posterior inferior en la que hay cinco vértebras lumbares.

lumen An open space, such as within a blood vessel, the intestine, a needle, a tube, or an examining instrument.
lumen Espacio abierto, como en el interior de un vaso sanguíneo, el intestino, una aguja, un tubo o un instrumento para examinar.

luteinizing hormone (LH) A hormone produced by the pituitary gland that promotes ovulation.
hormona luteinizante (LH) Hormona que produce la glándula pituitaria y que promueve la ovulación.

luxation Dislocation of a bone from its normal anatomical location.
luxación Dislocación de un hueso de su ubicación anatómica normal.

lymphadenopathy Any disorder of the lymph nodes or lymph vessels.
linfadenopatía Cualquier trastorno de los nódulos o de los vasos linfáticos.

macromolecules The molecules needed for metabolism: carbohydrates, lipids, proteins, and nucleic acids.
macromoléculas Moléculas que se necesitan para el metabolismo: carbohidratos, lípidos, proteínas y ácidos nucleicos.

magnetic resonance imaging (MRI) An imaging modality that uses a magnetic field and radiofrequency pulses to create computer images of both bones and soft tissues, in multiple planes.
formación de imágenes por resonancia magnética (MRI) Modalidad de formación de imágenes en la que se usa un campo magnético y pulsos de radiofrecuencia para crear imágenes computarizadas, tanto de huesos como de tejidos blandos, en planos múltiples.

malignant Cancerous.
maligno Canceroso.

manipulation Moving or exercising a body part by an externally applied force.
manipulación Mover o ejercitar una parte del cuerpo por medio de la aplicación de una fuerza externa.

mastectomy Surgical removal of the breast that usually includes excision of lymph nodes in the axillary region.
mastectomía Eliminación quirúrgica del seno que por lo general incluye la escisión de los nódulos linfáticos de la región axilar.

mediastinum The space in the center of the chest, under the sternum.
mediastino Espacio en el centro del pecho, bajo el esternón.

medullary cavity The inner portion of the diaphysis, containing bone marrow.
cavidad medular Porción interna de la diafisis que contiene la médula ósea.

melena Black, tarry stool containing digested blood and usually the result of bleeding in the upper GI tract.
melena Deposición negra y alquitranada que contiene sangre digerida y por lo general es le resultado de una hemorragia en el tracto gastrointestinal superior.

metabolite A substance produced by metabolism.
metabolito Sustancia producida por el metabolismo.

microcephaly Small size of the head in relation to the rest of the body.
microcefalia Tamaño pequeño de la cabeza en relación con el resto del cuerpo.

microorganism An organism of microscopic or submicroscopic size.
microorganismo Organismo de tamaño microscópico o sub-microscópico.

miotic Any substance or medication that causes contraction of the pupil.
miótico Cualquier sustancia o medicamento que produce una contracción de la pupila.

mock To imitate or practice.
simular Imitar o practicar.

molecule A group of like or different atoms held together by chemical forces.
molécula Grupo de átomos iguales o diferentes que se mantiene unido por fuerzas químicas.

mononuclear white blood cell A leukocyte having an unsegmented nucleus; monocytes and lymphocytes in particular.
glóbulo blanco mononuclear Leucocito que tiene un núcleo sin segmentar; en particular los monocitos y linfocitos.

mons pubis The fat pad that covers the symphysis pubis.
monte del pubis Almohadilla de grasa que cubre la sínfisis púbica.

multiparous Pertaining to women who have had two or more pregnancies.
multípara Perteneciente o relativo a la mujer que ha tenido dos o más embarazos.

murmur An abnormal sound heard when auscultating the heart. It may or may not be pathologic.
murmullo Sonido anómalo que se escucha al auscultar el corazón y que puede ser patológico o no.

myelography Fluoroscopic examination of the spinal canal with spinal injection of an iodine contrast medium.
mielografía Examen fluoroscópico del canal espinal con una inyección espinal de un medio de contraste yodado.

myelomeningocele A herniation of a portion of the spinal cord and its meninges that protrudes through a congenital opening in the vertebral column.
mielomeningocele Hernia de una parte de la médula espinal y sus meninges que sale hacia fuera a través de una abertura congénita en la columna vertebral.

myocardial Pertaining to the heart muscle.
miocárdico Perteneciente o relativo al músculo cardiaco.

myocardium The heart muscle.
miocardio Músculo cardiaco.

myoglobinuria Abnormal presence in the urine of a hemoglobin-like chemical of muscle tissue, which is the result of muscle deterioration.
mioglobinuria Presencia anómala en la orina de una susbtancia química del tejido muscular parecida a la hemoglobina; es el resultado de una deterioración muscular.

nanometer One billionth (10^{-9}) of a meter.
nanómetro Una mil millonésima parte (10^{-9}) de metro.

naturopathy An alternative to conventional medicine in which holistic methods are used, as well as herbs and natural supplements, with the belief that the body will heal itself. Naturopathic physicians can currently be licensed in twelve states.
naturopatía Alternativa a la medicina convencional en la que se usan métodos holísticos, así como hierbas y suplementos naturales, con la creencia de que el cuerpo sanará por sí mismo. En la actualidad, los médicos naturópatas pueden obtener la licencia en doce estados.

necrosis Pertaining to the death of cells or tissue.
necrosis Perteneciente o relativo a la muerte de células o tejidos.

networking The exchange of information or services among individuals, groups, or institutions; meeting and getting to know individuals in the same or similar career fields, and sharing information about available opportunities.
interconexión Intercambio de información o servicios entre individuos, grupos o instituciones; conocer a individuos del mismo campo profesional o de campos similares y compartir información acerca de oportunidades de empleo.

neural tube defect Any of a group of congenital anomalies involving the brain and spinal column that are caused by the failure of the neural tube to close during embryonic development.
defecto del tubo neural Cualquiera de las anomalías congénitas que afectan al cerebro y a la médula espinal y que tienen su origen en que el tubo neural no logró cerrarse durante el desarrollo embrionario.

nodule A small lump, lesion, or swelling felt when palpating the skin.
nódulo Pequeña protuberancia, herida o hinchazón que se siente al tocar la piel.

nomogram A graph on which variables are plotted so that a particular value can be read on the appropriate line.
nomograma Gráfica en la que las variables están presentadas de tal manera que se puede leer un valor específico en la línea adecuada.

nosocomial infection Infection acquired during hospitalization or in a healthcare setting. It is often due to E. coli, hepatitis viruses, pseudomonas, and staphylocci microorganisms.
infección nosocomial Infección adquirida en un establecimiento de atención sanitaria o durante una hospitalización. Con frecuencia se debe a E. coli, virus de hepatitis, pseudomonas y estafilococos.

nosocomial Pertaining to or originating in the hospital, said of an infection not present or incubating prior to admission to the hospital.
nosocomial Perteneciente o relativo al hospital, incubado en el hospital, dícese de la infección que no estaba presente ni en estado de incubación antes de ser ingresado al hospital.

NSAIDs Non-steroidal antiinflammatory drugs.
NSAID Medicamentos antiinflamatorios no esterioides.

nuclear medicine An imaging modality that uses radioactive materials injected or ingested into the body to provide information about the function of organs and tissues.
medicina nuclear Modalidad de la formación de imágenes que usa materiales radioactivos inyectados en el cuerpo o ingeridos para obtener información acerca del funcionamiento de órganos y tejidos.

obesity An excessive accumulation of body fat (usually defined as more than 20 percent above the recommended body weight).
obesidad Acumulación excesiva de grasa en el cuerpo (se suele definir como más del 20 por ciento del peso recomendado).

oblique projection Radiographic view in which the body or part is rotated so that the projection is neither frontal nor lateral.
proyección oblicua Vista radiográfica en la cual que cuerpo o parte del cuerpo se gira de forma que la proyección no es frontal ni lateral.

obturator A disk or plate that closes an opening.
obturador Disco o placa que cierra una abertura.

obturator A metal rod with a smooth rounded tip that is placed into hollow instruments to decrease destruction of the body tissues during insertion.
obturador Varilla de metal con un extremo redondeado que se coloca en el interior de instrumentos huecos para disminuir la destrucción de los tejidos corporales durante su inserción.

occlusion The complete blocking off of an opening.
oclusión Cierre completo de una abertura.

opaque Not translucent or transparent.
opaco Que no es translúcido ni transparente.

OPIM (other potentially infectious material) Substances or material other than blood (body fluids such as, urine, semen, etc., for example) which have the potential to carry infectious pathogens
OPIM (otras materias potencialmente peligrosas) Sustancias o materias además de la sangre (como, por ejemplo, los fluidos corporales, la orina, el semen, etc.).

opportunistic infection Infection caused by a normally nonpathogenic organism in a host whose resistance has been decreased.
infección oportunista Infección en una persona con una resistencia a las enfermedades más baja de lo normal, provocada por un organismo que en condiciones normales no resulta patógeno.

optic disc Region at the back of the eye where the optic nerve meets the retina. It is considered the blind spot of the eye because it contains only nerve fibers and no rods or cones, and thus is insensitive to light.
papila óptica Región en la parte posterior del ojo donde el nervio óptico se une con la retina. Se considera el punto ciego del ojo, ya que allí sólo hay fibras nerviosas y no bastoncillos ni conos, y por tanto es insensible a la luz.

optic nerve The second cranial nerve, which carries impulses for the sense of sight.
nervio óptico Segundo nervio del cráneo que transporta impulsos para el sentido de la vista.

organelle A differentiated structure within a cell, such as a mitochondrion, vacuole, or chloroplast, that performs a specific function.
organelo Estructura diferenciada dentro de una célula, como un mitocondrio, vacuola o cloroplasto que realiza una función específica.

orthopnea Difficulty breathing when in a supine position. The individual must sit or stand to breathe comfortably.
ortopnea Dificultad para respirar estando en posición supina. El individuo debe estar sentado o de pie para respirar con comodidad.

orthostatic (postural) hypotension A temporary fall in blood pressure when a person rapidly changes from a recumbent position to a standing position.
hipotensión ortostática (relacionada con la postura) Baja temporal de la presión sanguínea cuando una persona cambia con rapidez de una posición recostada a una posición en pie.

osteopathy A medical discipline based primarily on the manual diagnosis and holistic treatment of impaired function resulting from loss of movement in all kinds of tissues.
osteopatía Disciplina médica que se basa primordialmente en el diagnóstico manual y el tratamiento holístico de funciones deterioradas como resultado de la pérdida de movilidad en todo tipo de tejidos.

osteoporosis The loss of bone density. Lack of calcium intake is a major factor in its development.
osteoporosis Disminución de la densidad de los huesos. La falta de consumo de calcio es uno de los factores principales de su desarrollo.

otitis externa Inflammation or infection of the external auditory canal.
otitis externa Inflamación o infección del canal auditivo externo.

otosclerosis The formation of spongy bone in the labyrinth of the ear, often causing the auditory ossicles to become fixed and unable to vibrate when sound enters the ears.
otosclerosis Formación de huesos parecidos a esponjas en el laberinto del oído, a menudo causando que los huesecillos auditivos queden fijos y que no puedan vibrar cuando el sonido entra en los oídos.

ototoxic Pertaining to a substance or medication that damages the eighth cranial nerve or the organs of hearing and balance.
ototóxico Perteneciente o relativo a una sustancia o medicamento que daña el octavo nervio craneal o los órganos auditivos y del equilibrio.

over-the-counter drugs Medications legally sold without a prescription.
medicinas de venta libre Medicinas que se venden sin receta legalmente.

oxytocin A hormone secreted by the posterior pituitary gland that stimulates smooth muscle contractions of the uterus or mammary glands.
oxitocina Hormona que segrega la glándula pituitaria posterior y que estimula las contracciones del útero o de las glándulas mamarias.

palliative An agent that relieves or alleviates symptoms without curing the disease; something that alleviates or eases a painful situation without curing it.
paliativo Agente que calma o alivia los síntomas sin curar la enfermedad; algo que alivia o hace más soportable una situación dolorosa sin curarla.

pandemic Affecting the majority of the people in a country or a number of countries.
pandémico Que afecta a la mayoría de la población de un país o de varios países.

papilledema Bulging of the optic disk and dilated retinal veins seen by ophthalmoscopic examination of the retina. Papilledema is a sign of increased intracranial pressure.
edema papilar Abultamiento de la papila óptica y de las venas retinianas dilatadas que se ven en un examen oftalmoscópico de la retina. La emeda papilar es una señal de un aumento en la presión intracraneal.

parenteral Referring to injection or introduction of substances into the body through any route other than the digestive tract, such as subcutaneous, intravenous, or intramuscular administration.
parenteral Inyección o introducción de sustancias en el cuerpo a través de cualquier otra vía que no sea el tracto digestivo, como administración subcutánea, intravenosa o intramuscular.

paresthesia An abnormal sensation of burning, prickling, or stinging.
parestesia Sensación anómala de ardor, escozor o aguijoneo.

paroxysmal Pertaining to a sudden, recurrent spasm of symptoms.
paroxístico Perteneciente o relativo a espasmos repentinos recurrentes o a sus síntomas.

parturition The act or process of giving birth to a child.
parto Acción o proceso de dar a luz un niño.

patency The condition of a body cavity or canal that is open or unobstructed.
abertura Estado abierto de un cuerpo, cavidad o canal.

pathogen An agent that causes disease, especially a living microorganism such as a bacterium or fungus; a **disease**-causing **microorganism.**
patógeno Agente que causa enfermedades, especialmente microorganismos vivos como bacterias u hongos; **microorganismos** causantes de **enfermedades**.

pathogenic Pertaining to disease-causing microorganisms.
patogénico Perteneciente o relativo a los microorganismos causantes de enfermedades.

pathophysiology The study of biological and physical manifestations of disease as they are related to system abnormalities and physiologic disturbances.
patofisiología Estudio de las manifestaciones biológicas y físicas de las enfermedades y cómo se relacionan con las anomalías del sistema y las alteraciones fisiológicas.

perceiving The process of an individual looking at information and seeing it as real.
percibir Proceso en el cual un individuo mira la información y la ve como real.

pericardium The membranous sac that encloses the heart.
pericardio Saco membranoso que envuelve el corazón.

periosteum The thin, highly innervated, membranous covering of a bone.
periostio Membrana fina y sin nervios que recubre un hueso.

peristalsis The wavelike movement by which the gastrointestinal tract moves food downward.
peristalsis Movimiento ondulatorio por el cual el tracto gastrointestinal mueve la comida hacia abajo.

permeable Allowing a substance to pass or soak through.
permeable Permite el paso o penetración de una sustancia.

pertinent Having a clear, decisive relevance to the matter at hand.
pertinente Que tiene una importancia clara y decisiva en el asunto que se está tratando.

petechiae Small, purplish hemorrhagic spots on the skin.
petequia Pequeñas manchas en la piel, hemorrágicas y de color violeta.

phenylalanine An essential amino acid found in milk, eggs, and other foods.
fenilalanina Aminoácido esencial que se encuentra en la leche, los huevos y otros alimentos.

phlebotomy The invasive procedure used to obtain a blood specimen for testing, experimentation, or diagnosis of disease.
flebotomía Procedimiento invasivo que se usa para obtener un espécimen de sangre para analizar, experimentar o diagnosticar una enfermedad.

phosphors Fluorescent crystals that give off light when exposed to x-rays.
fósforos Cristales fluorescentes que alumbran cuando se exponen a los rayos X.

photometer An instrument for measuring the intensity of light, specifically to compare the relative intensities of different lights or their relative illuminating power.
fotómetro Instrumento para medir la intensidad de la luz, específicamente para comparar las intensidades relativas de luces diferentes o su poder de iluminación relativo.

photophobia Abnormal visual sensitivity to light.
fotofobia Sensibilidad visual anómala a la luz.

pipette A cylindrical glass or plastic tube used to deliver fluids.
pipeta Tubo cilíndrico de vidrio o plástico que se usa para distribuir fluidos.

pitch The property of a sound, especially a musical tone, that is determined by the frequency of the waves producing it; the highness or lowness of sound; the relative level, intensity, or extent of some quality or state.
tono Propiedad de un sonido, especialmente de un tono musical, que está determinada por la frecuencia de las ondas que lo producen; cualidad alta o baja de un sonido; nivel, intensidad o extensión relativos de alguna cualidad o estado.

plaque An abnormal accumulation of a fatty substance.
placa Acumulación anómala de una sustancia grasa.

plasma The liquid portion of whole blood that contains active clotting agents.
plasma Parte líquida de la sangre completa que contiene agentes coagulantes activos.

polycythemia vera A condition marked by an abnormally large number of red blood cells in the circulatory system.
policitemia vera Afección que se caracteriza por una cantidad anómalamente elevada de glóbulos rojos en el sistema circulatorio.

polydipsia Excessive thirst.
polidipsia Sed excesiva.

polymorphonuclear white blood cells Leukocytes having a segmented nucleus; also known as PMN (polymorphonuclear neutrophils) or segmented neutrophils.
glóbulos blancos polimorfonucleares Leucocitos que tienen un núcleo segmentado; también se conocen como PMN (neutrófilos polimorfonucleares) o neutrófilos segmentados.

polyphagia Excessive appetite.
polifagia Aumento del apetito.

polyps Tumors on stems frequently found in or on mucous membranes and in the mucosal lining of the colon.
pólipos Tumores en racimos que se encuentran con frecuencia en las membranas mucosas y en el recubrimiento mucoso del colon.

polyuria Excessive urine production; excretion of an unusually large amount of urine.
poliuria Producción y excreción de orina excesivas.

portal hypertension Increased venous pressure in the portal circulation caused by cirrhosis or compression of the hepatic vascular system.
hipertensión portal Aumento de la presión venosa en la circulación portal causado por cirrosis o compresión del sistema vascular hepático.

posterioanterior (PA) Frontal projection in which the patient is prone or facing the x-ray film or image receptor.
posterioanterior (PA) Proyección frontal en la que el paciente está boca abajo o de frente a la película de rayos X o al receptor de imagen.

present illness The chief complaint, written in chronological sequence with dates of onset.
enfermedad actual Problema principal, descrito en secuencia cronológica con las fechas de cada acceso.

preservatives Substances added to a specimen to prevent deterioration of cells or chemicals.
preservativos Sustancias añadidas a un espécimen para prevenir el deterioro de células o sustancias químicas.

professional behaviors Those actions that identify the Medical Assistant as a member of a healthcare profession, including dependability, respectful patient care, initiative, positive attitude, and teamwork.
comportamientos profesionales Características que identifican al asistente médico como profesional de la atención sanitaria, incluyendo confiabilidad, trato respetuoso a los pacientes, iniciativa, actitud positiva y disposición para trabajar en equipo.

prokaryote A unicellular organism that lacks a membrane-bound nucleus
procaryota Organismo unicelular cuyo núcleo no está unido por una membrana.

prolactin (PRL) A hormone secreted by the anterior pituitary gland that stimulates the development of the mammary gland.
prolactina (PRL) Hormona que segrega la glándula pituitaria anterior y que estimula el desarrollo de la glándula mamaria.

prosthesis The artificial replacement for a body part.
prótesis Pieza artificial para reemplazar una parte del cuerpo.

proteins Organic compounds, occurring in plants and animals, that contain the major elements carbon, hydrogen, oxygen, and nitrogen and the amino acids essential for life maintenance.
proteínas Compuestos orgánicos que existen en plantas y animales y que contienen los elementos principales: carbón, hidrógeno, oxígeno y nitrógeno y los aminoácidos esenciales para el mantenimiento de la vida.

psoriasis A usually chronic, recurrent skin disease marked by bright red patches covered with silvery scales.
psoriasis Enfermedad recurrente de la piel, por lo general crónica, caracterizada por manchas de color rojo brillante cubiertas por escamas plateadas.

psychosocial Pertaining to a combination of psychological and social factors.
psicosocial Perteneciente o relativo a una combinación de factores psicológicos y sociales.

pulmonary consolidation In pneumonia, the process by which the lungs become solidified as they fill with exudates.
solidificación pulmonar Proceso por el cual los pulmones se vuelven rígidos a medida que se llenan con exudados en los casos de pulmonía.

pulse deficit When the radial pulse is less than the apical pulse. It may indicate peripheral vascular abnormality.
déficit del pulso Cuando el pulso radial es menor que el apical. Puede indicar una anomalía vascular periférica.

pulse pressure The difference between the systolic and the diastolic blood pressures (less than 30 points or more than 50 points is considered normal)
presión del pulso Diferencia entre las presiones sanguíneas sistólica y diastólica (menos de 30 puntos o más de 50 puede considerarse normal).

pure culture A bacterial or fungal culture that contains a single organism.
cultivo puro Cultivo de bacterias u hongos que contiene un solo organismo.

putrefaction The decomposition of organic matter that results in a foul smell.
putrefacción Descomposición de materia orgánica que da como resultado un olor fétido.

pyemia The presence of pus-forming organisms in the blood.
piemia Presencia en la sangre de organismos formadores de pus.

rad The conventional unit of absorbed radiation dose.
rad Unidad convencional de dosis de radiación absorbido.

radiograph An x-ray image.
radiografía Imagen obtenida con el uso de rayos X.

radiographer A person qualified to perform radiographic examinations.
técnico de radiología Persona cualificada para realizar exámenes radiológicos.

radiography Making diagnostic images using x-rays.
radiografía Proceso de diagnosticar imágenes usando rayos X.

radiologist A physician specialist in medical imaging and/or therapeutic applications of radiation.
médico radiólogo Médico especialista en formación de imágenes o en aplicaciones terapéuticas de la radiación.

radiolucent Describing a substance that is easily penetrated by x-rays; these substances appear dark on radiographs.
transparente a la radiación Término que se aplica a una substancia que puede ser penetrada con facilidad por los rayos X; estas substancias aparecen oscuras en las radiografías.

radiopaque Describing a substance that can be easily visualized on an x-ray image; describing a substance that is not easily penetrated by x-rays; these substances appear light on radiographs.
opaco a la radiación Sustancia que puede visualizarse con facilidad en la imagen de rayos X. Término que se aplica a una substancia que no puede ser penetrada con facilidad por los rayos X; estas substancias aparecen claras en las radiografías.

rales Abnormal or crackling breath sounds during inspiration.
estertores Sonidos respiratorios o crujidos anómalos durante la inspiración.

ramifications Consequences produced by a cause or following from a set of conditions.
ramificaciones Consecuencias producidas por una causa o que siguen a una serie de estados.

rapport A relationship of harmony and accord between the patient and the health care professional.
concordia Relación de armonía y acuerdo entre el paciente y el profesional de la atención sanitaria.

Raynaud's phenomenon Intermittent attacks of ischemia in the extremities resulting in cyanosis, numbness, tingling, and pain.
fenómeno de Raynaud Ataques intermitentes de isquemia en las extremidades, resultando en cianosis, entumecimiento, picazón y dolor.

rectify To correct by removing errors.
rectificar Corregir eliminando errores.

reduction The return to correct anatomical position, as in the reduction of a fracture.
reducción Regreso a la posición anatómica correcta, como en el caso de reducción de una fractura.

referral (reference) laboratory A private or hospital-based laboratory that performs a wide variety of tests, many of them specialized. Physicians often send specimens collected in the office to referral laboratories for testing.
laboratorio de referencia Laboratorio privado o de un hospital que realiza una amplia gama de análisis, muchos de ellos especializados. Con frecuencia los médicos envían especímenes recogidos en la consulta a estos laboratorios para ser analizados.

reflection The process of considering new information and internalizing it to create new ways of examining information.
reflexión Proceso de estudiar información nueva e interiorizarla para crear formas nuevas de examinar información.

refractile Capable of causing light rays to bend thus thus altering or distorting an image.
refractante Capaz de provocar la refracción de la luz, desviación alterando o distorcionando una imagen.

registered dietitian (RD) A professionally certified person with a bachelor's degree in food and nutrition who is concerned with the maintenance and promotion of health and the treatment of diseases through proper diet.
dietista registrado (RD) Profesional certificado persona con titulación universitaria en alimentos y nutrición y que se preocupa del mantenimiento y la promoción de la salud y el tratamiento de las enfermedades a través de la dieta adecuado.

relapse The recurrence of disease symptoms after apparent recovery.
recaída Recurrencia de los síntomas de una enfermedad tras una aparente recuperación.

rem The dose of ionizing radiation equivalent to one roentgen of x-ray exposure.
rem La dosis de radiación ionizante equivalente a un roentgen de exposición a rayos X.

remission A decrease in the severity of a disease or symptoms; the partial or complete disappearance of the clinical and subjective characteristics of a chronic or malignant disease.
remisión Disminución de la gravedad de una enfermedad o sus síntomas; desaparición parcial o total de las características clínicas y subjetivas de una enfermedad crónica o maligna.

remittent fever Fever in which temperature fluctuates greatly but never falls to the normal level.
fiebre remitente Fiebre en la cual la temperatura fluctúa mucho pero nunca baja al nivel normal.

renal threshold The level above which a substance cannot be reabsorbed by the renal tubules and is thus excreted in the urine
umbral renal Nivel por encima del cual una sustancia no puede ser reabsorbida por los túbulos renales y por lo tanto es excretada en la orina.

resolution The ability of the eye to distinguish two objects that are very close together; the sharpness of an image.
resolución Capacidad del ojo para distinguir dos objetos que están muy cerca uno del otro; nitidez de una imagen.

rhinitis Inflammation of the mucous membranes of the nose.
rinitis Inflamación de las membranas mucosas de la nariz.

rhonchi Abnormal rumbling sounds during expiration that indicate airway obstruction caused by thick secretions or spasms; continuous dry rattling in the throat or bronchial tube due to partial obstruction.
ronquido Ruido sordo y anómalo durante la expiración que indica obstrucción de las vías respiratorias debido a secreciones espesas o a espasmos; ruido seco y continuo en la garganta o en el tubo bronquial debido a una obstrucción parcial.

rods Structures located in the retina of the eye that form the light-sensitive elements.
bastoncillos Estructuras que están en la retina del ojo y constituyen los elementos sensibles a la luz.

Roentgen (R) The conventional unit of radiation exposure.
Roentgen (R) Unidad convencional de exposición a radiación.

sagittal plane The plane that divides the body into right and left halves.
plano sagital Plano que divide el cuerpo en la mitad derecha y la mitad izquierda.

sanitization Reducing the number of potentially harmful **microorganisms** to a relatively safe level.
saneamiento Reducción del número de **microorganismos** a un nivel relativamente seguro.

sclera The wite part of the eye that encloses the eyeball.
esclerótica Parte blanca del ojo que encierra el globo ocular.

scleroderma An autoimmune disorder that affects the blood vessels and connective tissue, causing fibrous degeneration of the major organs.
escleroderma Trastorno autoinmune que afecta a los vasos sanguíneos y los tejidos conectivos provocando degeneración en las fibras de los órganos principales.

sclerotherapy The injection of sclerosing (hardening) solutions to treat hemorrhoids, varicose veins, or esophageal varices.
escleroterapia Inyección de soluciones de esclerosis (endorecedores) para tratar hemorroides, venas varicosas o varices esofágicas.

scoliosis Abnormal lateral curvature of the spine.
escoliosis Curvatura lateral anómala de la columna.

scored tablet A drug tablet manufactured with an indentation that allows it to be broken or cut into equal parts.
tableta con hendidura Tableta que se fabrica con una hendidura que permite dividirla o romperla en partes iguales.

screen Something that shields, protects, or hides; to select or eliminate products or applicants by comparing them to a set of desired criteria.
pantalla Algo que actúa como escudo, que protege u oculta para permitir un proceso de selección.

seborrhea Excessive discharge of sebum from the sebaceous glands, forming greasy scales on the skin or cheesy plugs in skin pores.
seborrea Descarga excesiva de sebo de las glándulas sebáceas, formando escamas de grasa en la piel o tapones con aspecto de queso en los poros de la piel.

secondary hypertension Elevated blood pressure caused by another medical condition.
hipertensión secundaria Presión sanguínea elevada causada por otra enfermedad o afección médica.

serous Pertaining to thin, watery, serumlike drainage.
seroso Perteneciente o relativo a una materia poco espesa, acuosa, parecida al suero.

serum The portion of whole blood that remains liquid after the blood has clotted.
suero La porción de la sangre que queda líquida después de la coagulación.

sheath The covering surrounding the axon of the nerve cell that acts as an electrical insulator to speed the conduction of nerve impulses.
película Recubrimiento que rodea los axones de la célula nerviosa y que se comporta como aislante eléctrico para aumentar la velocidad de conducción del impulso nervioso.

Sievert (Sv) International unit of radiation dose equivalent.
Sievert (Sv) Unidad internacional de dosis equivalentes de radiación.

sinoatrial (SA) node The pacemaker of the heart, located in the right atrium.
nódulo sinoauricular (SA) Marcapasos del corazón que se halla en la aurícula derecha.

sinus arrhythmia Irregular heartbeat originating in the sinoatrial (pacemaker) node.
arritmia de seno Ritmo cardiaco irregular que tiene su origen en el nódulo sinoauricular (marcapasos).

sonography An imaging modality that uses sound waves to produce images of soft tissues; also called diagnostic ultrasound.
sonografía Modalidad de formación de imágenes que usa ondas sonoras para producir imágenes de los tejidos blandos; también se conoce como ultrasonido de diagnóstico.

specimen A sample of body fluid, waste product, or tissue that is collected for analysis and diagnosis.
espécimen Muestra de un fluido corporal, residuo o tejido que se usa para análisis y diagnósticos.

spirometer An instrument that measures the volume of inhaled and exhaled air.
espirómetro Instrumento que sirve para medir el volumen del aire inhalado y exhalado.

spores Thick-walled reproductive cells formed within bacteria and capable of withstanding unfavorable environmental conditions; thick-walled dormant forms of bacteria that are very resistant to **disinfection** measures.
esporas Células reproductoras de paredes gruesas que se forman dentro de las bacterias y son capaces de resistir condiciones ambientales adversas; tipos de bacterias letárgicas de paredes gruesas que son muy resistentes a las medidas de **desinfección**.

stat Medical abbreviation for immediately or at this moment; an order found on a laboratory requisition indicating that the test must be done immediately (from the Latin word *statin,* meaning "at once"); immediately.
stat Abreviatura usada en medicina que significa inmediatamente o ahora mismo. Orden encontrada en un pedido de laboratorio que indica que el análisis debe llevarse a cabo inmediatamente (de la palabra latina *statin,* que significa "ahora"); inmediatamente.

stereotactic An x-ray procedure to guide the insertion of a needle into a specific area of the breast.
estereotáctico Procedimiento de rayos X para guiar la inserción de una aguja en zonas específicas del pecho.

sterilization Complete destruction of all forms of microbial life.
esterilización Destrucción total de toda forma de vida microbiana.

stertorous Describing strenuous respiratory effort that has a snoring sound.
estertóreo Esfuerzo respiratorio penoso que tiene el sonido de un ronquido.

stressors Stimuli that cause stress.
estresantes Dícese de los estímulos que causan estrés.

stridor A shrill, harsh respiratory sound heard during inhalation during laryngeal obstruction.
estridor Sonido respiratorio estridente que se oye durante la inhalación en los casos de obstrucción laríngea.

stroke Sudden paralysis and/or loss of consciousness caused by extreme trauma or injury to an artery in the brain.
apoplejía Súbita pérdida de conocimiento y parálisis causada por una lesión o daño grave de una arteria del cerebro.

stylus A metal probe inserted into or passed through a catheter, needle, or tube that is used for clearing purposes or to facilitate passage into a body orifice.
punzón Sonda metálica que se inserta o pasa por medio de un catéter, aguja o tubo y que se usa para limpiar o para facilitar el paso a un orificio del cuerpo.

subluxation Incomplete dislocation of a bone from its normal anatomical location
subluxación Dislocación incompleta de un hueso desde su posición anatómica normal.

subluxations Slight misalignments of the vertebrae, or a partial dislocation.
subluxaciones Alineamientos ligeramente defectuosos o dislocaciones parciales de las vértebras.

subtle Difficult to understand or perceive; having or marked by keen insight and the ability to penetrate deeply and thoroughly.
sutil Difícil de comprender o percibir; que tiene perspicacia y la capacidad de penetrar a fondo y en toda su extensión en un asunto.

suppurative Forming and/or discharging of pus.
supuración Formación o emisión de pus.

surrogate A substitute; put in place of another.
subrogado Sustituto; puesto en lugar de otro.

syncope Fainting; a brief lapse in consciousness
síncope Desmayo; lapso breve en estado de consciencia.

syndrome A group of signs and symptoms related to a common cause or presenting a clinical picture of a disease or an inherited abnormality.
síndrome Conjunto de signos y síntomas relacionados con una causa común o que presentan el cuadro clínico de una enfermedad o una anomalía heredada.

synopsis A condensed statement or outline.
sinopsis Declaración resumida; resumen.

synovial fluid Clear fluid found in joint cavities that facilitates smooth movements and nourishes joint structures.
fluido sinovial Fluido claro que se halla en las cavidades de las articulaciones y que facilita los movimientos suaves y nutre las estructuras articulatorias.

tachycardia Rapid but regular heart rate exceeding 100 beats per minute.
taquicardia Ritmo cardiaco rápido pero regular que sobrepasa los 100 latidos por minuto.

tachypnea Respiration that is rapid and shallow; hyperventilation.
taquipnea Respiración rápida y profunda; hiperventilación.

target organ The organ that is affected by a particular hormone.
órgano objetivo Órgano afectado por una hormona específica.

target tissue A group of cells that are affected by a particular hormone.
tejido objetivo Grupo de células afectadas por una hormona específica.

tendon A tough band of connective tissue connecting muscle to bone.
tendón Banda resistente de tejido conectivo que conecta los músculos con los huesos.

teratogen Any substance that interferes with normal prenatal development.
teratógeno Cualquier sustancia que interfiere con el desarrollo prenatal normal.

teratogenic A substance that is known to cause birth defects.
teratogénico Sustancia que se sabe que provoca defectos de nacimiento.

thanatology The description or study of the phenomena of death and of psychological methods of coping with death.
tanatología Descripción o estudio del fenómeno de la muerte y de los métodos psicológicos para hacerle frente.

thixotropic gel A material that appears to be a solid until subjected to a disturbance such as centrifugation, when it becomes a liquid.
gel tisotrópico Material que parece ser sólido hasta el momento en que se somete a una alteración como la centrifugación, cuando se convierte en líquido.

thoracic Pertaining to the region of the back containing 12 thoracic vertebrae, between the neck and low back.
torácica Perteneciente o relativo a región de la espalda entre el cuello y la región lumbar inferior en la que hay 12 vértebras torácicas.

thready pulse Pulse that is scarcely perceptible.
pulso débil Pulso que es apenas perceptible.

thrombus Blood clot.
trombo Cóagulo de sangre.

thyroid stimulating hormone (TSH) A hormone secreted by the anterior lobe of the pituitary gland that stimulates the secretion of hormones produced by the thyroid gland.
hormona estimulante de la tiroides (TSH) Hormona que segrega el lóbulo anterior de la glándula pituitaria y que estimula la secreción de hormonas producidas por la glándula tiroides.

tinea Fungal skin disease that results in scaling, itching, and inflammation.
tinea Enfermedad de la piel causada por hongos y que produce descamación, picazón e inflamación.

tissue culture The technique or process of keeping tissue alive and growing in a culture medium.
cultivo de tejidos Técnica o proceso de mantener un tejido vivo y en fase de crecimiento en un medio de cultivo.

toxemia An abnormal condition of pregnancy characterized by hypertension, edema, and protein in the urine.
toxemia Característica anómala del embarazo, con presencia de hipertensión, edema y proteínas en la orina.

tracer A radioactive substance administered to a patient undergoing a nuclear medicine imaging procedure.
trazador Sustancia radioactiva que se administra al paciente para someterlo a procedimientos de formación de imágenes en medicina nuclear.

tracheostomy A surgical opening through the neck into the trachea, to facilitate breathing.
traqueotomía Abertura realizada quirúrgicamente en el cuello a la altura de la tráquea para facilitar la respiración.

transducer The part of the sonography machine in contact with the patient that sends high frequency sound waves and receives the sound echoes that return from the patient's body.
transductor Parte de una máquina de sonografía que está en contacto con el paciente envía ondas sonoras de alta frecuencia y recibe los ecos de los sonidos que regresan del cuerpo del paciente.

transection A cross-section, division by cutting across.
sección transversal División cortando a través.

transient ischemic attack Temporary neurological symptoms caused by gradual or partial occlusion of a cerebral blood vessel.
ataque isquémico transitorio Síntomas neurológicos temporales causados por una oclusión gradual o parcial de un vaso sanguíneo del cerebro.

transillumination Inspection of a cavity or organ by passing light through its walls.
diafanoscopia Inspección de una cavidad u órgano haciendo pasar luz a través de sus paredes.

transport medium A medium used to keep an organism alive during transport to the laboratory.
medio para transporte Medio usado para mantener un organismo vivo durante el transporte al laboratorio.

transverse plane Plane that divides the body into superior and inferior parts.
plano transversal Plano que divide el cuerpo en parte superior e inferior.

trauma Physical injury or wound caused by an external force or violence.

trauma Lesión física o herida causada por una fuerza externa o violencia.

triglycerides Fatty acids and glycerols that are bound to proteins and form high- and low-density lipoproteins.

triglicéridos Ácidos grasos y gliceroles que se unen a las proteínas y forman lipoproteínas de alta y baja densidad.

truss An elastic, canvas, or metallic device for retaining a reduced hernia within the abdominal cavity.

braguero Malla elástica o dispositivo metálico para retener una hernia reducida dentro de la cavidad abdominal.

turgor Resistance of the skin to being grasped between the fingers and released; normal skin tension that is decreased in dehydration and increased with edema.

turgor Resistencia de la piel a ser pellizcada; tensión normal de la piel que disminuye con la deshidratación y aumenta con el edema.

type and cross match Tests performed to assess the compatibility of blood to be transfused.

prueba de tipo y RH Análisis que se realizan para evaluar la compatibilidad de la sangre que va a ser usada en una transfusión.

unequal pulses Pulses in which the beats vary in intensity.

pulso desigual Pulso en el cual los latidos varían en intensidad.

unit dose A method used by the pharmacy to prepare individual doses of medications. **dosis unitaria** Método usado por la farmacia para preparar dosis individuales de medicamentos.

upper GI series Fluoroscopic examination of the esophagus, stomach, and duodenum using oral administration of barium sulfate as a contrast medium.

serie GI superior Examen fluoroscópico del esófago, estómago y duodeno usando una administración oral de sulfato de bario como medio de contraste.

urea The major nitrogenous end-product of protein metabolism and the chief nitrogenous component of the urine.

urea Principal producto final nitrogenado del metabolismo de las proteínas y el principal componente nitrogenado de la orina.

urease An enzyme that catalyzes the hydrolysis of urea to form ammonium carbonate.

ureasa Enzima que cataliza la hidrólisis de la urea para formar carbonato de amonio.

uremia A toxic renal condition characterized by an excess of urea, creatinine, and other nitrogenous end-products in the blood.

uremia Enfermedad renal tóxica que se caracteriza por un exceso de urea, creatinina y otros productos finales en la sangre.

urgency A sudden, compelling desire to urinate and the inability to control its release.

urgencia Deseo repentino y apremiante de orinar y la incapacidad de controlarlo.

urticaria A skin eruption creating inflamed wheals; hives.

urticaria Erupción cutánea que produce ampollas imflamadas.

Valsalva's maneuver Occurs when one strains to defecate and urinate, uses the arms and upper trunk muscles to move up in bed, or strains during laughing, coughing, or vomiting. It causes a trapping of blood in the great veins, preventing it from entering the chest and right atrium, which may cause heart attack and death.

maniobra de Valsalva Ocurre cuando uno hace fuerza para defecar y orinar, usa los brazos y los músculos de la parte superior del tronco para levantarse de la cama, o hace fuerza al reír, toser o vomitar. Causa una retención de sangre en las venas mayores, impidiendole que entre en el pecho y la aurícula derecha y puede provocar un ataque al corazón y la muerte.

vasodilation Increase in the diameter of a blood vessel.

vasodilatación Aumento en el diámetro de un vaso sanguíneo.

vector An organism, such as an insect or tick, that transmits the causative organisms of disease.

vector Organismos, tales como un insecto o garrapata, que transmite los organismos que provocan enfermedades.

ventricles The two lower chambers of the heart.
ventrículos Las dos cavidades inferiores del corazón.

veracity Devotion to or conformity with the truth.
veracidad Compromiso o conformidad con la verdad.

vertigo Dizziness; a sensation of faintness or an inability to maintain normal balance.
vértigo Mareo; sensación de desmayo o de incapacidad de mantener el equilibrio normal.

viable Capable of living, developing, or germinating under favorable conditions.
viable Capaz de vivir, desarrollarse o germinar bajo condiciones favorables.

virulent Exceedingly pathogenic, noxious, or deadly.
virulento Excesivamente patógeno, nocivo o mortal.

viscosity The quality of being thick and lacking the capability of easy movement.
viscosidad Cualidad de espeso e incapaz de moverse con facilidad.

vocation The work in which a person is regularly employed.
profesión Trabajo en el que una persona está empleada regularmente.

volatile Referring to a flammable substance's capacity to vaporize at a low temperature. Easily aroused; tending to erupt in violence.
volátil Referente a la capacidad de una sustancia flamable para evaporarse a baja temperatura. Que reacciona con facilidad y tiene tendencia a entrar en erupción de forma violenta.

vulva The external female genitalia, which begins at the mons pubis and terminates at the anus.
vulva Zona genital exterior femenina que comienza en el monte púbico y termina en el ano.

wet mount A slide preparation in which a drop of liquid specimen for example, protected by a coverslip and observed with a microscope.
montaje húmedo Preparación de una lámina en la que una gota de espécimen líquido por ejemplo, se protege con una cubierta de vidrio y se observa con un microscopio.

wheal Localized area of edema, or a raised lesion.
roncha Área localizada de un edema o una lesión protuberante.

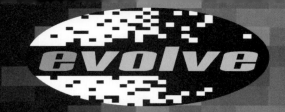

The Latest Evolution in Learning.

Evolve provides online access to free learning resources and activities designed specifically for the textbook you are using in your class. The resources will provide you with information that enhances the material covered in the book and much more.

Visit the Web address listed below to start your learning evolution today!

▶ **LOGIN:** *http://evolve.elsevier.com/Kinn/*

Evolve Student Learning Resources for Morton: Student Study Guide to accompany *Kinn's The Clinical Medical Assistant: An Applied Learning Approach* offer the following features:

- **Content Updates**
  The latest content updates from the authors of the textbook to keep you current with recent developments in medical assisting, updated procedures, and more!

- **Online Quizzes**
  Quizzes for each chapter are set up for instant feedback, any time you want a little practice.

- **WebLinks**
  An exciting resource that lets you link to hundreds of websites carefully chosen to supplement the content of the textbook and student study guide. The Weblinks are regularly updated, with new ones added as they develop.

- **Chapter Resources**
  Additional materials, including chapter summaries & suggested readings, to enhance each chapter.

- **Study Tips**
  Get advice on how to maximize study time and review material for optimal results. Discover your individual learning style and find out how it applies to your ability to learn new material.

Think outside the book...evolve

Credits

Pages 625-626 constitute an extension of the copyright page. The illustrations that appear on the pages listed below are from the following sources.

From Barkaukas VH, Baumann, LC, and Darling-Fisher, CS: *Health and Physical Assessment,* 3rd ed., St. Louis, 2002, Mosby.
Pages 47-49, 78-79, 92-94, 96-97, 100, 106, 116, 123-124, 128, 134, 138, 156-159, 166-167, 187, 190

From Buck CJ: *Saunders 2002 ICD-9-CM volumes 1, 2, & 3 and HCPCS level II,* Philadelphia, 2002, WB Saunders.
Pages 98-99, 110, 122, 132, 142, 170, 179, 191-192, 200

From Davis N, Lacour M: *Introduction to health information technology,* Philadelphia, 2002, WB Saunders.
Pages 283-286

From Doucette LJ: *Basic mathematics for the health-related professions,* Philadelphia, 2000, WB Saunders.
Pages 75, 77, 80, 231-232, 235-236, 256

From Hunt SA, Zonderman JH: *Saunders fundamentals of medical assisting: student mastery manual,* Philadelphia, 2002, WB Saunders.
Pages 225, 232, 248-249, 271-274

From Hunt SA, Zonderman JH: *Saunders medical assisting pocket pal,* Philadelphia, 2002, WB Saunders.
Page 30

From Kinn ME, Woods, M: *The medical assistant: administrative and clinical,* 8th ed., Philadelphia, 1999, WB Saunders.
Pages 44-47, 214, 289

From Lilly AL, Kinn ME, Woods, M: *Student mastery manual for the medical assistant: administrative and clinical,* 8th ed., Philadelphia, 1999, WB Saunders.
Page 157

From Young T, Kennedy D: *Kinn's the medical assistant: an applied learning approach,* 9th ed., Philadelphia, 2003, Elsevier Science (USA).
Pages 10, 31, 37

From Sole ML, Lamborn ML, Hartshorn JC: *Introduction to critical care nursing,* 3rd ed., Philadelphia, 2001, WB Saunders.
Pages 187, 189, 196, 213-216

From Swisher L: *Study guide to accompany Thibodeau and Patton the human body in health & disease,* 3rd ed., 2002, Mosby.
Pages 213, 223, 240-241, 243-244, 255, 257, 261-264